THE 5 INGREDIENT EXERCISE BOOK

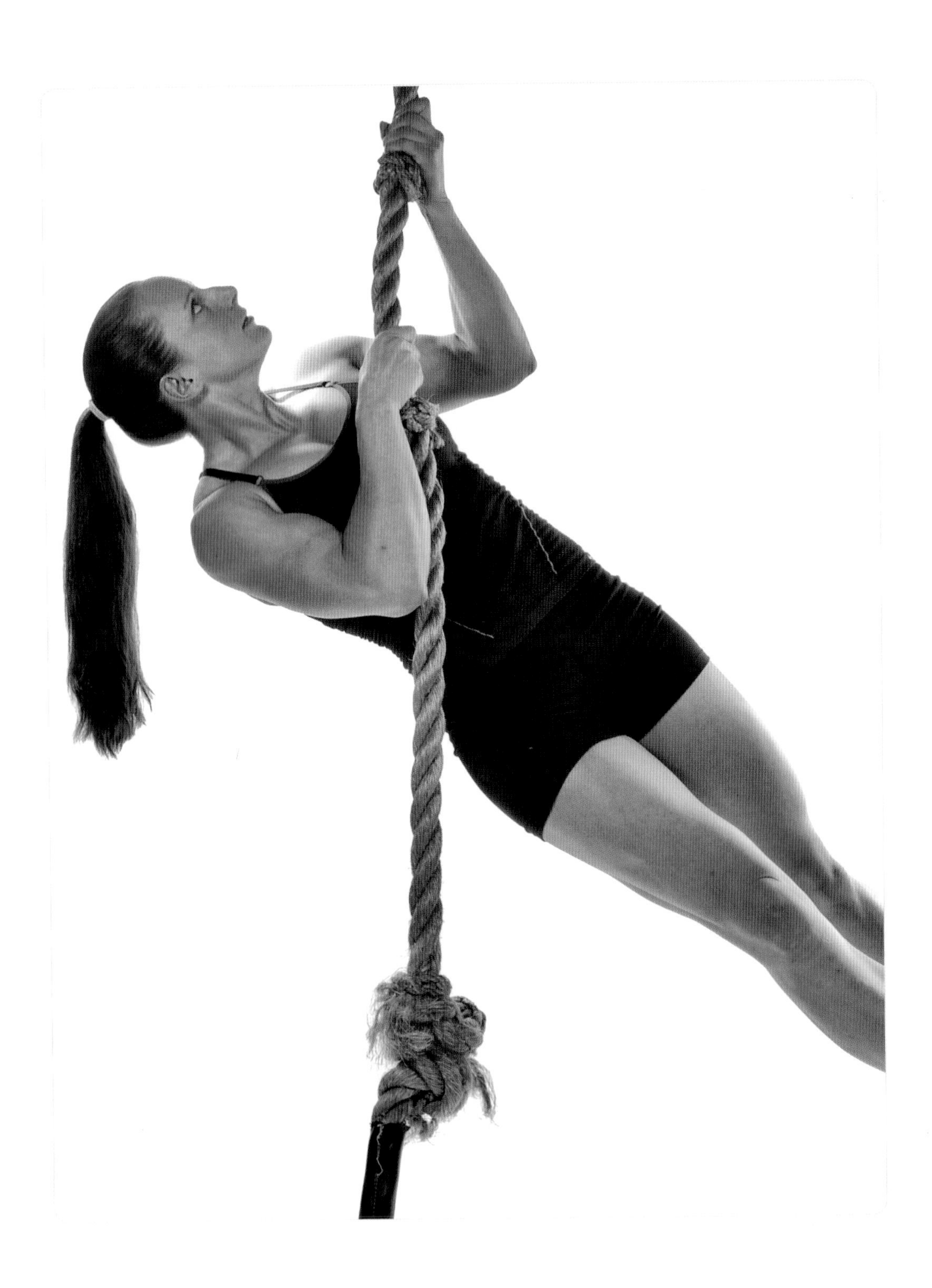

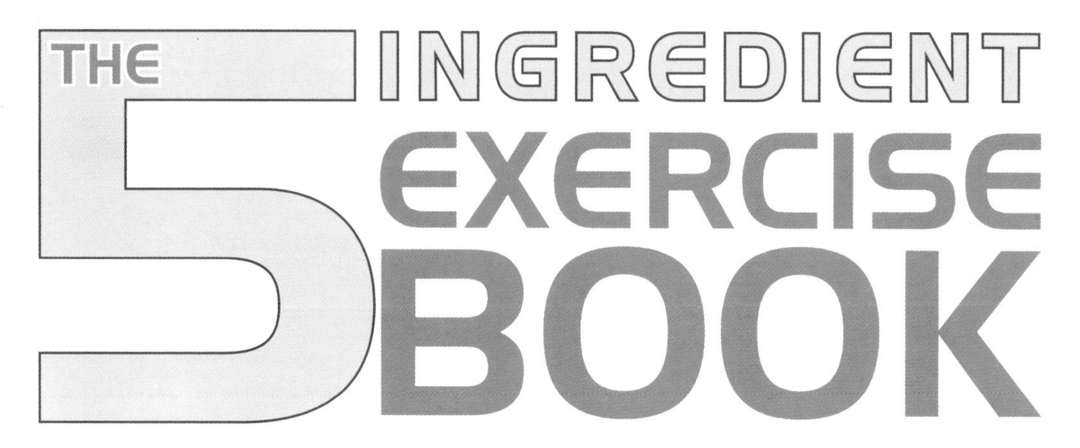

A TRAINER'S INSIDE GUIDE TO YOUR WORKOUT

PAT MANOCCHIA

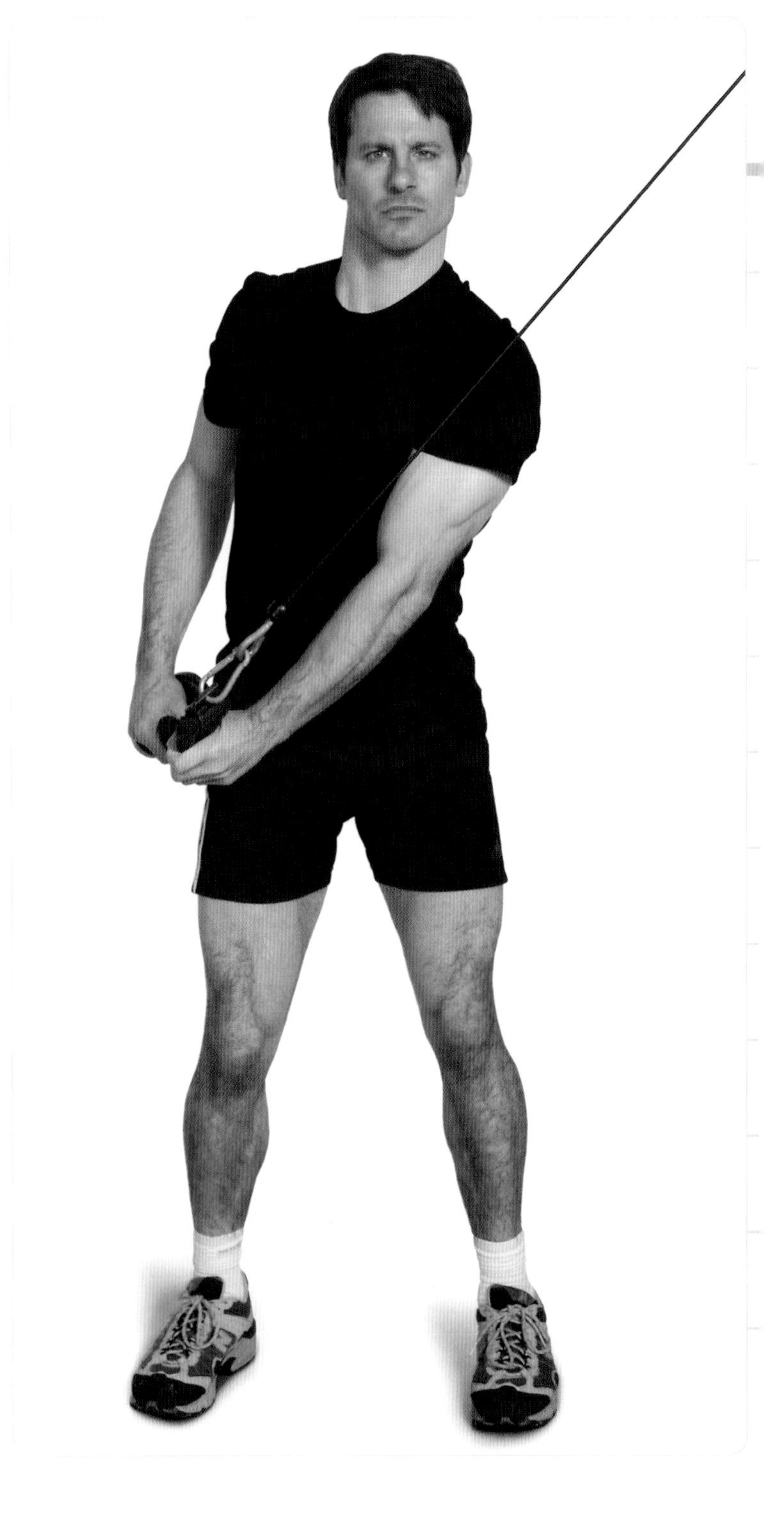

Published by Hinkler Books Pty Ltd
45–55 Fairchild Street
Heatherton Victoria 3202 Australia
www.hinklerbooks.com

Cover Design: Graphic Print Group
Typesetting and Repro: MPS Limited

ISBN: 978 1 7418 4386 6

Printed and bound in China

CONTENTS

INTRODUCTION

In Rhode Island, we call it "gravy." Most other places in the world refer to it as "tomato sauce." Whatever the name, there is just one thing that determines whether it is worthy of a perfectly cooked rigatoni and a giant Barolo. The one thing that truly separates the ordinary from the extraordinary: Ingredients. Of course, there is always an element of skill included, but all the skill in the world cannot substitute for stale olive oil and unripe tomatoes.

In the realm of exercise, I believe there is simply too little attention given to the actual "ingredients" of a training program. For overall physiological health, in my opinion, there are 5 Ingredients:

- Rest and Recovery
- Diet/Nutrition
- Cardiovascular Training
- Sport Specific Skill or Technique Training
- Musculoskeletal Conditioning

As it happens, each of these components also has within them five basic ingredients. This book focuses on the five ingredients for musculo-skeletal conditioning, which consists of all of the muscles, bones, joints, ligaments, and tendons of the body.

This book will include visual and verbal representations of each of the 5 Ingredients as well as variations that can be made in order to adjust for skill level and intensity when using them. I've also included a basic matrix of conditioning programs (or "recipes") depicting some different ways in which they may be used. Whether cooking or training, there are many many, ways to skin the proverbial cat. Consequently, an almost unlimited variety of programs can be created by mixing and matching elements from each exercise category.

One must understand that the end result will depend upon "how" these ingredients are used as well. Even with the best tomatoes, if the heat is too high, the garlic will stick to the pan, resulting in a burnt flavor permeating the gravy—and a very, very sad situation for those perfect tomatoes. The "how," or variables, that need to be manipulated for these exercises are time, intensity, and frequency, or, more specifically, reps, sets, weights, sessions per week, and increments of progression.

There are many excellent books on how to use these variables for a given desired effect, ranging from increased overall endurance and range of motion to absolute strength and the ability to generate power (force at high speeds), so I will not address anything in this book to that level of specificity. This book is designed to give anyone an understanding of the necessary elements of musculoskeletal conditioning and to guide you on how they should be used, with some basic programs as examples.

I also would like to be crystal clear from the beginning regarding the commitment required to be successful with a conditioning program: There are NO SHORTCUTS! I in no way want the reader to assume that this is a "7 minutes a day" deal. That is simply not ever the case. I am, and have always been, vehemently opposed to the idea of shortening or condensing the time required to become healthy and fit. It simply does not work like that. This book is ultimately about process, and the focus is specifically on how to maximize the quality of the process by organizing it and simplifying it. I sincerely hope that the information here sheds some light on how to efficiently craft an exercise program for musculoskeletal conditioning, whether you are a rank beginner or elite athlete.

FULL BODY ANATOMY

FRONT

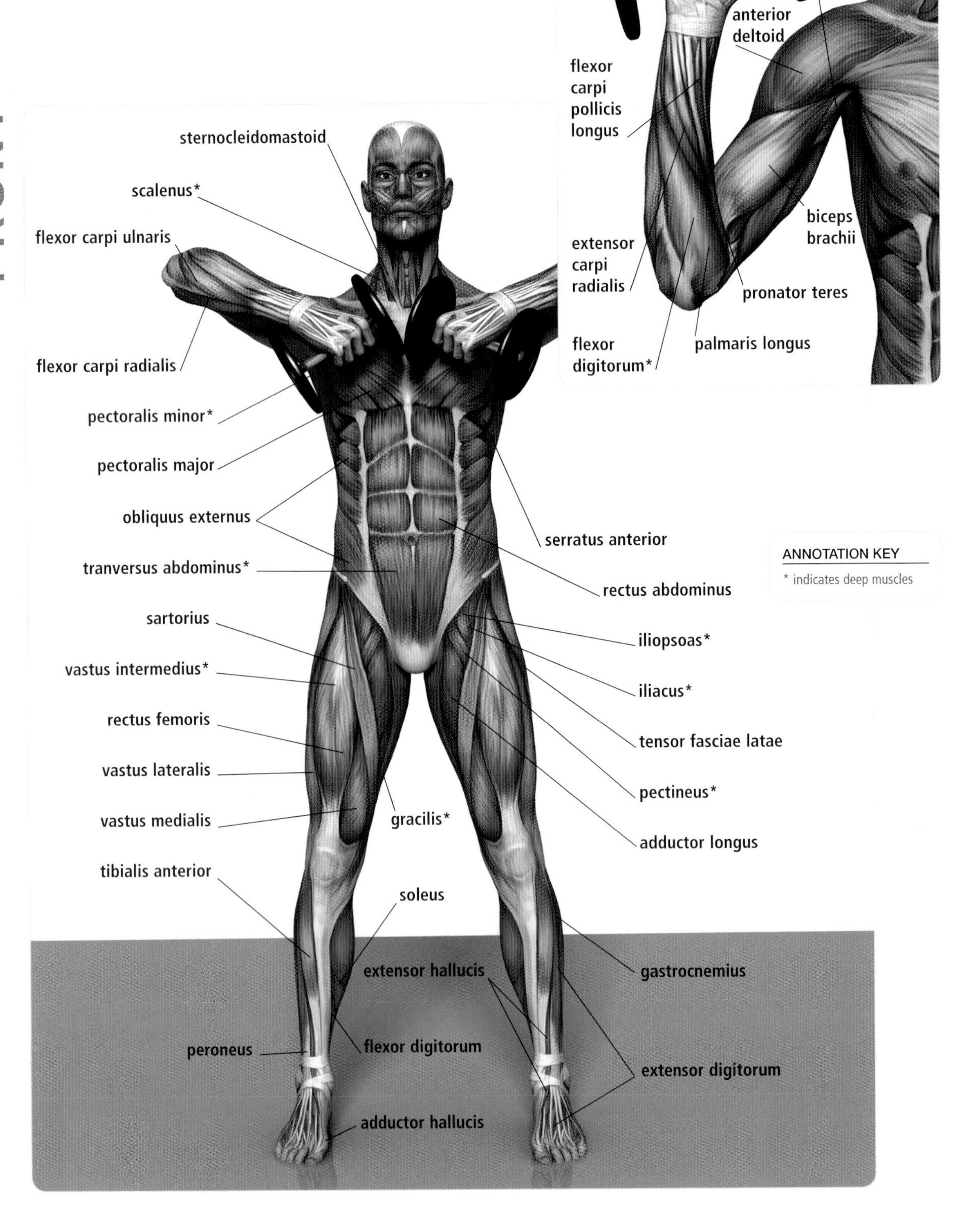

ANNOTATION KEY

* indicates deep muscles

BACK

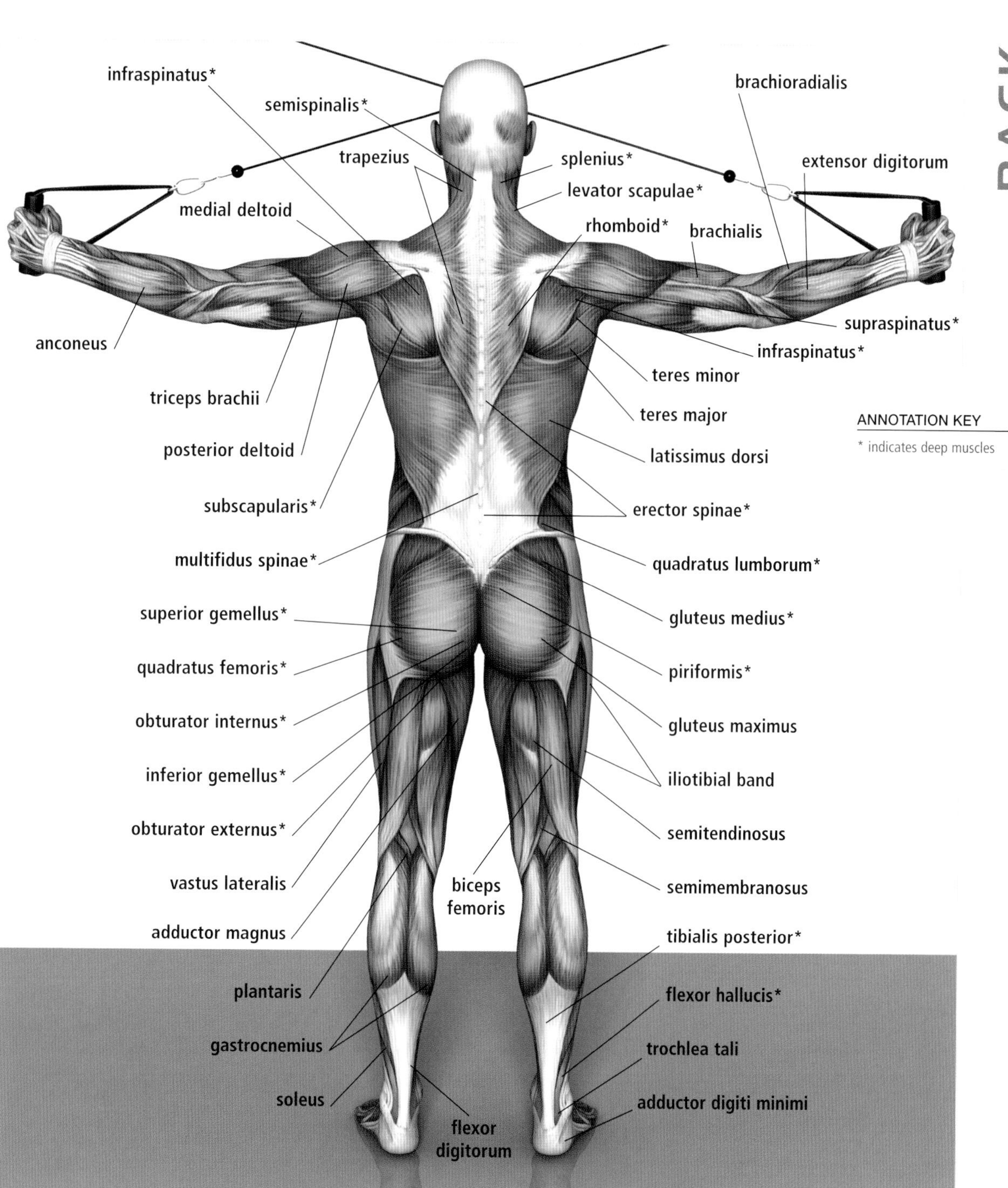

ANNOTATION KEY

* indicates deep muscles

THE 5 INGREDIENTS

When broken down into movements, the body basically does only five things: *flexion* (bending of a joint), *extension* (straightening of a joint), *adduction* (moving limb toward the body), *abduction* (moving limb away from body), and *rotation* (turning or twisting). In this book I've created categories of exercises that represent each and, in some cases, combine two different ones, depending upon the joint being activated.

The categories provide a five-exercise regimen that addresses each of the body's movements.

The exercises are:

1. DEAD LIFT

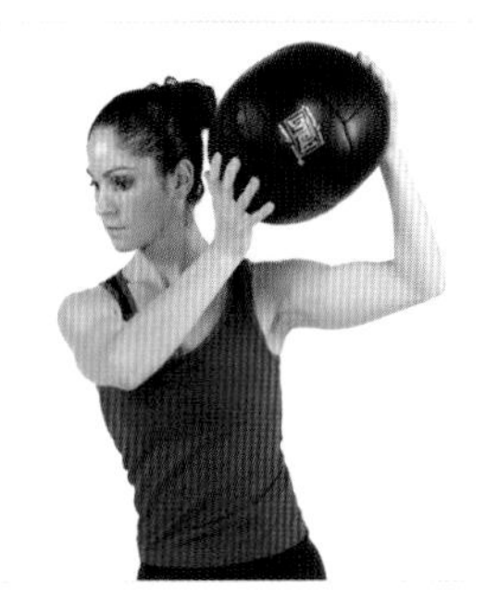

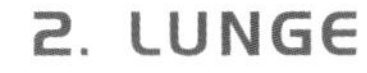

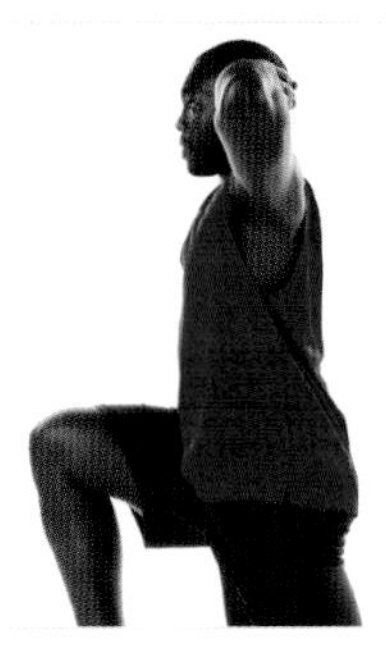

3. PUSH-UP

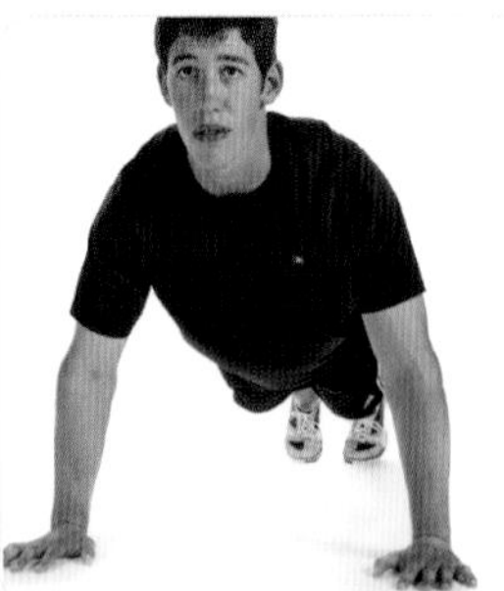

4. CHIN-UP

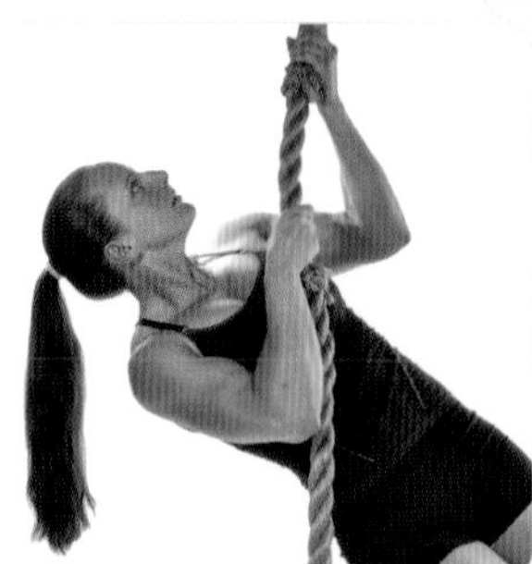

5. AB WHEEL

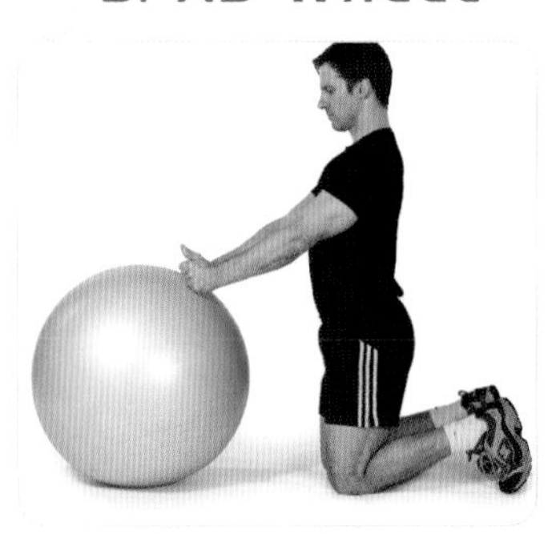

I've included approximately 10 to 15 variations of each exercise, all of which makes the specific category address slightly different aspects of the body's function.

The primary muscles and movements addressed in each exercise category are:

EXERCISE	JOINTS	FUNCTION
1. Dead Lift	Hip, Back, Knee	Extension
2. Lunge	Hip, Knee	Extension, Adduction, Abduction
3. Push-up	Shoulder, Elbow	Flexion, Adduction, Extension
4. Chin-up	Shoulder, Elbow	Extension, Flexion
5. Ab Wheel	Hip, Back, Knee	Flexion

In this book, the rotational aspect of movements is basically addressed by either creating a rotational torque using unilateral resistance or by using the same basic movement in a different plane.

Any level of conditioning can be effectively built on these five movements with a very modest, very basic set of equipment.

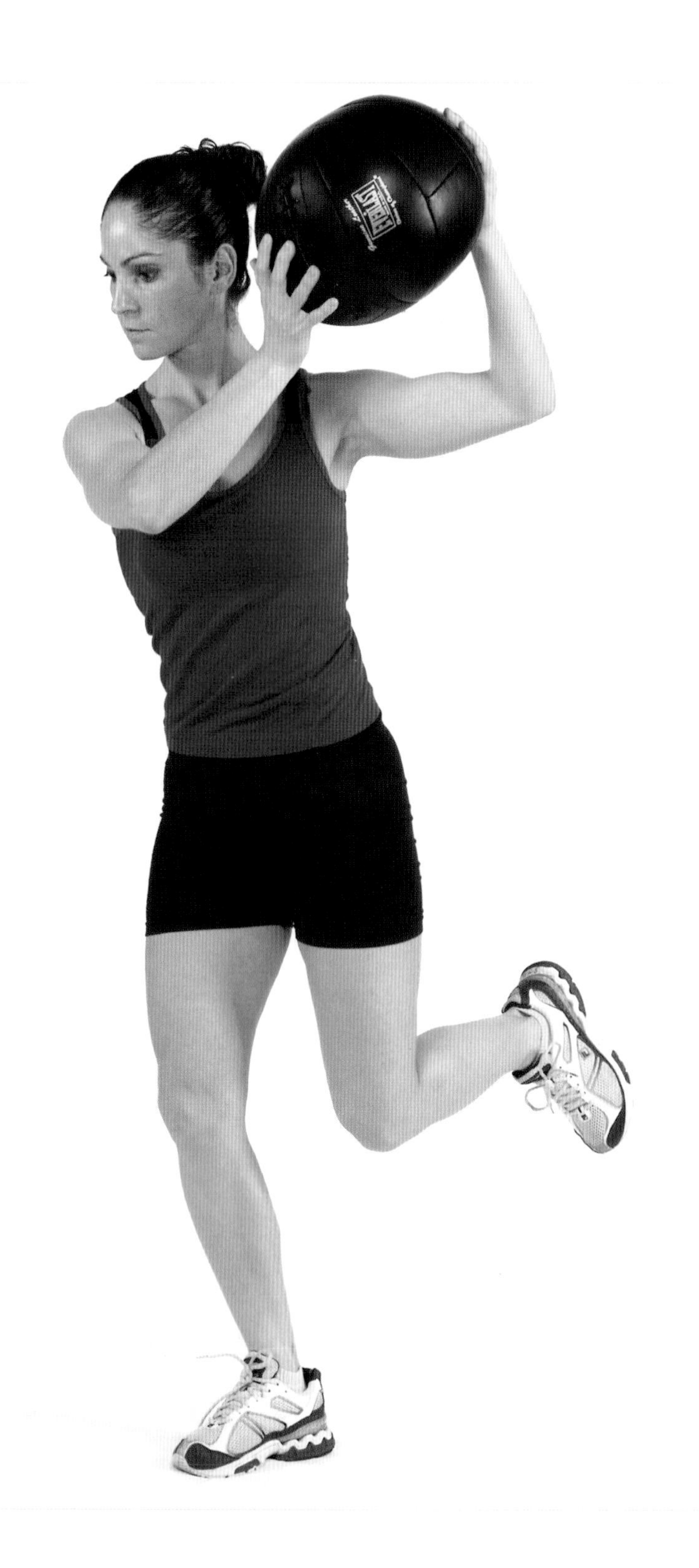

DEAD LIFT

Of all the traditional movements that people perform while exercising, the dead lift is arguably the most important of them all. Why? Because it is the most translatable into everyday life: it is something we do every single day, young and old, rich and poor, weak and strong. From picking up our laundry bags to carrying our briefcases, this movement, and variations of it, *must* be a cornerstone of any exercise program.

The joints involved are the ankle, knee, hip, spine, and shoulder (and wrist isometrically). The primary muscles are hamstrings, glutes, calves, lower, middle and upper back, shoulders, and forearms. In this movement all of these muscles function primarily as extensors.

Primary benefits are hip, leg, and low back strength, as well as improved spinal position (posture) and range of motion (flexibility).

DEAD LIFT

1

Starting Position: With the barbell on the ground and your feet shoulder-width apart, stand so that your shins contact the bar. Grasp the bar with an alternating grip (with one palm facing toward you and the other away) or with palms facing inward (toward your body). Keep your spine neutral, positioned at a 45-degree angle to perpendicular. Drop and retract your hips so that your upper legs are parallel to the ground (or as close to parallel as your flexibility will allow). Position your shoulder joints directly over the bar. Make sure that your feet are flat and your weight is evenly distributed. Pull your chest, head, and rib cage up and your abdominal muscles up and in. Inhale at the bottom of the position.

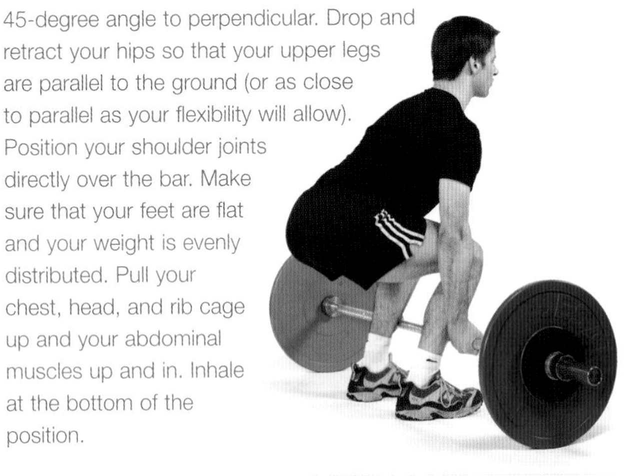

2

Action: Exhale, and drive your torso up and backward and your hips up and forward. Push your feet into the ground, extending your knees and pulling backward on the bar with your upper back and shoulders until you arrive at a vertical position.

3

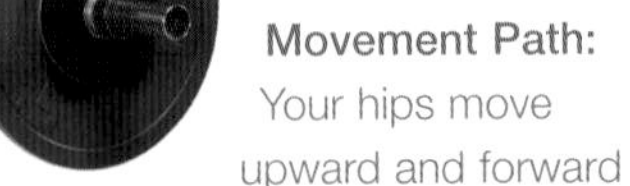

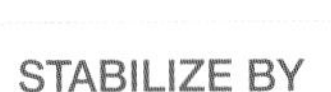

Movement Path: Your hips move upward and forward while your spine and torso move upward and backward, your knees extend, and your entire body moves upward and away from the floor.

LOOK FOR

- The angle of your spine to never drop below 45 degrees during the movement
- A slight arch in your back throughout the movement
- All of your joints to move at the same time and at the same rate

AVOID

- Straightening your knees prior to extending your back and hips
- Rounding your back
- Elevating your shoulders or lowering your head
- Allowing your knees to migrate either inward or outward

STABILIZE BY

- Keeping your rib cage high and your head up
- Pushing your shoulders down and back, with your shoulder blades flat on your rib cage
- Keeping your knees directly over your feet

ANNOTATION KEY
Black text indicates active muscles
Gray text indicates stabilizing muscles
* indicates deep muscles

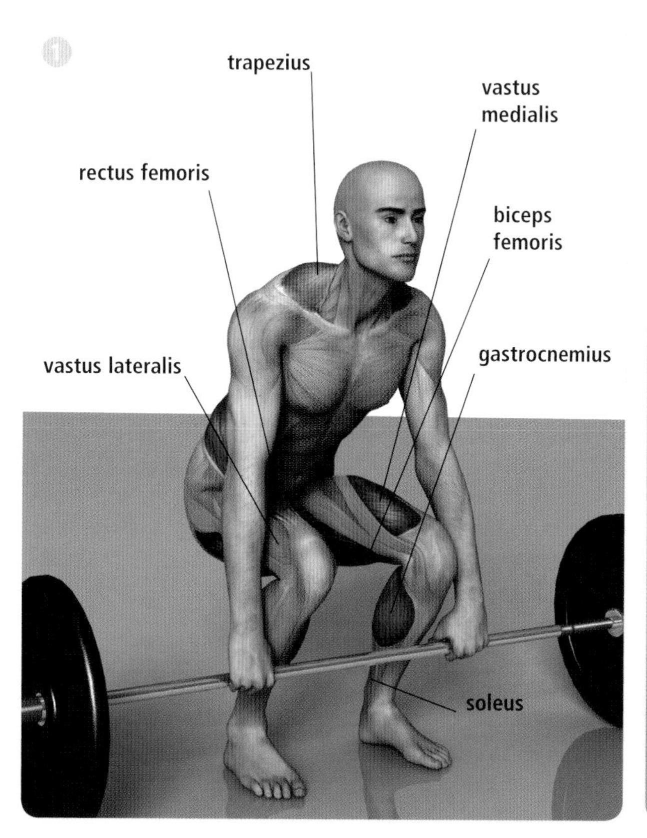

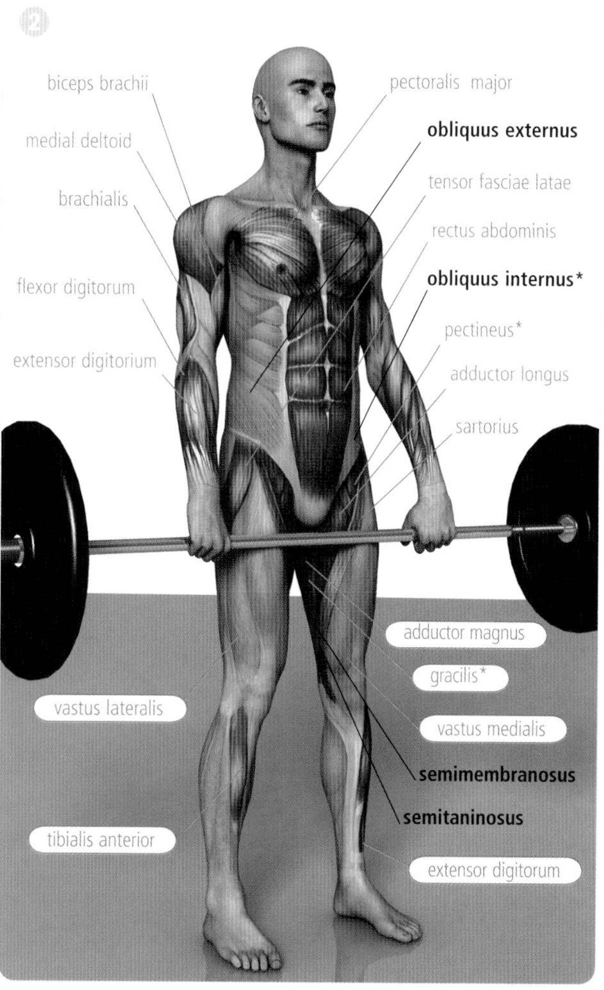

MODIFICATIONS

Similar Difficulty: Start with the dumbbells on ground adjacent to outside of feet. Grasp dumbbells with palms facing inward. Follow same action and movement path.

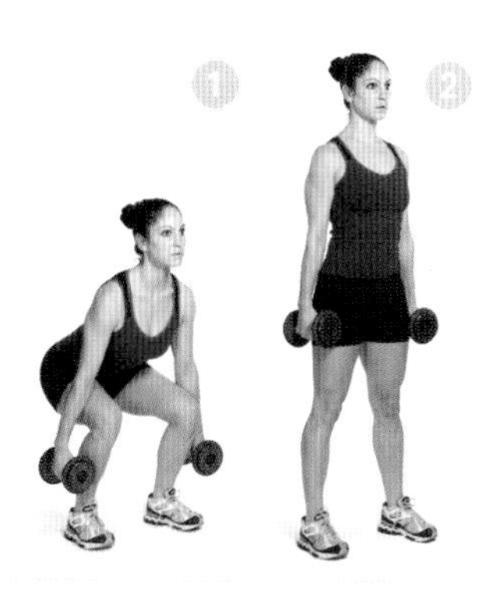

MUSCLES USED

- biceps femoris
- erector spinae
- gluteus maximus
- latissimus dorsi
- levator scapulae
- obliquus externus
- quadradus lumborum
- rectus femoris
- rhomboid
- semimembranosus
- semitendinosus
- soleus
- trapezius
- vastus lateralis
- vastus medialis

STRAIGHT-LEG WITH BARBELLS

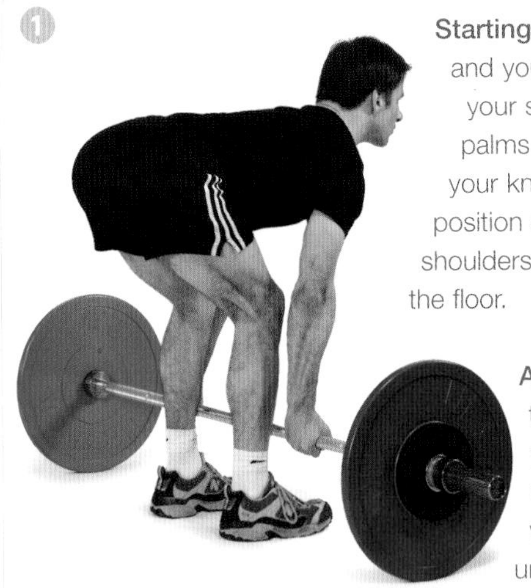

Starting Position: With the barbell on the ground and your feet shoulder-width apart, stand so that your shins contact the bar. Grasp the bar with an palms facing outward (away from your body). Bend your knees slightly, keeping your spine in a neutral position and your hips elevated, so that your head, shoulders, and hips are in a straight line and parallel to the floor.

Action: Create tension from your hands through the back of your body, all the way to your heels. Drive your back up and your hips forward, drawing the bar in a straight line vertically adjacent to your shins, and continue until you are in a full standing position.

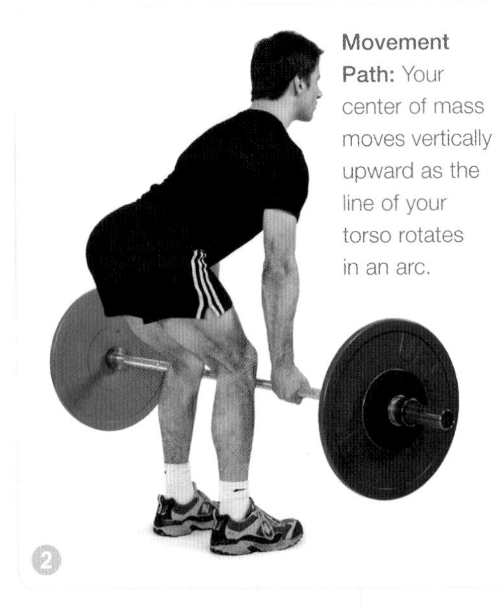

Movement Path: Your center of mass moves vertically upward as the line of your torso rotates in an arc.

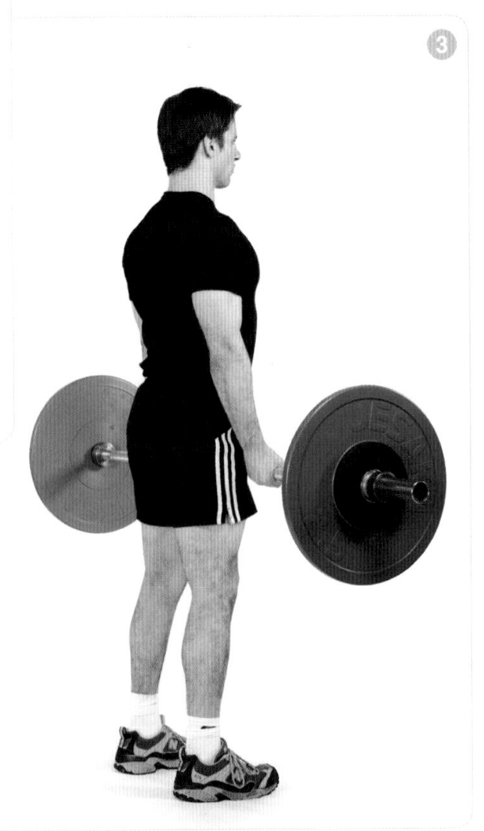

LOOK FOR

- All movement to happen at the same time
- Your spine to remain completely stable from hips to head
- Your head to be up, with your eyes forward and looking upward

AVOID

- Allowing your spine to round (by flexing forward)
- Allowing your spine to change position in segments as it moves
- Bending so that your hips are above your shoulders during the movement
- Bending your elbows or shrugging your shoulders
- Allowing your weight to rest in the front part of the foot or the bar to be forward of the toe line

STABILIZE BY

- Keeping your rib cage high, your head up, and your shoulders down and back, with your shoulder blades flat on your rib cage

STRAIGHT-LEG WITH BARBELLS • DEAD LIFT

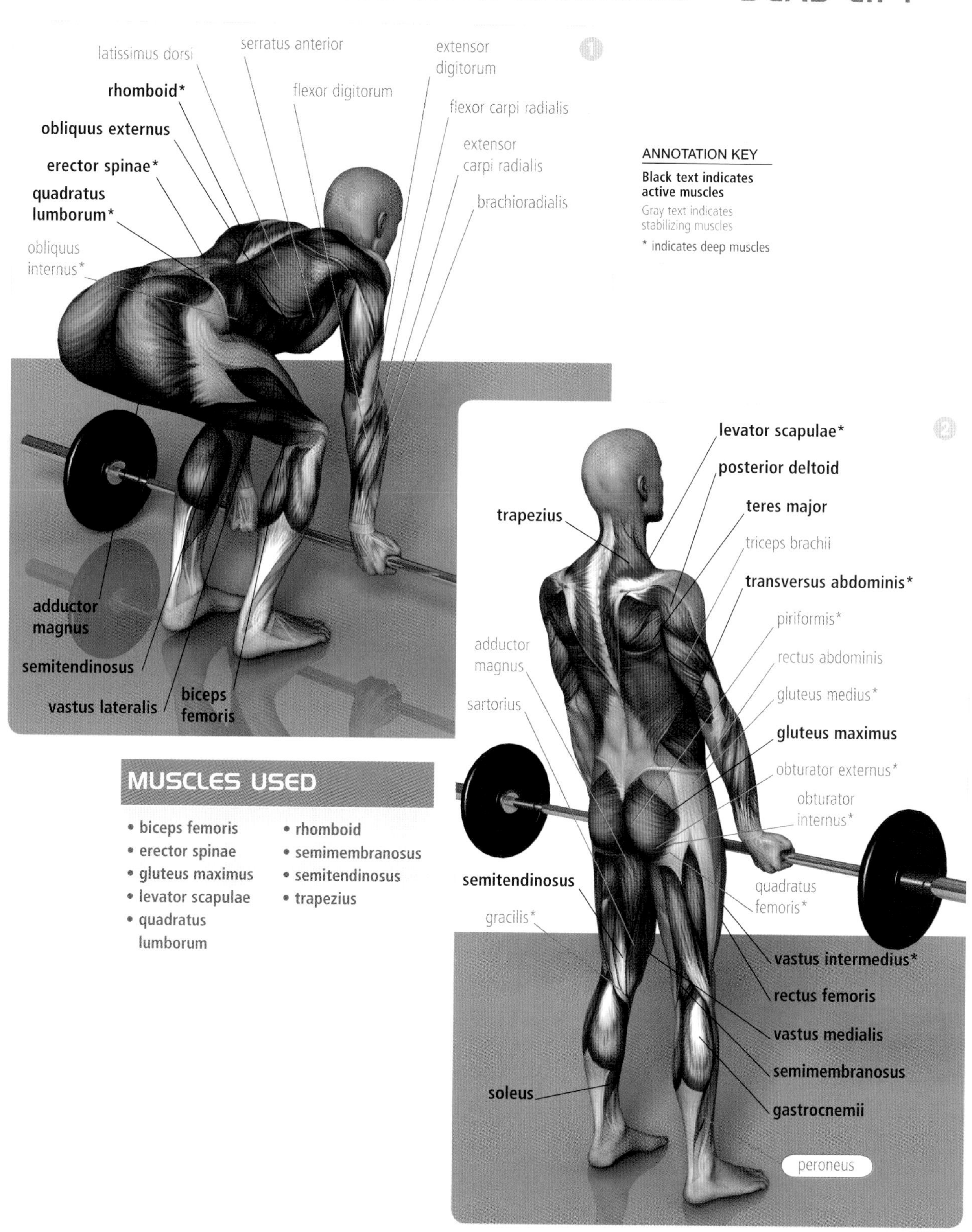

ANNOTATION KEY

Black text indicates active muscles

Gray text indicates stabilizing muscles

* indicates deep muscles

MUSCLES USED

- biceps femoris
- erector spinae
- gluteus maximus
- levator scapulae
- quadratus lumborum
- rhomboid
- semimembranosus
- semitendinosus
- trapezius

SUMO WITH KETTLEBELL

Starting Position: With the kettlebell on the ground and your feet slightly wider than shoulder-width apart, toes and knees pointed outward at 45-degree angles, grasp the bell with palms facing toward you. Your knees are bent so that your toes are directly over your feet. Keep your spine in a neutral position, positioned at a 45-degree angle to perpendicular. Your hips are dropped and retracted so that your upper legs are parallel to the ground (or as close to parallel as your flexibility will allow). Position your shoulder joints directly over the bell. Make sure that your feet are flat and your weight is evenly distributed. Pull your chest, head, and rib cage up and your abdominal muscles up and in. Inhale at the bottom of the position.

1

STABILIZE BY
- Keeping your rib cage high and your head up
- Pushing your shoulders down and back, with your shoulder blades flat on your rib cage
- Keeping your knees directly over your feet

Action: Exhale and drive your torso up and backward and your hips up and forward. Push your feet into the ground, extending your knees so that they move in a scissorlike action inward, and pull backward on the kettlebell with your upper back and shoulders until you arrive at a vertical position.

2

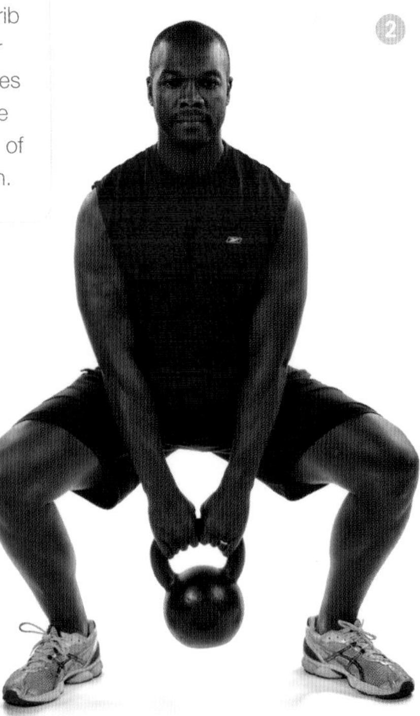

LOOK FOR
- The angle of your spine to never drop below 45 degrees during the movement
- A slight arch in your back throughout the movement
- All of your joints to move at the same time and at the same rate

AVOID
- Straightening your knees prior to extending your back and hips
- Rounding your back
- Elevating your shoulders or lowering your head
- Allowing your knees to migrate either inward or outward

Movement Path: Your hips move upward and forward, while your spine and torso move upward and backward, your knees extend and move inward, and your entire body moves upward and away from the floor.

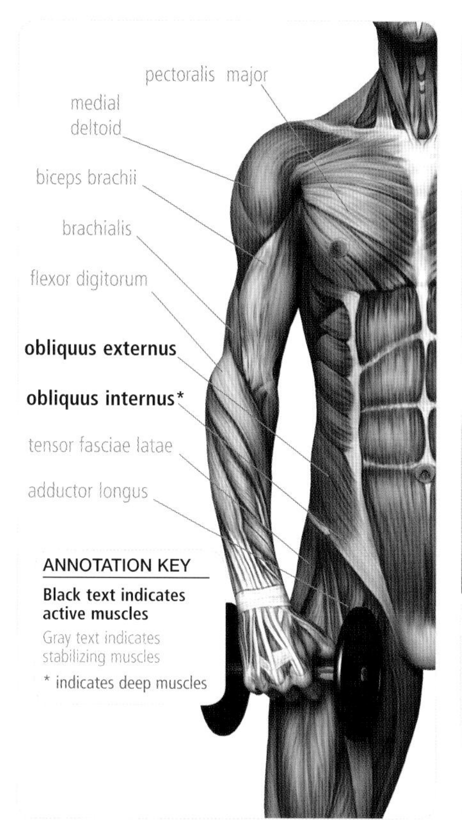

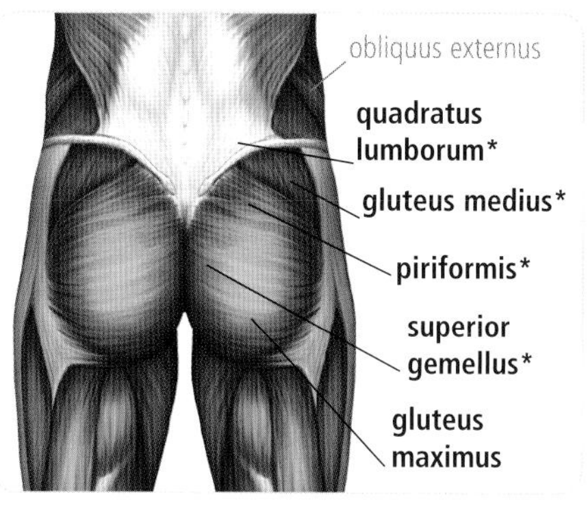

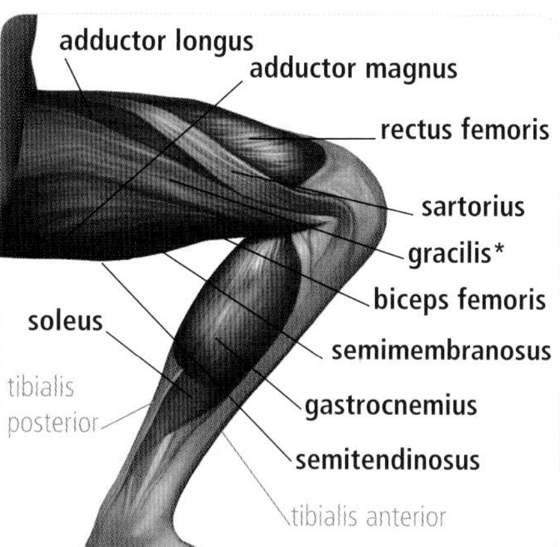

MODIFICATIONS

More Difficult: Holding the kettlebell directly in front of you, with arms extended, straddle boxes or blocks in the movement, going as deeply as you can while still maintaining spinal position.

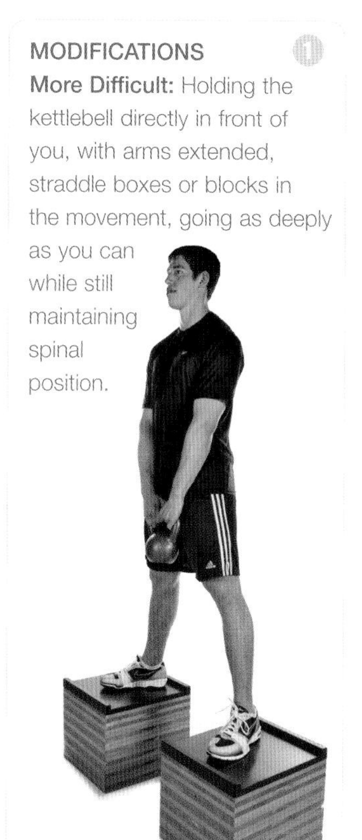

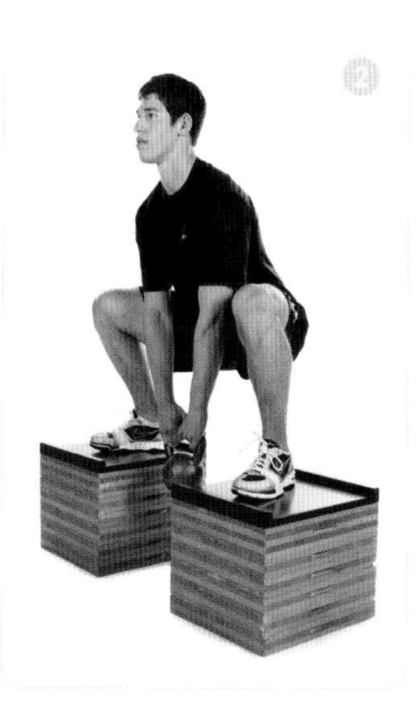

MUSCLES USED

- quadratus lumborum
- rectus femoris
- soleus
- biceps femoris
- semitendinosus
- semimembranosus
- gastrocnemius
- adductor magnus
- adductor longus
- gracilis
- adductor brevis
- gluteus maximus
- rectus abdominis
- obliquus internus
- obliquus externus
- trapezius
- levator scapulae
- vastus lateralis
- vastus medialis
- vastus intermedius

More Difficult: With two kettlebells on the ground and your feet slightly wider than shoulder-width apart, toes and knees pointed outward at 45-degree angles, grasp the pair of kettlebells. Follow same action and movement path as with single kettlebell.

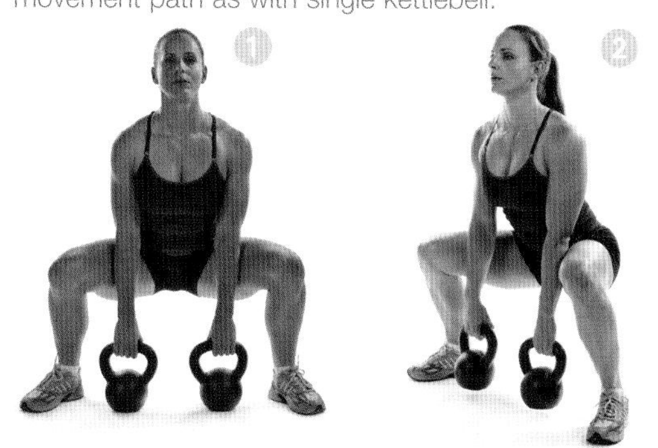

FULL SINGLE-LEG WITH DUMBBELLS

1

Starting Position: Stand on your right leg, and bend your left leg to a 90-degree angle. Keep your torso upright, and squeeze your shoulder blades together. Hold dumbbells in both hands.

Movement Path: Your center of mass descends vertically, and your torso moves in an arc, as though rotating around the center of a circle.

STABILIZE BY
- Maintaining a focus on balance—it is key! Look and focus on a spot in front of you as you bend over, balancing on one leg
- Contracting your quadriceps on the eccentric movement and your hamstrings and gluteals on the concentric movement

Action: Bend your right leg slightly as you bend over from your hip and reach the dumbbells toward the floor. Keep your chest up and your back slightly arched. Your left leg remains bent at 90 degrees throughout the exercise. Once you've touched the floor or gone as deep as you can, squeeze your gluteals and shoulder blades as you stand up again.

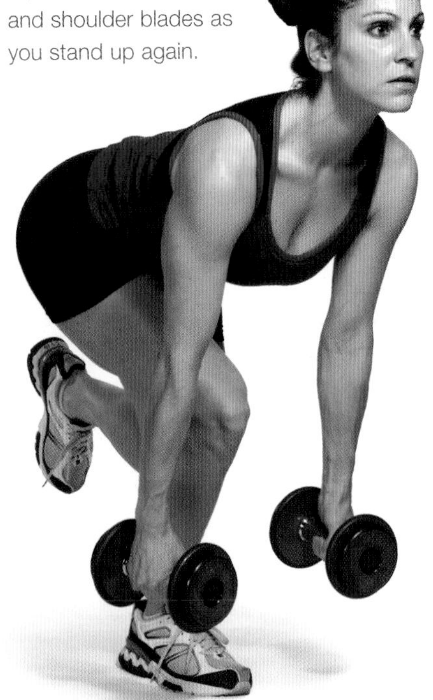

2

LOOK FOR
- Your spine to remain in a constant position throughout the movement
- Your torso to flex forward from the hip joint
- Your hamstring to stretch; allow your pelvis to rotate forward from below the waist

AVOID
- Improper form. Correct posture is extremely important: make sure that your chest is up and your back is slightly arched. If you can't bend over very far in this position, that's okay. It is better to have proper posture than greater range of motion.
- Rounding your back
- Allowing your shoulder blades to slip forward

FULL SINGLE-LEG WITH DUMBBELLS • DEAD LIFT

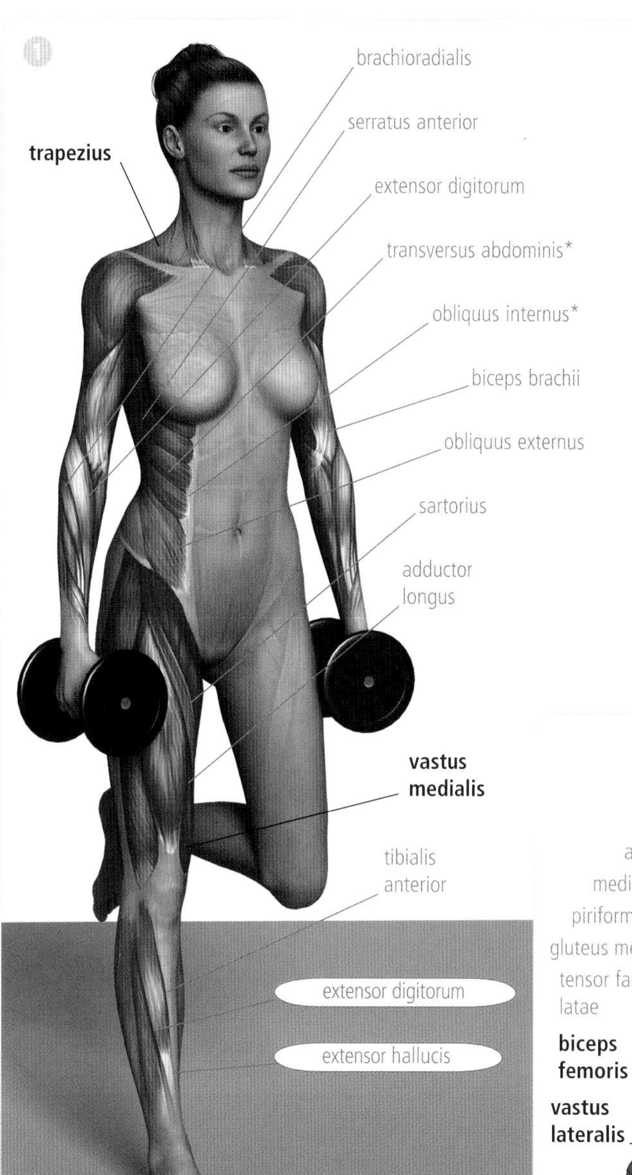

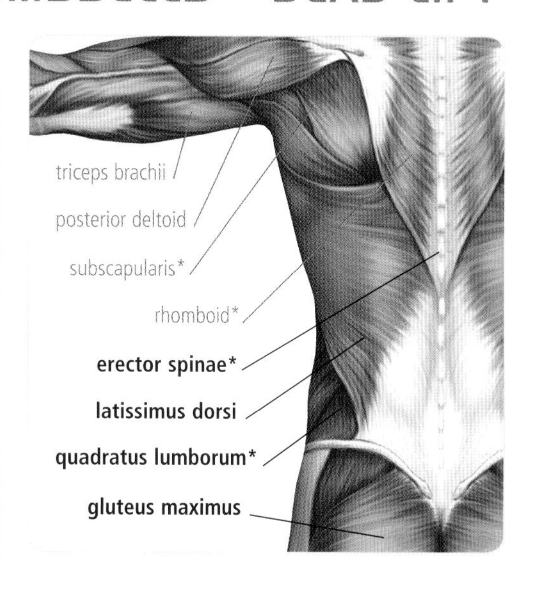

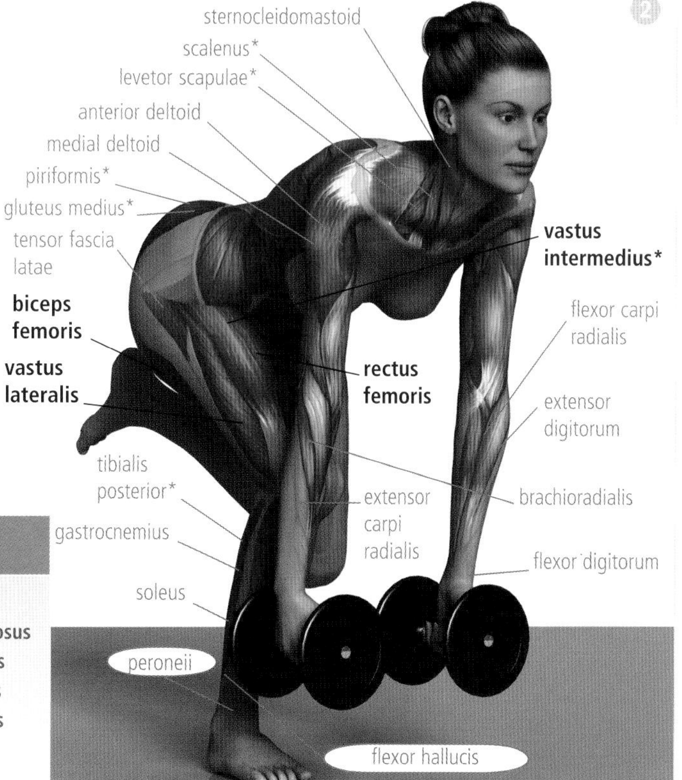

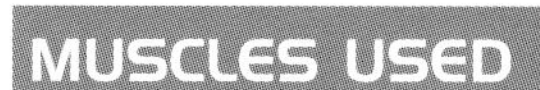

MUSCLES USED

- biceps femoris
- erector spinae
- gluteus maximus
- latissimus dorsi
- quadradus lumborum
- rectus femoris
- semimembranosus
- semitendinosus
- vastus lateralis
- vastus medialis

STRAIGHT-LEG WITH DUMBBELL

Starting Position: Holding the dumbbell directly in front of one leg, and your feet shoulder-width apart, place the opposite hand behind your head elbow facing out to the side. Bend your knees slightly, keeping your spine in a neutral position and your hips elevated, so that your head, shoulders, and hips are in a straight line and parallel to the floor.

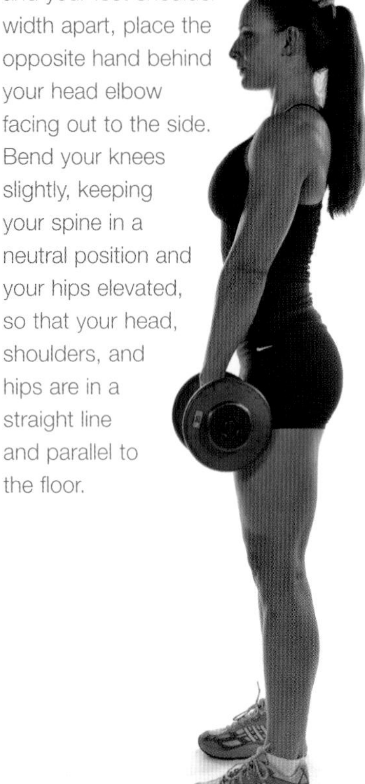

1

Action: Descend by retracting your hips and dropping your chest and rib cage forward. Create tension from your hands through the back of your body, all the way to your heels. Return by driving your back up and your hips forward, drawing the dumbbell in a straight line vertically adjacent to your shins, and continue until you are in a full standing position.

Movement Path: Push your feet into the ground, drive your shoulders back and up, and your hips forward simultaneously.

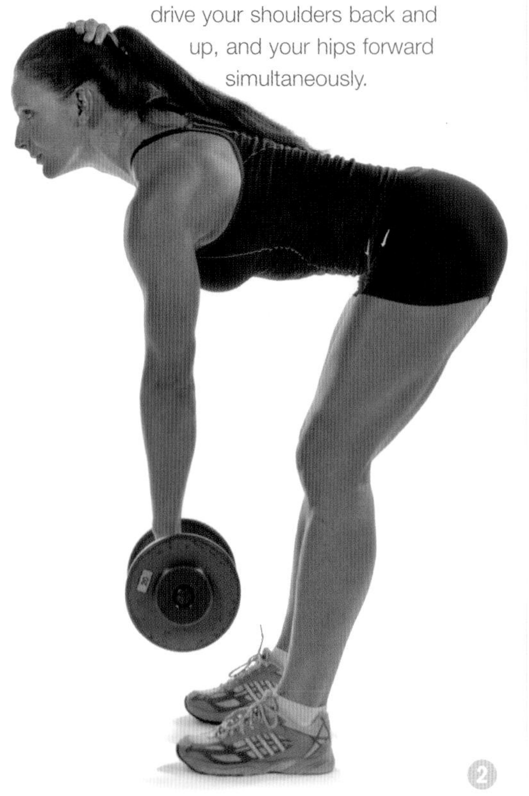

2

LOOK FOR

- Keeping weight evenly distributed through hips, legs, and feet into the ground
- All movement to happen at the same time
- Your spine to remain completely stable from hips to head
- Your head to be up, with your eyes forward and looking upward

AVOID

- Allowing your spine to round (by flexing forward) or change position in segments as it moves
- A rotation of any part of the spine or upper body
- Bending so that your hips are above your shoulders during the movement
- Bending your elbows or shrugging your shoulders
- Allowing your weight to rest in the front part of the foot or the dumb-bell to be forward of the toe line

STABILIZE BY

- Keeping your rib cage high, your head up, and your shoulders down and back, with your shoulder blades flat on your rib cage

STRAIGHT-LEG WITH DUMBBELL • DEAD LIFT

MUSCLES USED

- erector spinae
- rhomboids
- quadratus lumborum
- vastus lateralis
- vastus medialis
- vastus intermedius
- rectus femoris
- soleus
- adductor magnus
- biceps femoris
- semitendinosus
- semimembranosus
- gastrocnemii

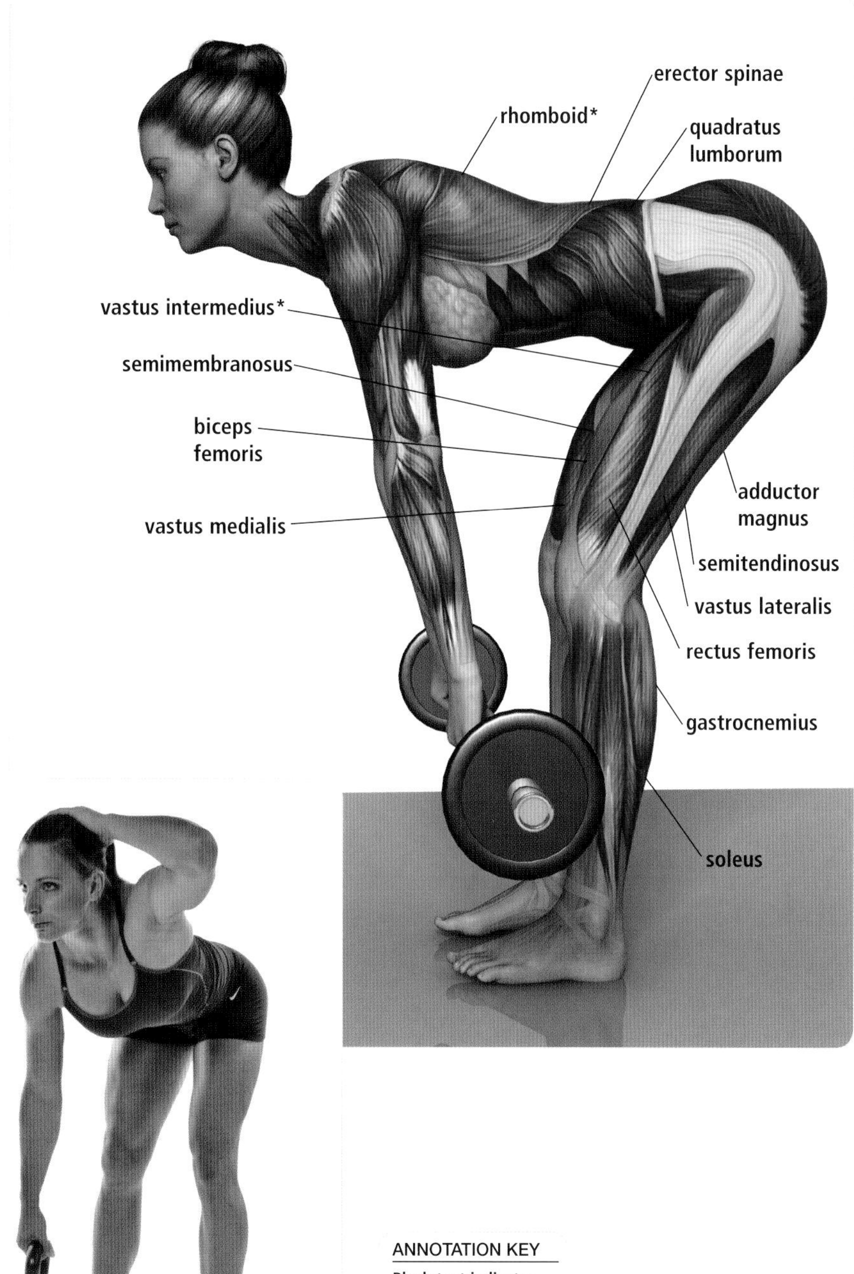

MODIFICATIONS

Similar Difficulty:
Replace the dumbbell with a kettlebell and maintain the same action and movement path.

ANNOTATION KEY

Black text indicates active muscles

Gray text indicates stabilizing muscles

* indicates deep muscles

SINGLE-LEG / STRAIGHT-LEG WITH KETTLEBELL

Starting Position: Stand on your right leg, and keep your left slightly behind your right heel, bearing little to no weight. Keep your torso upright, and squeeze your shoulder blades together. Hold the kettlebell in your left hand.

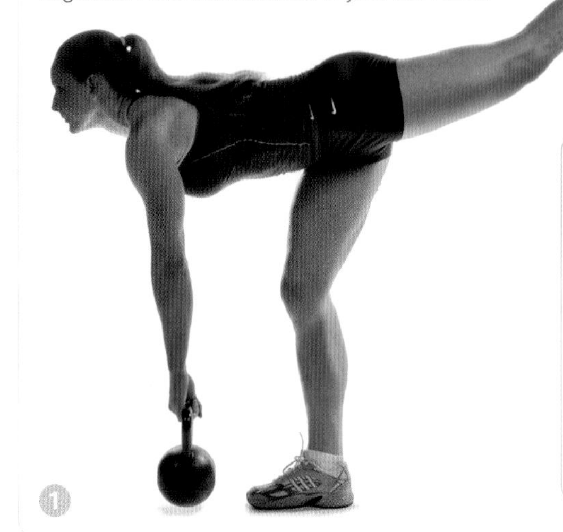

1

STABILIZE BY

- Maintaining a focus on balance—it is key! Look and focus on a spot in front of you as you bend over, balancing on one leg.
- Contracting your quadriceps on the eccentric movement and your hamstrings and gluteals on the concentric movement.
- Keeping your low back solid and keeping opposite leg straight and gluteus contracted.

LOOK FOR

- Spine to remain in a constant position throughout movement
- Torso to flex forward from the hip joint
- Hamstring to stretch and allow pelvis to rotate forward from below the belt
- Opposite leg to work as a counterbalance

AVOID

- Improper form. Correct posture is extremely important: make sure that your chest is up and your back is slightly arched. If you can't bend over as far in this position, that is OK. It is better to have proper posture than greater range of motion.
- Rounding the back/spine
- Allowing the shoulder blades to slip forward
- Not keeping opposite leg and spine in a straight line at all times

2

Action: Bend your right leg very slightly as you bend over from your hip, and reach the kettlebell toward the floor. Make sure that you keep your chest up and your back slightly arched. Your left leg remains in line with your spine throughout the exercise. Once you've touched the floor or gone as deep as you can, squeeze your gluteal hamstrings and shoulder blades as you stand up on your right leg, while your left leg returns to starting position.

Movement Path: The movement path consists of starting in an erect position and going into a bent over position, originating at the hip joint, and then returning to the erect position.

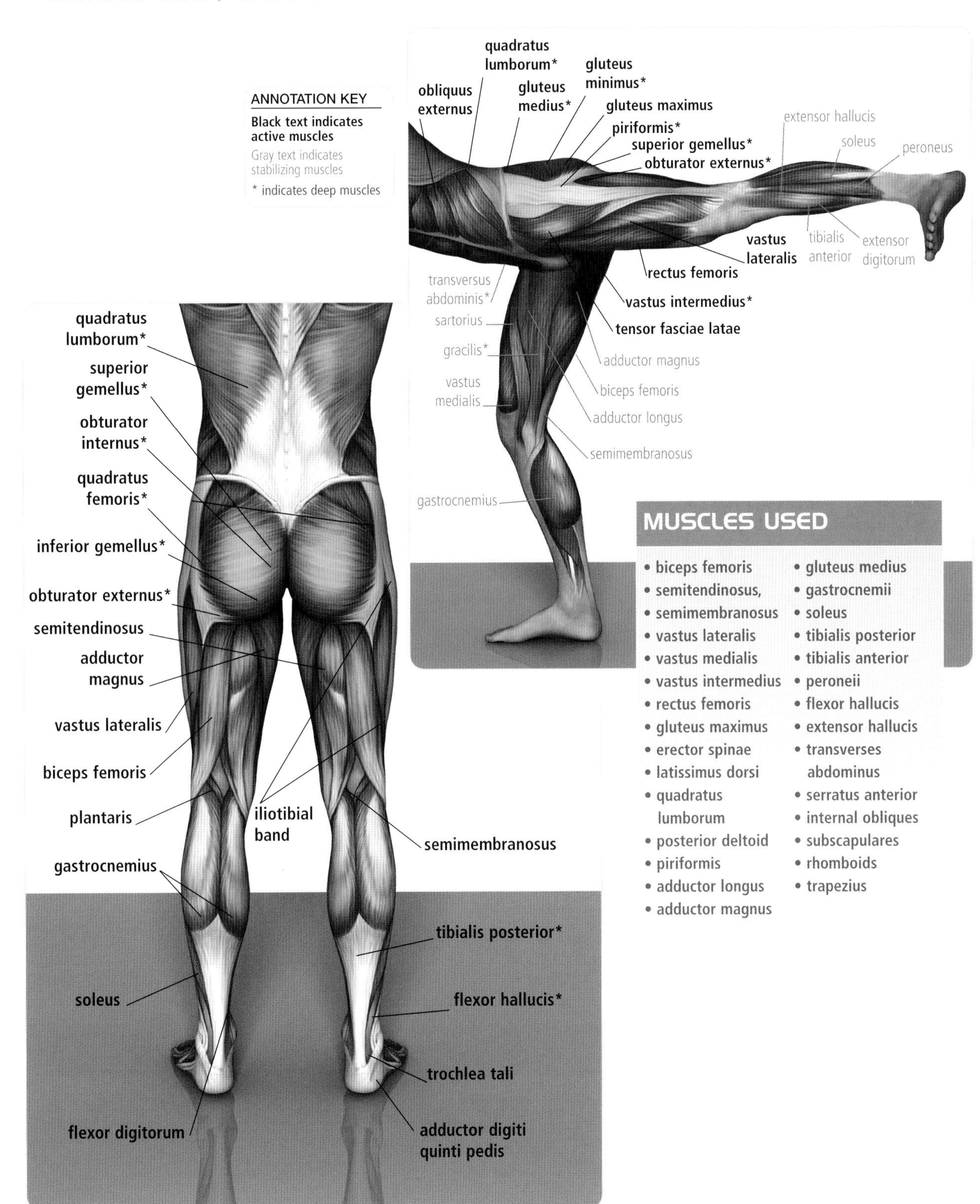

ANNOTATION KEY

Black text indicates active muscles

Gray text indicates stabilizing muscles

* indicates deep muscles

MUSCLES USED

- biceps femoris
- semitendinosus,
- semimembranosus
- vastus lateralis
- vastus medialis
- vastus intermedius
- rectus femoris
- gluteus maximus
- erector spinae
- latissimus dorsi
- quadratus lumborum
- posterior deltoid
- piriformis
- adductor longus
- adductor magnus
- gluteus medius
- gastrocnemii
- soleus
- tibialis posterior
- tibialis anterior
- peroneii
- flexor hallucis
- extensor hallucis
- transverses abdominus
- serratus anterior
- internal obliques
- subscapulares
- rhomboids
- trapezius

PNF RAISE WITH MEDICINE BALL

1

STABILIZE BY
- Pulling your abdomen up and in
- Distributing your weight evenly across your foot
- Using all muscles and joints in a coordinated, relaxed manner

Starting Position: Stand on one foot, bending the raised knee, and grasp a medicine ball just below and to the outside of the knee on the standing leg.

LOOK FOR
- Your knee and hip to extend and rise at the same time
- The ball to remain equidistant from your torso throughout the movement
- Your elbows to remain extended

AVOID
- Excessive flexion of your torso and spine
- Bringing the ball close to your body or lifting any part of your foot from the floor

2

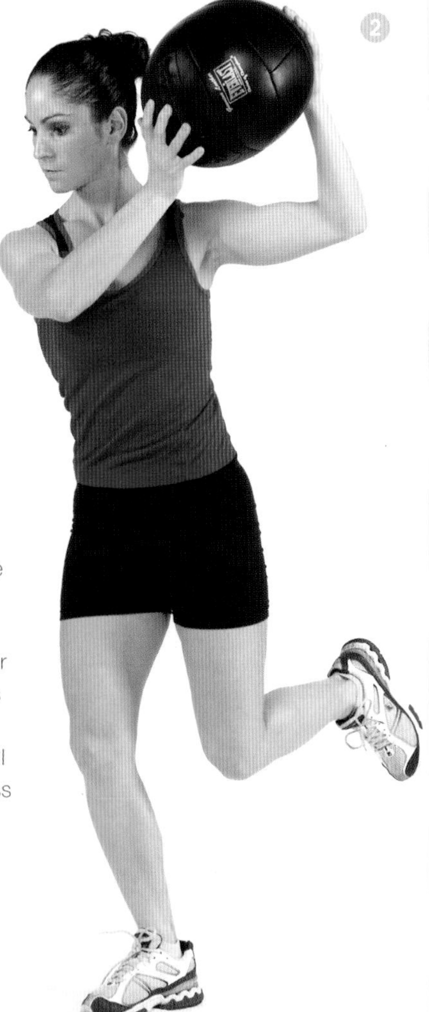

Action: Stand, extending your leg, while bringing the ball across your body to above and outside the opposite shoulder.

Movement Path: Your upper body rotates as your center of mass shifts upward. The ball moves in an arc across your body.

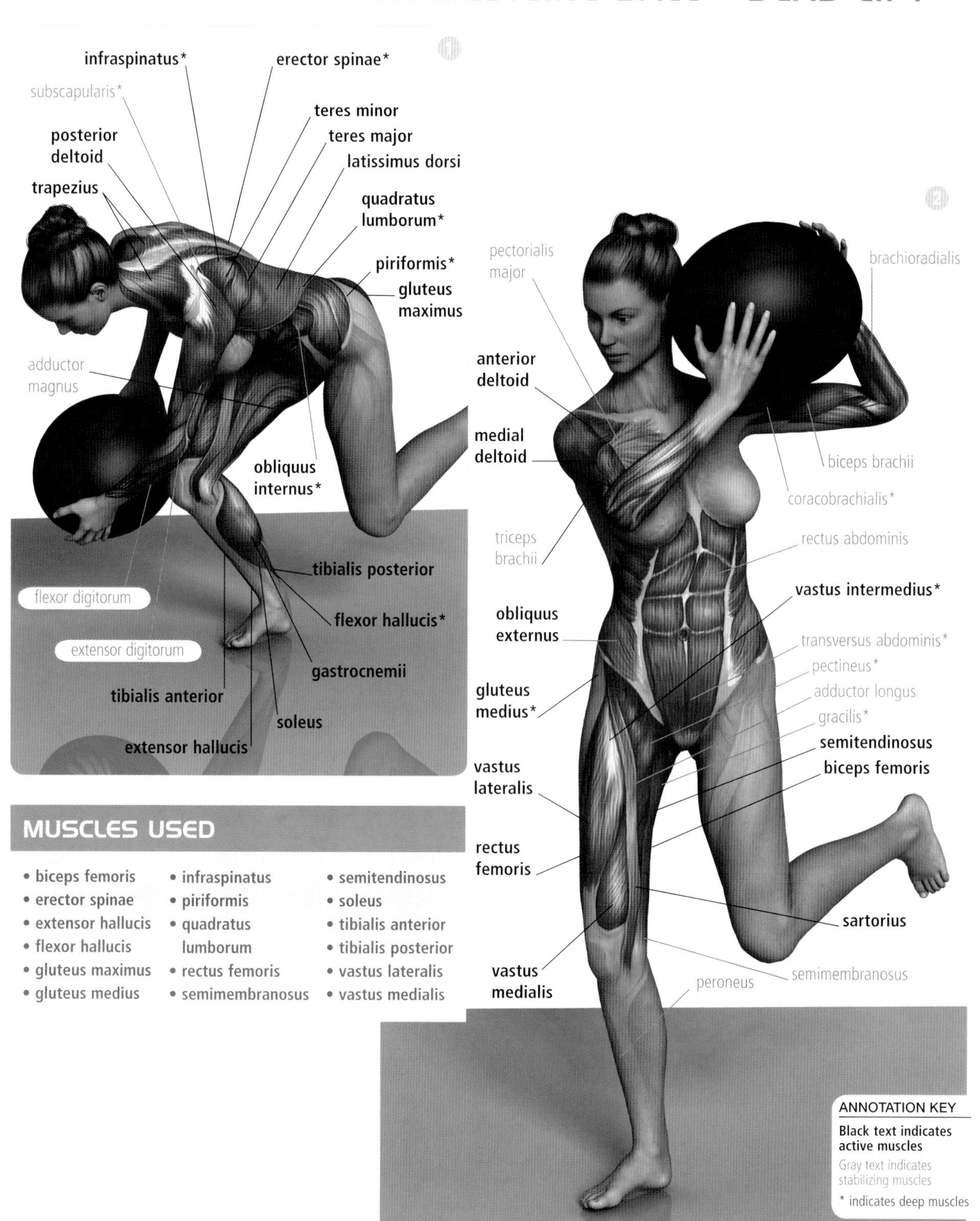

MUSCLES USED

- biceps femoris
- erector spinae
- extensor hallucis
- flexor hallucis
- gluteus maximus
- gluteus medius
- infraspinatus
- piriformis
- quadratus lumborum
- rectus femoris
- semimembranosus
- semitendinosus
- soleus
- tibialis anterior
- tibialis posterior
- vastus lateralis
- vastus medialis

FULL CABLE WITH ROTATION

Starting Position: Standing with feet slightly wider than shoulder-width, grasp the cable with both hands directly in front of you at your body's midline. See figure 1, page 31.

Action: Drop and retract your hips so that the tops of your legs are parallel to the ground (or as close to parallel as your flexibility will allow). Position your shoulder joints directly over your feet. Make sure that your feet are flat and your weight is evenly distributed. Pull your chest, head, and rib cage up and your abdominal muscles up and in. Inhale at the bottom of the position. Exhale and drive your torso up and backward and your hips up and forward. Push your feet into the ground, extending your knees until you arrive at a vertical position.

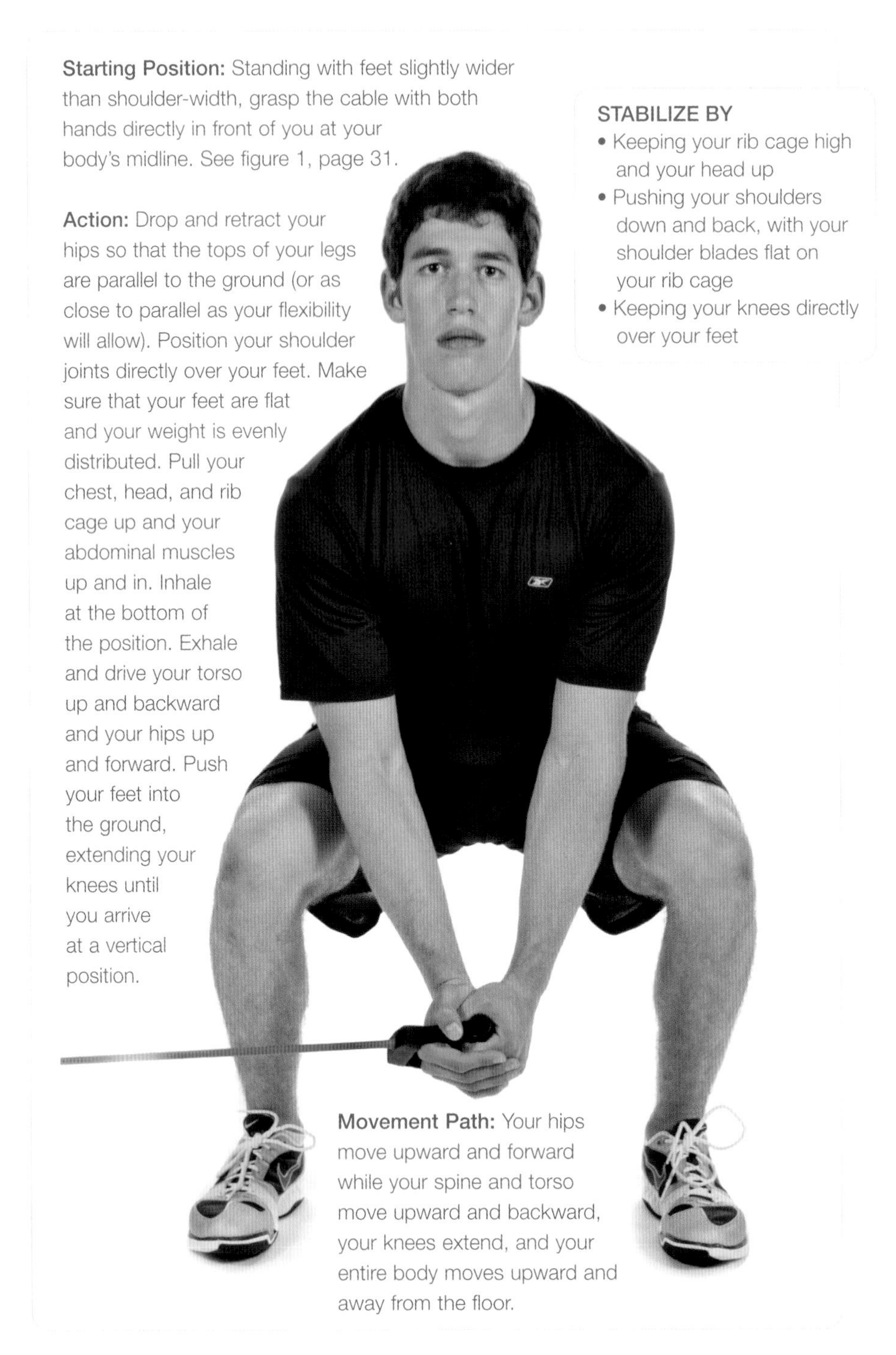

Movement Path: Your hips move upward and forward while your spine and torso move upward and backward, your knees extend, and your entire body moves upward and away from the floor.

STABILIZE BY
- Keeping your rib cage high and your head up
- Pushing your shoulders down and back, with your shoulder blades flat on your rib cage
- Keeping your knees directly over your feet

LOOK FOR
- The angle of your spine to never drop below 45 degrees during the movement
- A slight arch in your back throughout the movement
- All of your joints to move at the same time and at the same rate

AVOID
- Straightening your knees prior to extending your back and hips
- Rounding your back
- Elevating your shoulders or lowering your head
- Allowing your knees to migrate either inward or outward

MUSCLES USED

- erector spinae
- rhomboids
- latissimus dorsi
- teres major
- quadratus lumborum
- middle trapezius
- levator scapulae
- upper trapezius
- vastus lateralis
- vastus medialis
- vastus intermedius
- rectus femoris
- soleus
- biceps femoris
- semitendinosus
- semimembranosus
- gastrocnemius
- gluteus maximus
- rectus abdominis
- internal oblique
- external oblique
- flexor digitorum
- posterior deltoid
- adductor longus
- adductor magnus
- sartorius
- gracilis

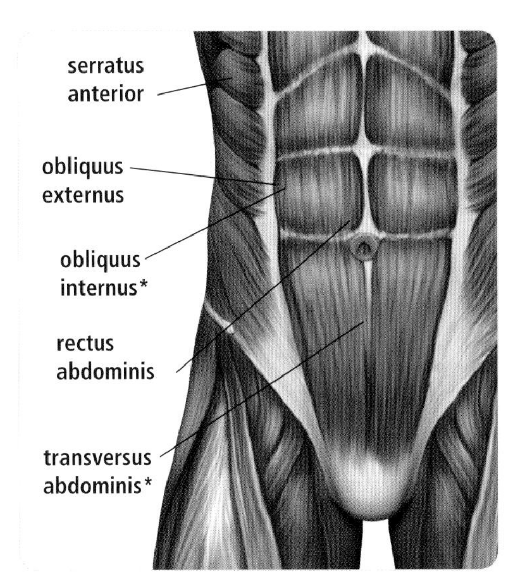

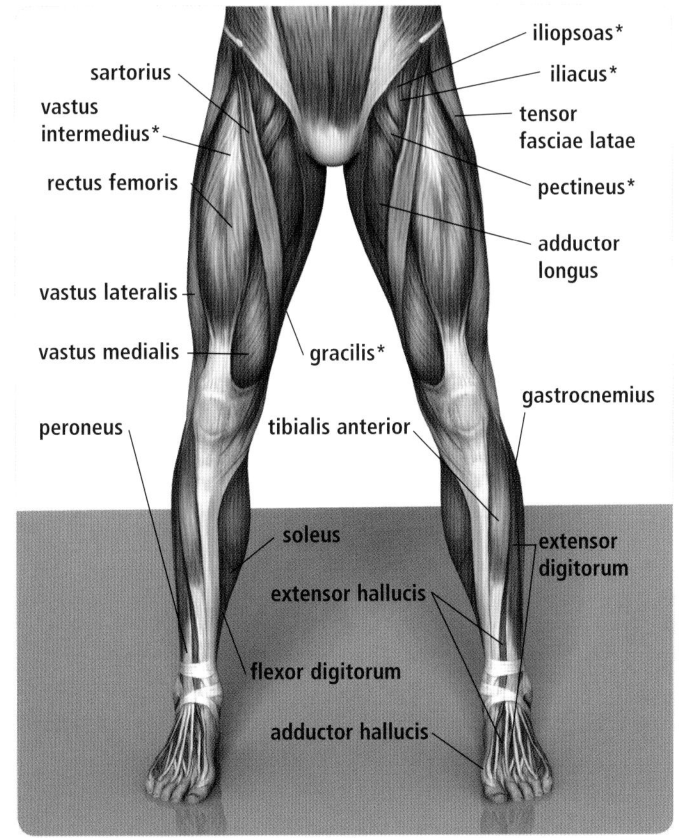

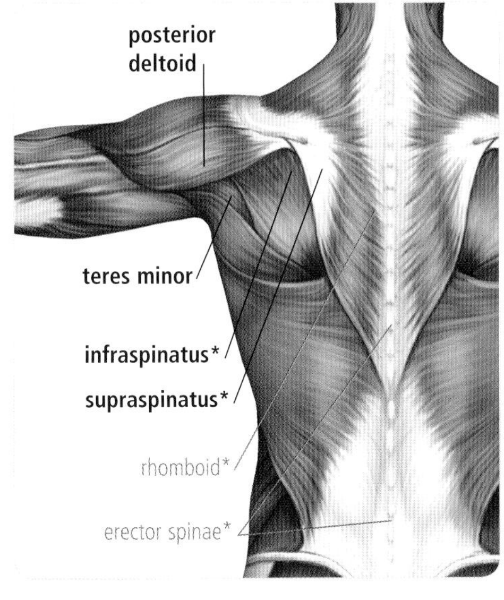

ANNOTATION KEY

Black text indicates active muscles

Gray text indicates stabilizing muscles

* indicates deep muscles

STRAIGHT-LEG CABLE DEAD LIFT

Starting Position: Grasp cable in one hand at your side so that the cable crosses the front of both legs. With your feet shoulder-width apart, place the opposite hand behind your head with elbow facing out to the side. Bend your knees slightly, keeping your spine in a neutral position and your hips elevated, so that your head, shoulders, and hips are in a straight line and parallel to the floor.

Action: Descend by retracting your hips and dropping your chest and rib cage forward. Create tension from your hand through the back of your body, all the way to your heels. Return by driving your back up and your hips forward, keeping your hand adjacent to your leg, your shoulder steady (continue until you are in a full standing position).

Movement Path: Push your feet into the ground, drive your shoulders back and up, and your hips forward simultaneously.

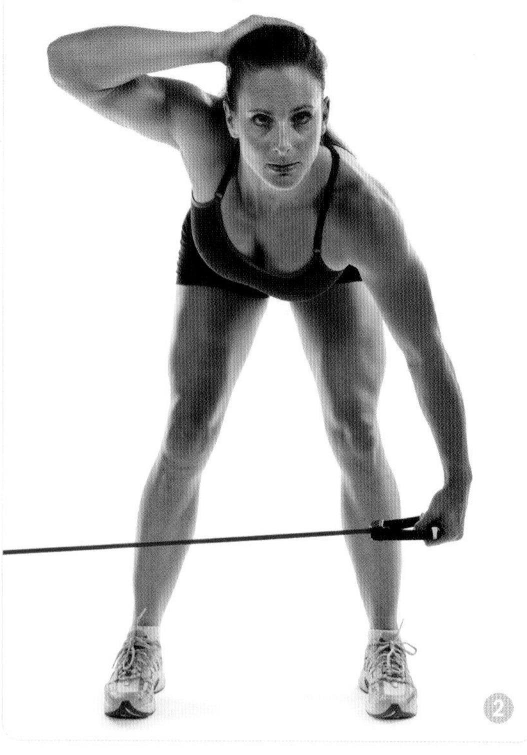

LOOK FOR
- Keeping weight evenly distributed through hips, legs, and feet into the ground
- All movement to happen at the same time
- Your spine to remain stable from hips to head with no rotation
- Your head to be up, with your eyes forward and looking upward
- Knees and hips to remain parallel

AVOID
- Rotation of any part of the spine or upper body
- Allowing your spine to round or change position in segments
- Bending so that hips are above your shoulders
- Bending your elbows or shrugging your shoulders
- Allowing your weight to rest in the front part of the foot or the cable to be forward of the toe line

STABILIZE BY
- Keeping your rib cage high, your head up, and your shoulders down and back with your shoulder blades flat on your rib cage, hand with cable solid and stable

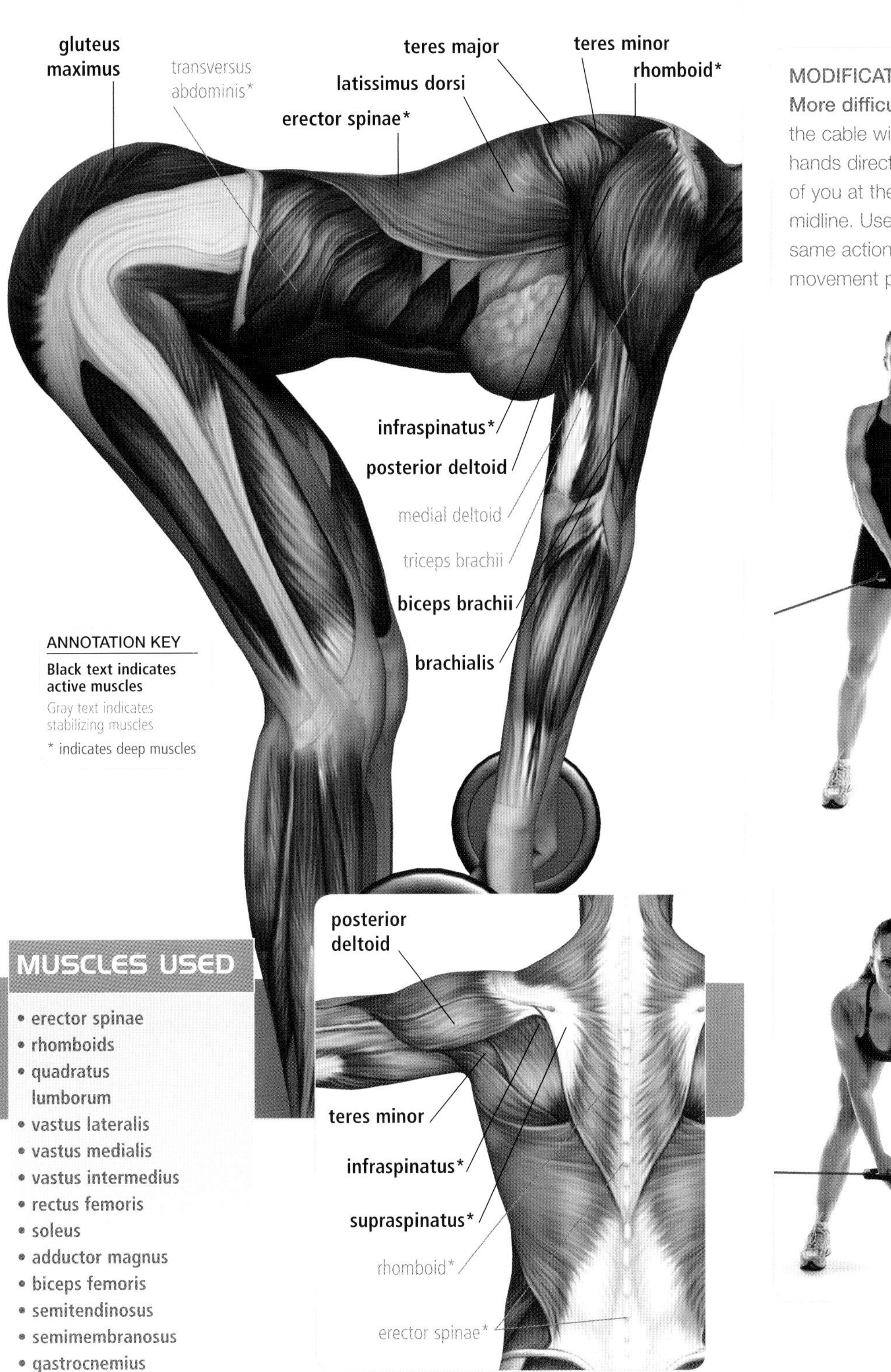

ANNOTATION KEY

Black text indicates active muscles

Gray text indicates stabilizing muscles

* indicates deep muscles

MUSCLES USED

- erector spinae
- rhomboids
- quadratus lumborum
- vastus lateralis
- vastus medialis
- vastus intermedius
- rectus femoris
- soleus
- adductor magnus
- biceps femoris
- semitendinosus
- semimembranosus
- gastrocnemius

MODIFICATIONS

More difficult: Grasp the cable with both hands directly in front of you at the body's midline. Use the exact same action and movement path.

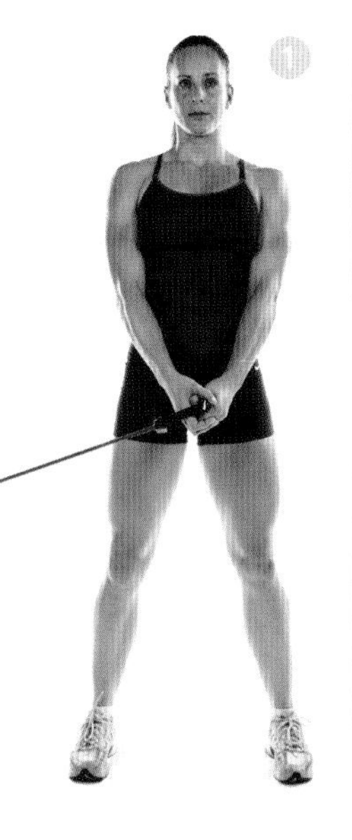

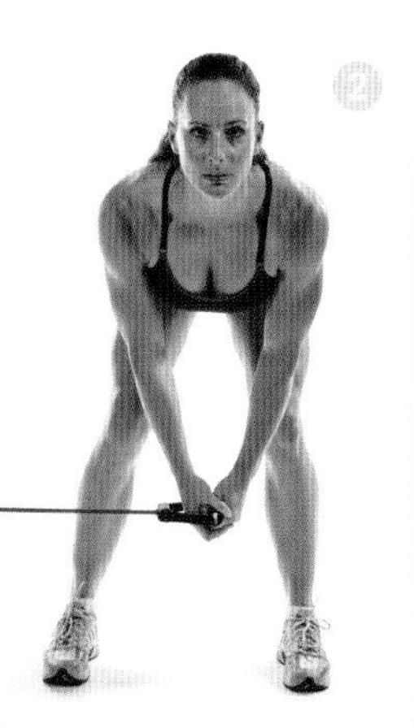

BAG FLIP

Starting Position: With the punching bag on the ground and your feet shoulder-width apart, grasp the bag with your palms facing each another. Bend your knees so that your toes are over your knees. Keep your spine in a neutral position, positioned at a 45-degree angle to perpendicular. Your hips are dropped and retracted so that the tops of your legs are parallel to the ground (or as close to parallel as your flexibility will allow). Position your shoulder joints directly over the bag. Make sure that your feet are flat and your weight is evenly distributed. Pull your chest, head, and rib cage up and your abdominal muscles up and in. Inhale at the bottom of the position.

Action: Exhale and drive your torso upward and your hips up and forward. Push your feet into the ground, extending your knees and pulling upward on the bag, forcefully and quickly, with your upper back, shoulders, and elbows. Elevate onto the toes and follow through with your hand upward and forward away from your body, releasing the bag all in one fluid movement.

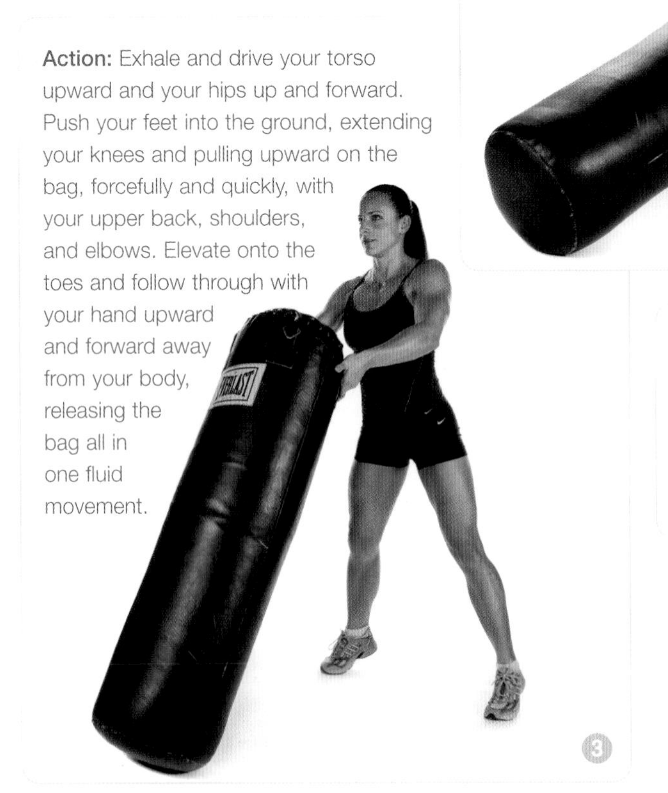

LOOK FOR
- The angle of your spine to never drop below 45 degrees during the movement
- A slight arch in back throughout the movement
- All of your joints to move at the same time and at the same rate

AVOID
- Straightening your knees prior to extending your back and hips
- Rounding your back
- Lowering your head
- Allowing your knees to migrate either inward or outward

STABILIZE BY
- Keeping your rib cage high and your head up
- Keeping your spine in a solid, neutral position
- Keeping your knees directly over your feet

BAG FLIP • DEAD LIFT

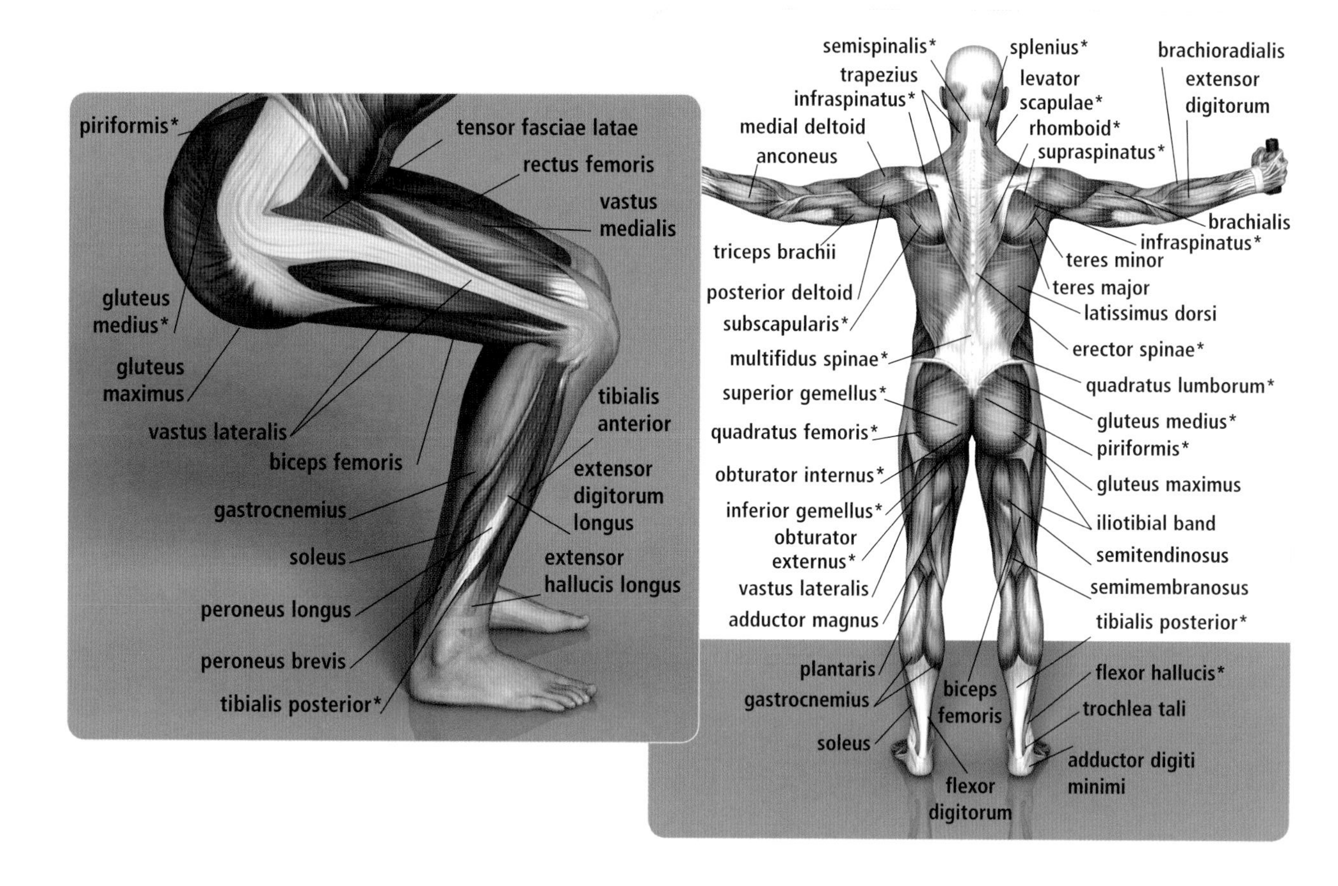

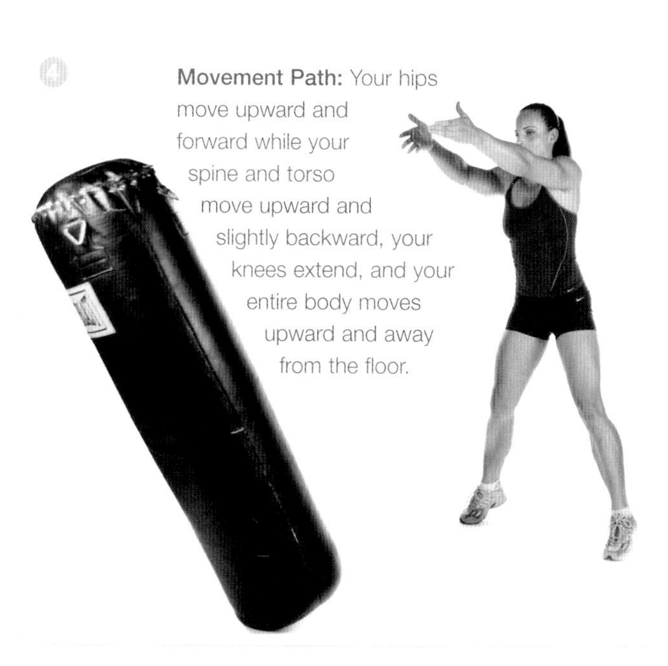

Movement Path: Your hips move upward and forward while your spine and torso move upward and slightly backward, your knees extend, and your entire body moves upward and away from the floor.

MUSCLES USED

- biceps femoris
- erector spinae
- gluteus maximus
- latissimus dorsi
- levator scapulae
- obliquus externus
- quadradus lumborum
- rectus femoris
- rhomboid
- semimembranosus
- semitendinosus
- soleus
- trapezius
- vastus lateralis
- vastus medialis

ANNOTATION KEY

Black text indicates active muscles

Gray text indicates stabilizing muscles

* indicates deep muscles

FULL WITH DUMBBELL

DEAD LIFT

Starting Position: With the dumbbell on the ground and your feet slightly wider than shoulder-width apart, grasp the dumbbell with palm facing toward you. Place the other hand behind your head, elbows pointing outward. Your knees are positioned so that they are directly over your toes. Keep your spine in a neutral position.

Action: Bend as deeply as you can while still maintaining spinal position. Your hips are dropped and retracted so that your upper legs are parallel to the ground (or as close to parallel as your flexibility will allow). Position your shoulder joints directly over your feet. Make sure that your feet are flat and your weight is evenly distributed. Pull your chest, head, and rib cage up and your abdominal muscles up and in. Inhale at the bottom of the position. Exhale and drive your torso up and backward and your hips up and forward. Push your feet into the ground, extending your knees and pulling upward on the dumbbell with your upper back and shoulders until you arrive at a vertical position.

STABILIZE BY

- Keeping your rib cage high and your head up
- Pushing your shoulders down and back, with your shoulder blades flat on your rib cage
- Keeping your knees directly over your feet

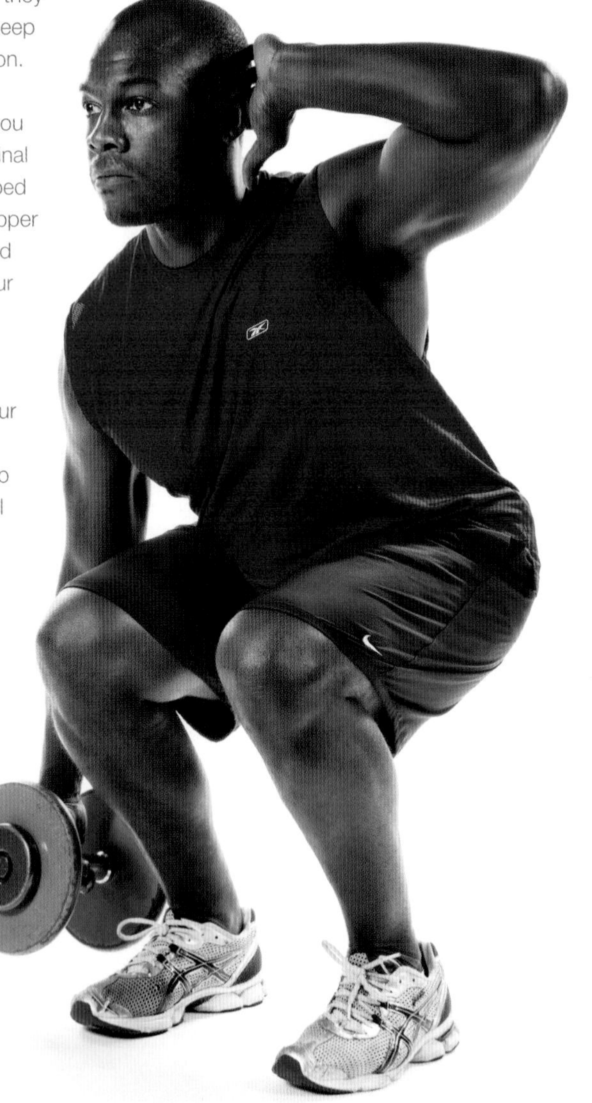

LOOK FOR

- The angle of your spine to never drop below 45 degrees during the movement
- A slight arch in your back throughout the movement
- All of your joints to move at the same time and at the same rate
- The dumbbell to drop in a straight vertical line

AVOID

- Straightening your knees prior to extending your back and hips
- Rounding your back
- Elevating your shoulders or lowering your head
- Allowing your knees to migrate either inward or outward
- Any rotation of the torso, hips, or shoulders

Movement Path: Your hips move upward and forward, while your spine and torso move upward and backward, your knees extend and move inward, and your entire body moves upward and away from the floor.

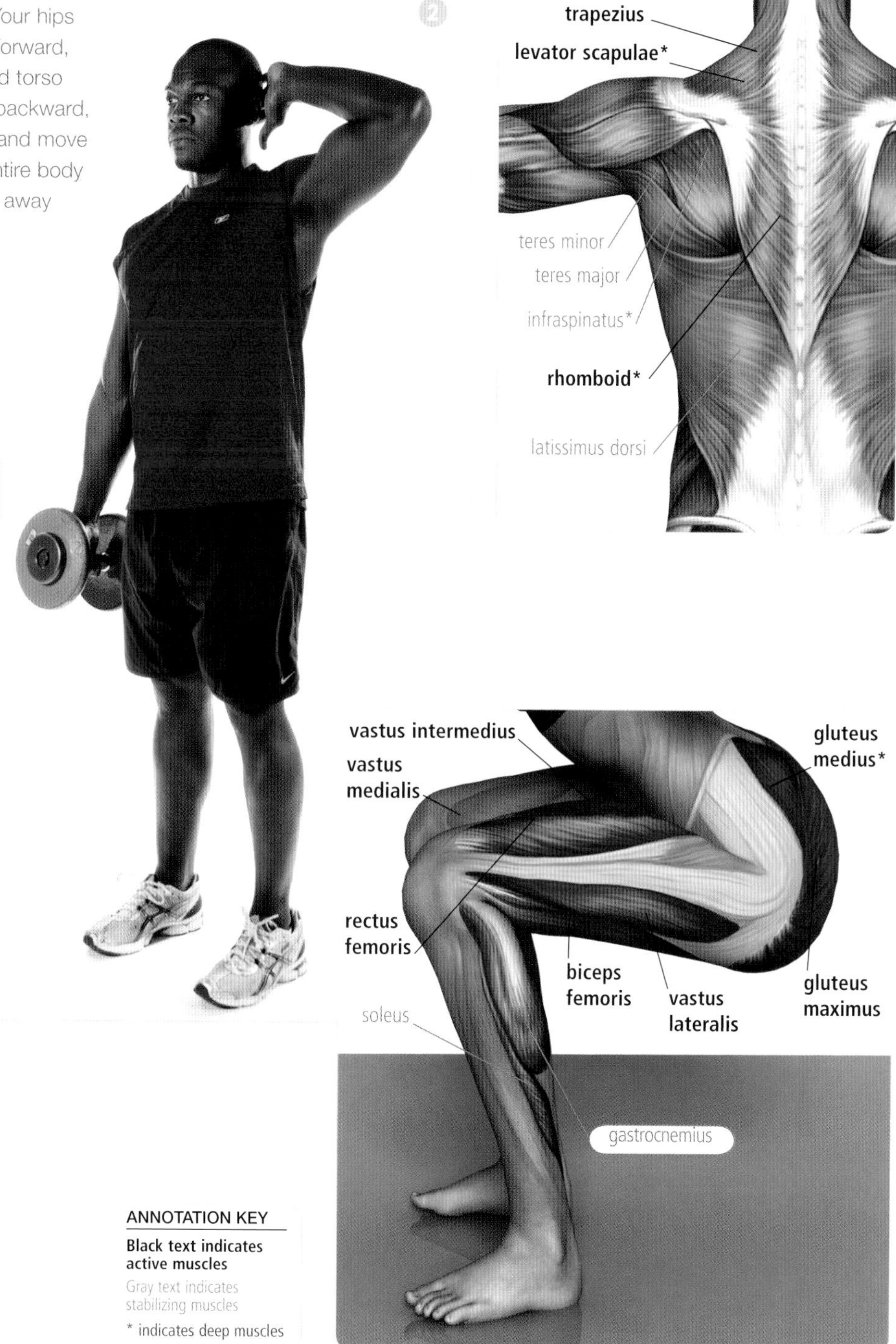

MUSCLES USED

- erector spinae
- rhomboids
- latissimus dorsi
- teres major
- quadratus lumborum
- middle trapezius
- levator scapulae
- upper trapezius
- vastus lateralis
- vastus medialis
- vastus intermedius
- rectus femoris
- soleus
- biceps femoris
- semitendinosus
- semimembranosus
- gastrocnemius
- adductor magnus
- adductor longus
- gracillus
- adductor brevis
- gluteus maximus
- rectus abdominis
- internal oblique
- external oblique
- flexor digitorum
- posterior deltoid
- latissimus dorsi
- obturator externus
- gluteus medius
- piriformis

ANNOTATION KEY

Black text indicates active muscles

Gray text indicates stabilizing muscles

* indicates deep muscles

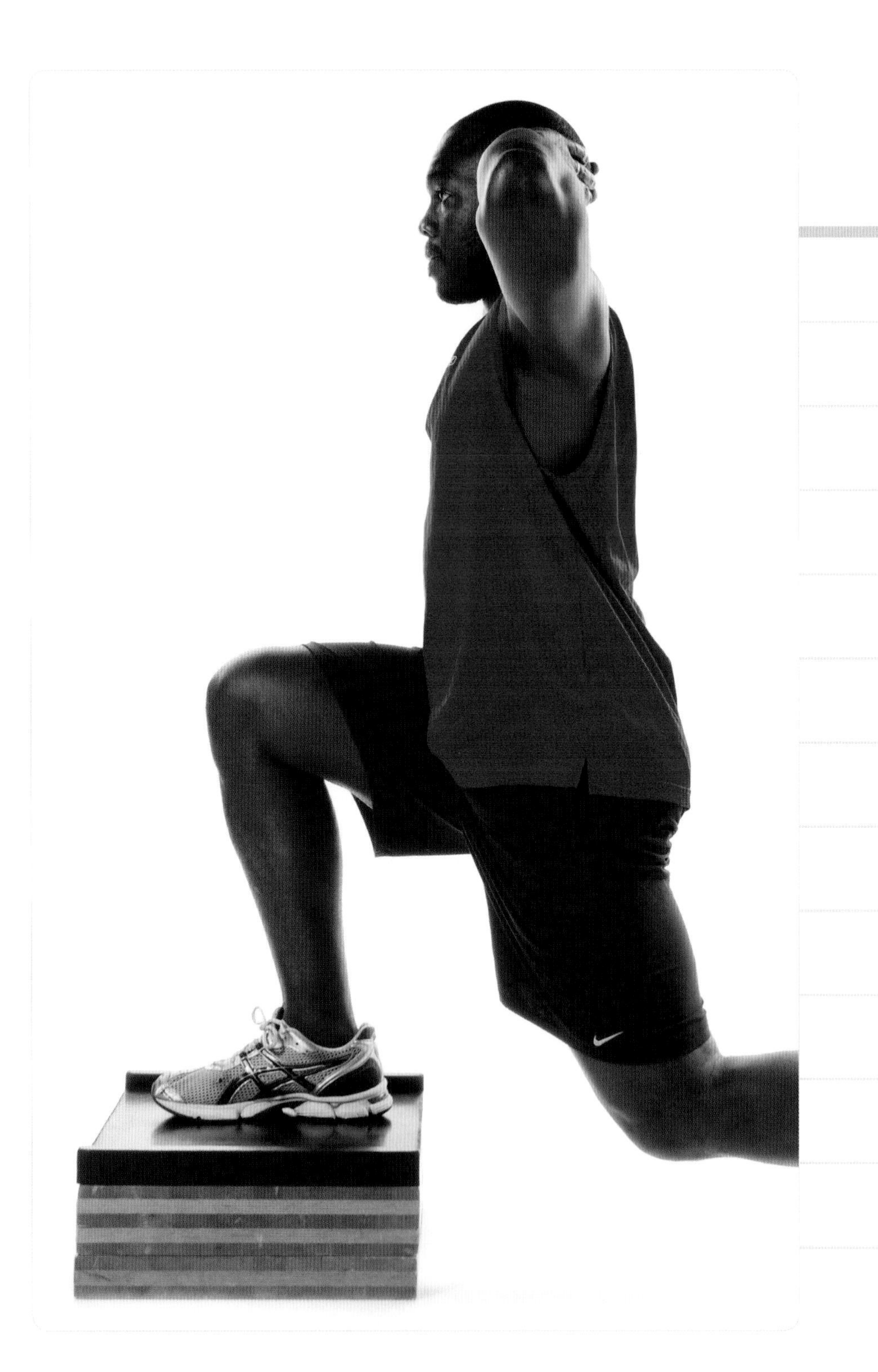

LUNGE

In order for the body to function properly, the legs, hips, and back must be strong, stable, and flexible. Lunges address all three of these body parts in one movement. Low-back and disc-related injuries are rampant, as are knee injuries (ACL, meniscus, patellofemoral, and Iliotibial Band Syndromes, etc.). A vast majority of these injuries stem from one of the following three issues: strength (imbalances), instability, and inflexibility, if not a combination of two or all of them at once. A steady diet of lunges will, without question, improve strength, stability, and flexibility and lower the possibility of related injuries.

Joints involved are ankle, knee, and hip. The muscles involved are legs (*all*), glutes, lower back, and stomach.

Primary benefits are leg and hip strength, flexibility, and balance.

STATIONARY LUNGE

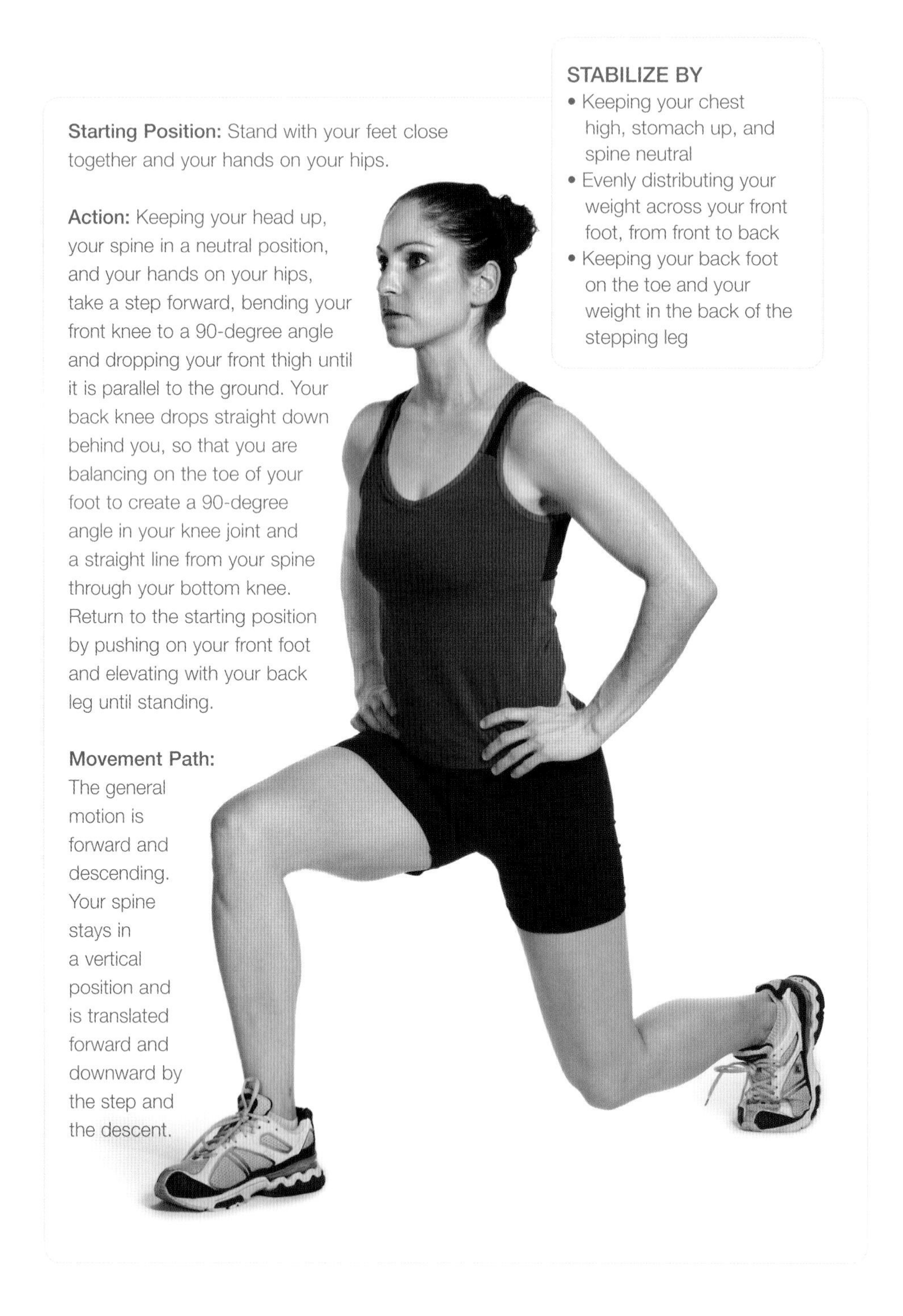

Starting Position: Stand with your feet close together and your hands on your hips.

Action: Keeping your head up, your spine in a neutral position, and your hands on your hips, take a step forward, bending your front knee to a 90-degree angle and dropping your front thigh until it is parallel to the ground. Your back knee drops straight down behind you, so that you are balancing on the toe of your foot to create a 90-degree angle in your knee joint and a straight line from your spine through your bottom knee. Return to the starting position by pushing on your front foot and elevating with your back leg until standing.

Movement Path: The general motion is forward and descending. Your spine stays in a vertical position and is translated forward and downward by the step and the descent.

STABILIZE BY
- Keeping your chest high, stomach up, and spine neutral
- Evenly distributing your weight across your front foot, from front to back
- Keeping your back foot on the toe and your weight in the back of the stepping leg

LOOK FOR
- No translation forward from the hips (do not bend)
- Your spine to remain in the same position as it moves down and up
- No lateral movement of your leg as you step, either landing or pushing

AVOID
- Raising the heel of your stepping foot off the ground or rotating your hips or torso

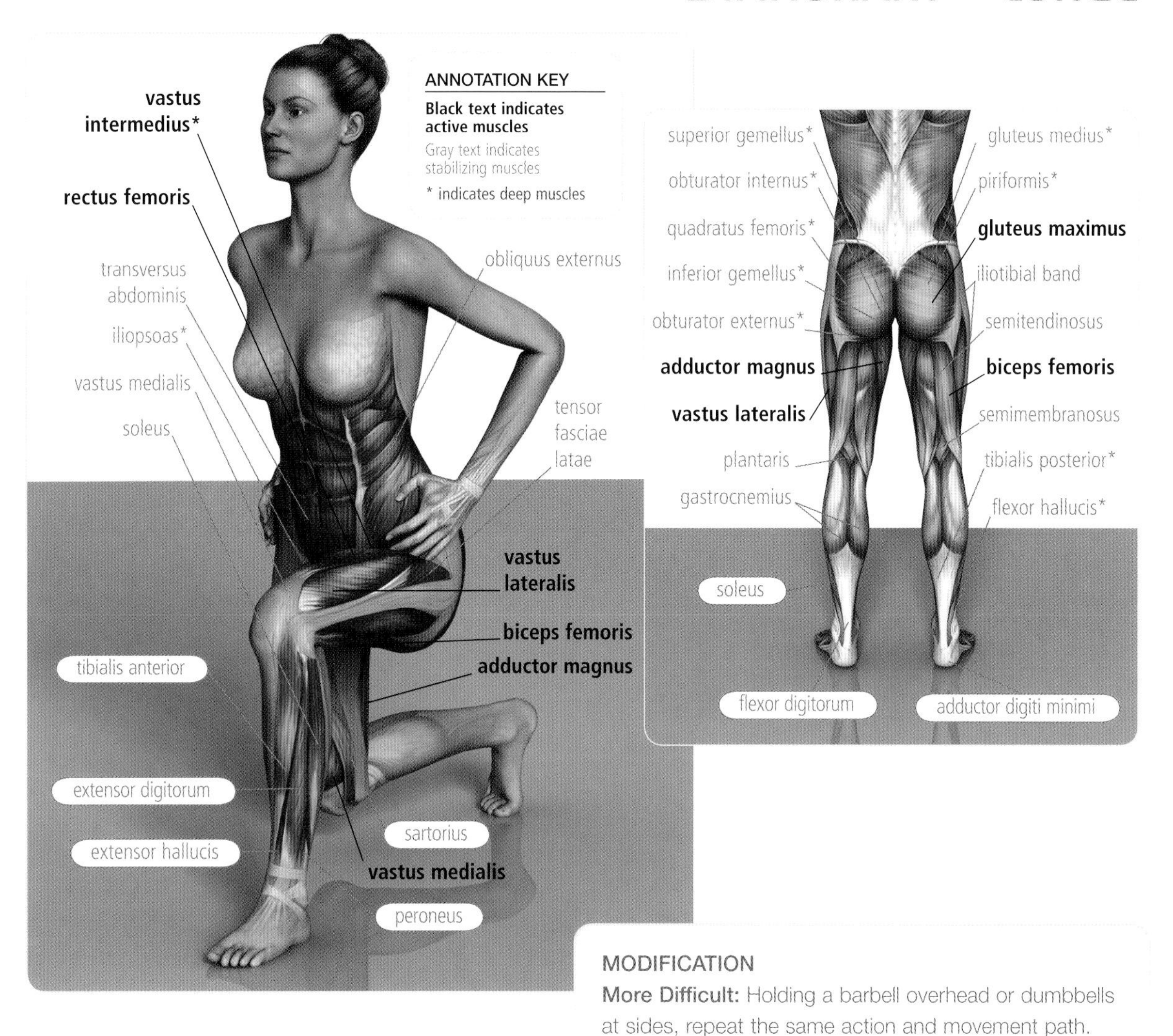

MODIFICATION

More Difficult: Holding a barbell overhead or dumbbells at sides, repeat the same action and movement path.

MUSCLES USED

- adductor magnus
- biceps femoris
- gluteus maximus
- rectus femoris
- vastus intermedius
- vastus lateralis
- vastus medialis

WALKING WITH ROTATION

STABILIZE BY

- Keeping your chest high, stomach up, and spine neutral
- Evenly distributing your weight across your front foot, from front to back
- Keeping your back foot on the toe and your weight in the back of the stepping leg

Starting Position: Stand with your feet close together and your hands on your hips. With palms facing each other and arms extended at chest height, grasp a medicine ball on the sides.

Action: Keeping your head up, your spine in a neutral position, and both hands in front of you, step forward, bending your front knee to a 90-degree angle and dropping your front thigh until it is parallel to the ground. Your back knee drops straight down behind you, so that you are balancing on the toe of your foot, to create a 90-degree angle in your knee joint and a straight line from your spine through your bottom knee. During the stepping-out process, simultaneously move the ball across your body 45 degrees to the side of the forward leg, keeping arms extended and level.

Movement Path: A forward motion and a descending motion. Your spine stays in a vertical position and is translated forward and down by the step and the deceleration. Return to the starting position by pushing on your front foot and elevating with your back leg while bringing the ball back to starting position. Repeat with other leg.

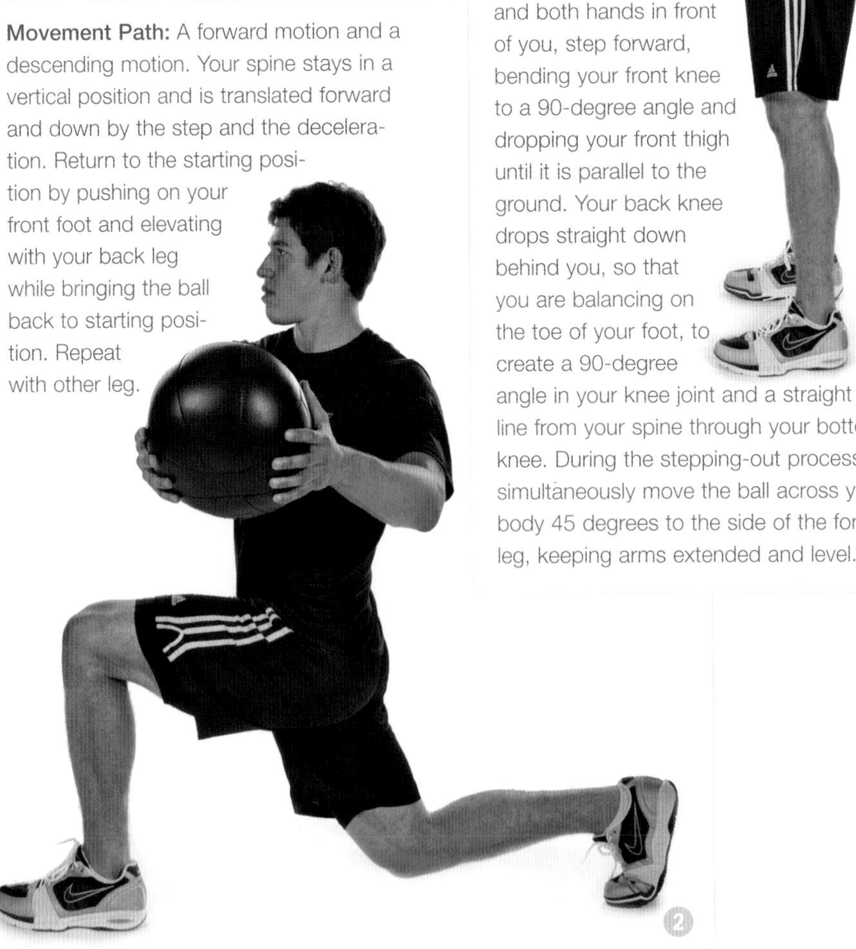

LOOK FOR

- No translation forward from the hips or your spine
- Your spine to remain in the same position as it moves down and up
- No lateral movement of your leg as you step, either landing or pushing

AVOID

- Raising the heel of your stepping foot off the ground or rotating your hips or torso

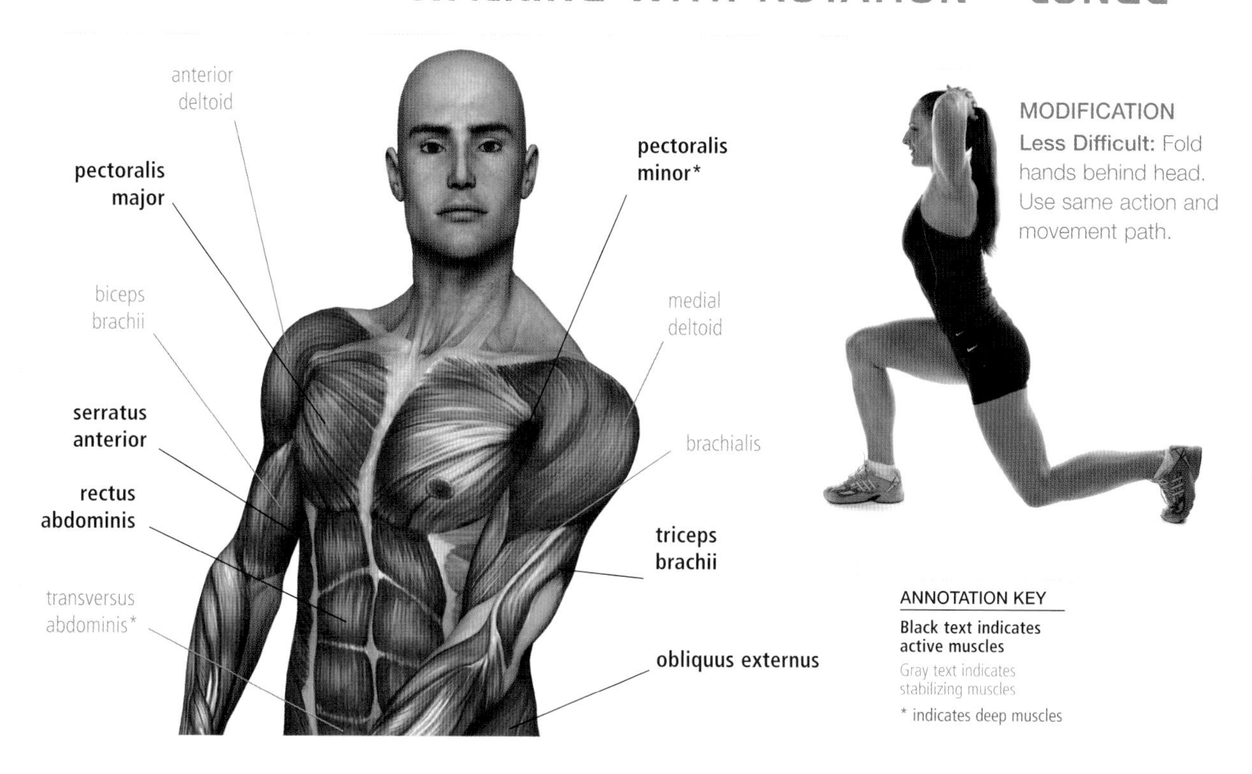

MODIFICATION

Less Difficult: Fold hands behind head. Use same action and movement path.

ANNOTATION KEY

Black text indicates active muscles

Gray text indicates stabilizing muscles

* indicates deep muscles

MUSCLES USED

- gluteus maximus
- vastus lateralis
- vastus medialis
- vastus intermedius
- biceps femoris
- rectus femoris
- adductor magnus
- erector spinae
- soleus
- tibialis anterior

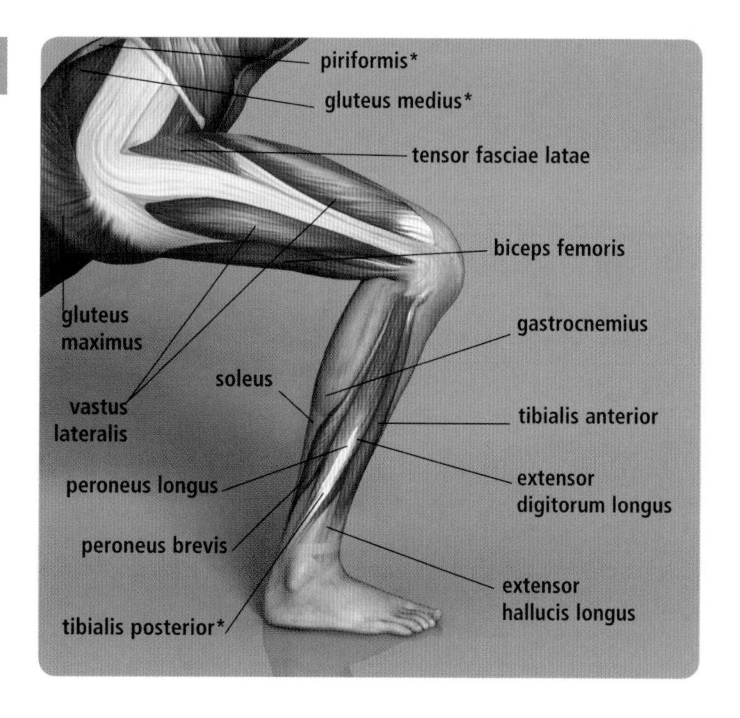

LATERAL

LUNGE

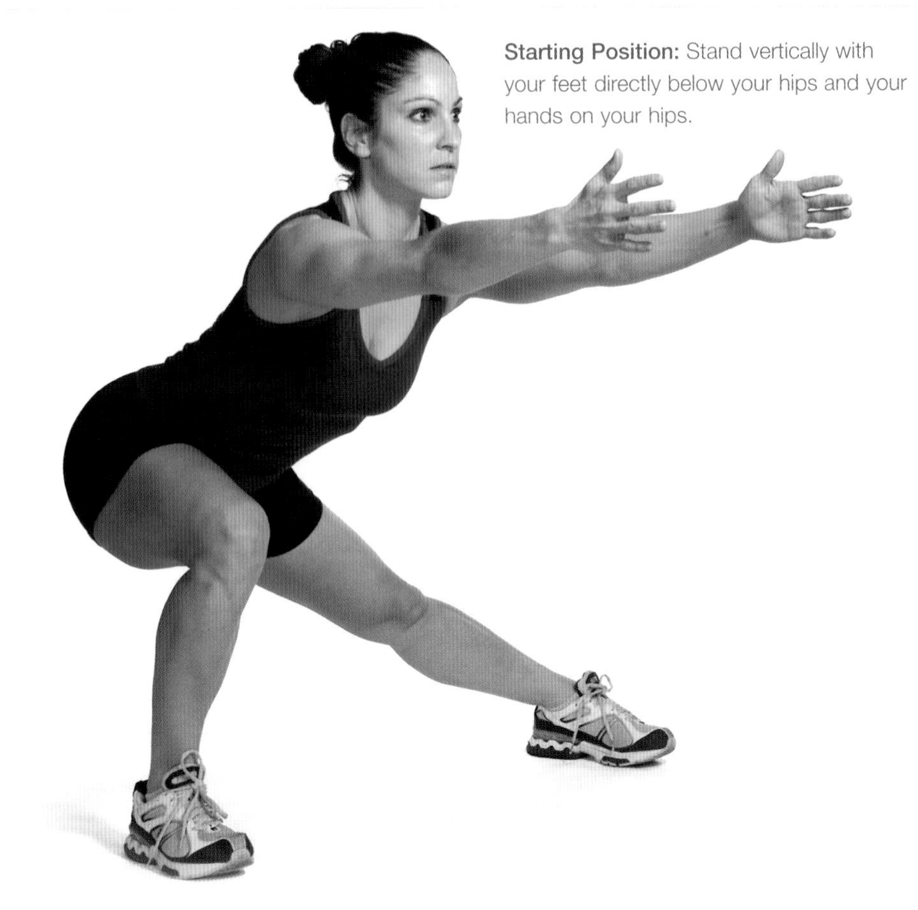

Starting Position: Stand vertically with your feet directly below your hips and your hands on your hips.

Action: Step directly out to the side at 180 degrees, retracting your hips and keeping your spine neutral. As your chest moves forward and your hips retract, extend your arms to ensure balance. Stop at the bottom of the movement when the upper thigh of your stepping leg is parallel to the ground. The opposite knee should be extended, your hips should be behind the stepping foot, and your knee should not exceed the toe line and should be directly over the foot. Your upper arms should be parallel to the ground. Pushing back off the stepping leg, return to the starting position.

Movement Path: You move laterally to the side; your arms go forward, and your hips go back. Your torso drops as your hips retract. Use one foot as both decelerator and accelerator. Use the standing or stationary foot as a balance lever.

STABILIZE BY

- Keeping your hips retracted, your chest up, and using your arms as a counterbalance to the retraction of your hips
- Keeping the opposite leg in contact with the floor, and maintain tension on your quadriceps and hamstrings, so that your knee is locked and extended

LOOK FOR

- A simultaneous movement of your arms and hips
- Your chest to remain up and your shoulders to remain down

AVOID

- Any part of the stepping foot leaving contact with the ground or your knee extending forward beyond your toe
- An excessive drop in torso angle beyond or below 45 degrees

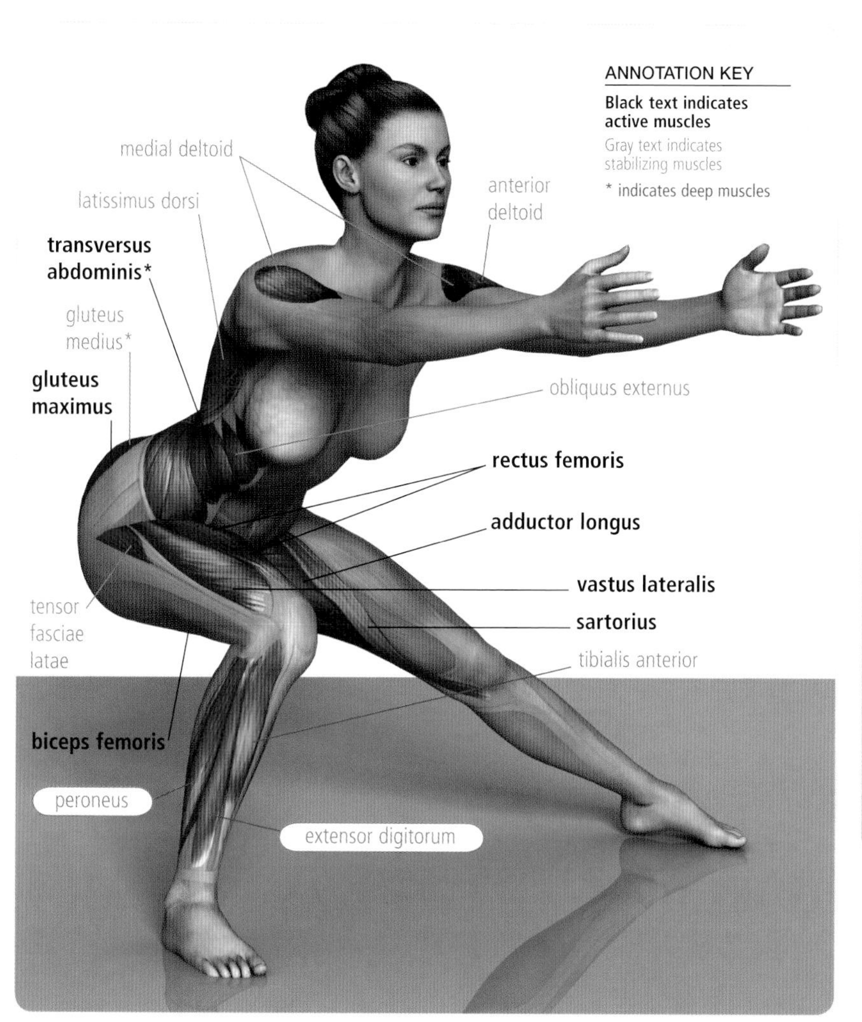

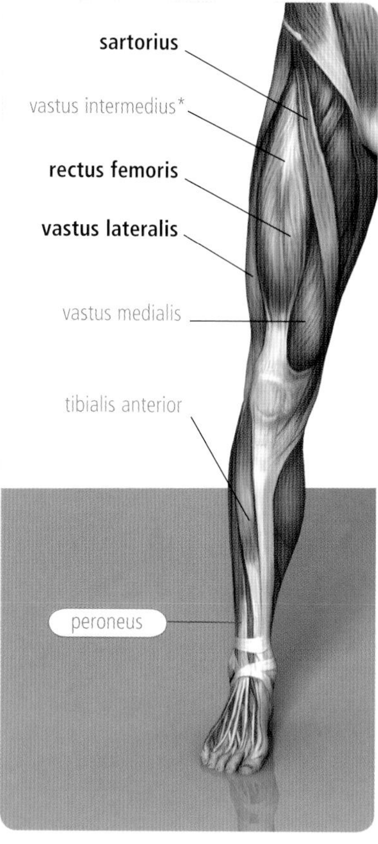

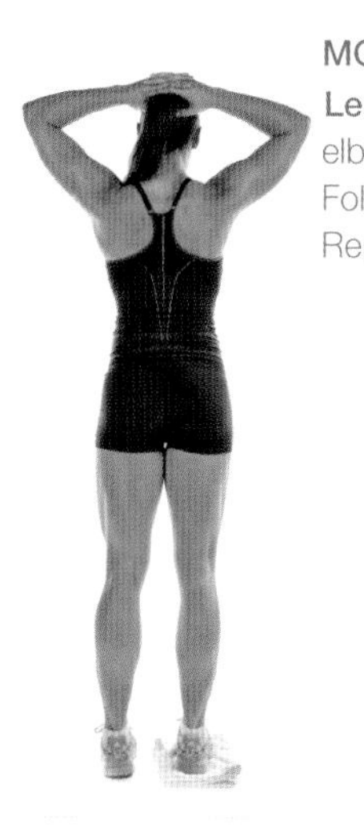

MODIFICATION

Less Difficult: Place hands behind head with elbows pointed wide and shoulders down. Follow same action and movement path. Repeat on other side.

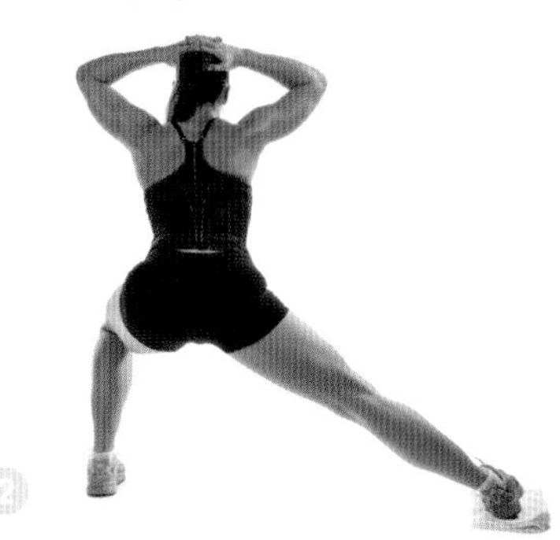

MUSCLES USED

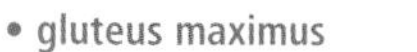

- adductor longus
- adductor magnus
- biceps fermoris
- gluteus maximus
- rectus femoris
- sartorius
- vastus lateralis

45° TOWEL SLIDE

Starting Position: With your hands placed behind your head, start with your feet close together, one foot centered on a small towel.

1

Action: Looking straight ahead, keep your head neutral and spine long. Now, slide the foot with the towel directly out to the side at a 45-degree angle. As you begin the movement, your chest should move forward and your hips backward. Retract your hips on the stationary leg while keeping your spine neutral. This should allow the upper thigh to be parallel to the ground. Stop at the bottom of the movement when the towel-sliding leg is fully extended. Return to the starting position by pushing into the ground with the standing foot and sliding the foot with the towel underneath back toward the stationary front foot, moving the hips forward and spine upward to vertical.

Movement Path: The general motion of the hips and pelvis is lateral downward and backward at a 45-degree angle. Your spine flexes slightly forward and arms extend, with weight focused on the nonmoving leg. The towel-sliding leg is moving with assistance from the towel. The towel foot bears little to no weight and is used primarily for balance. The stationary foot is the balance lever and prime mover.

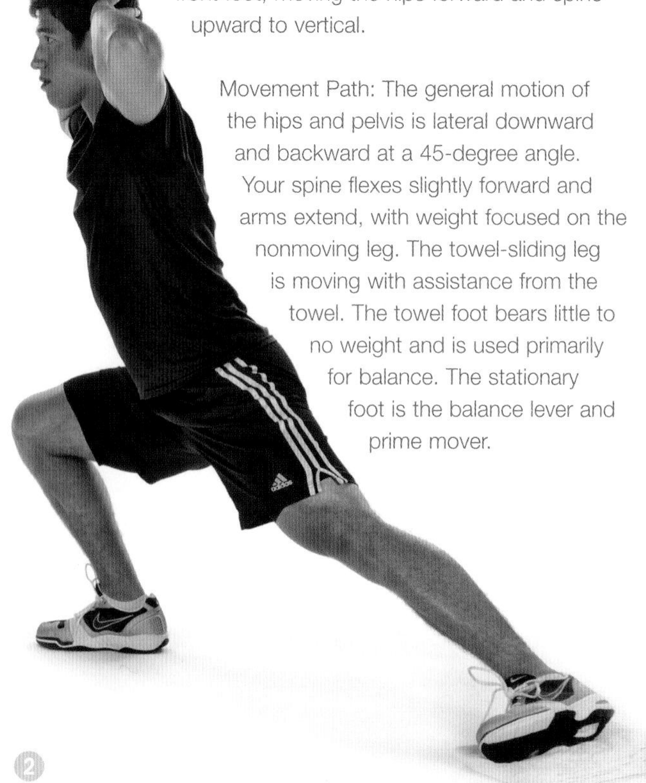

2

LOOK FOR

- Keeping the torso solid and chest up
- Keeping the hips and shoulders facing forward

AVOID

- Hips behind the stepping foot and knee directly over the foot
- A simultaneous movement of your legs and hips
- Your chest to remain up and your shoulders to remain down
- Spine to remain in a neutral position as it translates forward and backward
- Sliding leg to move backward and outward at a 45-degree angle to standing foot

STABILIZE BY

- Keeping the torso solid and chest up
- Keeping the hips and shoulders facing forward

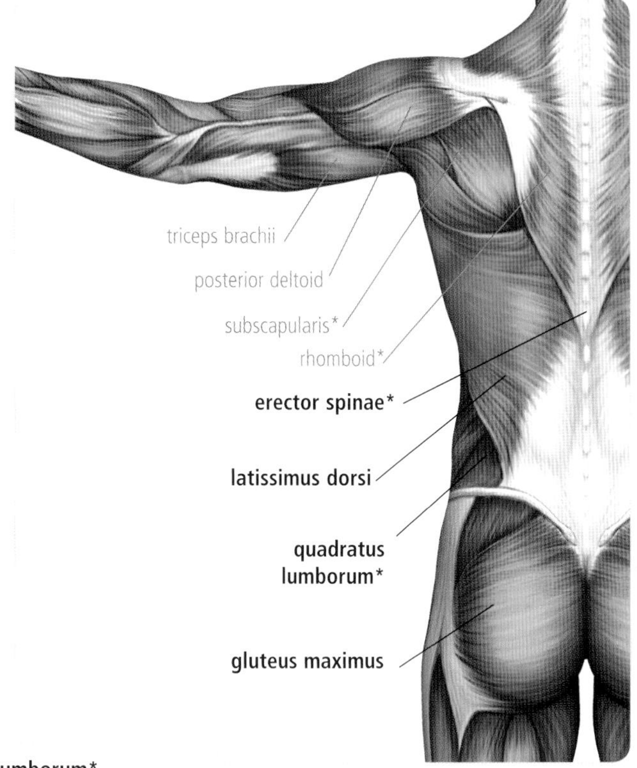

MUSCLES USED

- biceps fermoris
- vastus lateralis
- vastus medialis
- rectus femoris
- sartorius
- adductor magnus
- adductor longus
- erector spinae
- transversus abdominis
- trapezius
- rhomboid major
- gluteus medius
- gluteus minimus
- tibialis anterior
- erector spinae

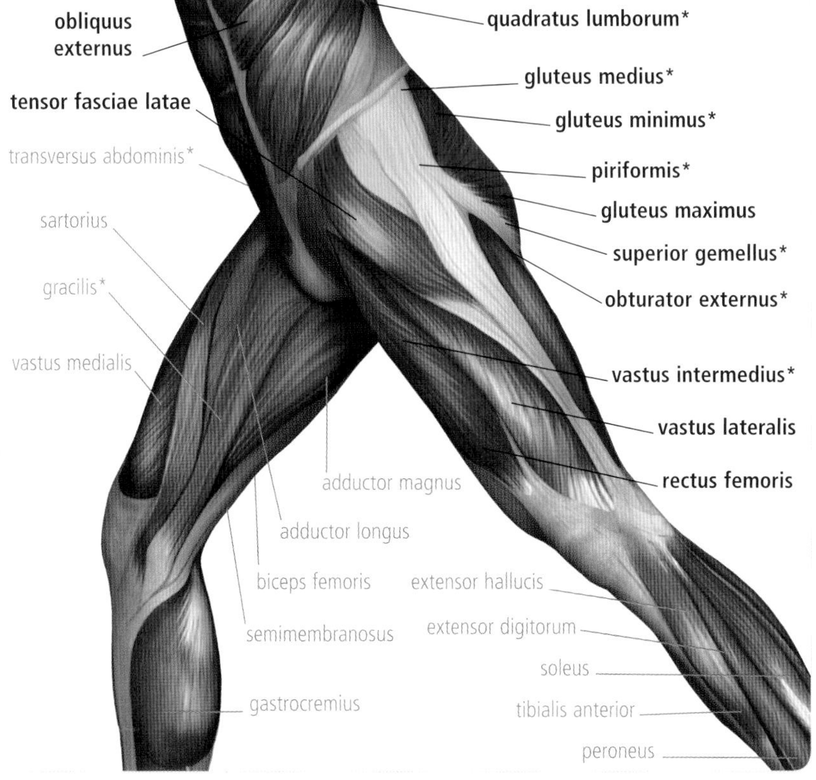

ANNOTATION KEY

Black text indicates active muscles

Gray text indicates stabilizing muscles

* indicates deep muscles

BACKWARD TOWEL SLIDE

1

Starting Position: Stand with your hands placed behind your head and your feet close together, one foot centered on a small towel, bearing little to no weight.

STABILIZE BY
- Keeping the torso solid and chest up
- Keeping the hips and shoulders facing forward

Action: Looking straight ahead, keep your head neutral and spine long. Now, slide the foot with the towel underneath behind and across your body, so that you are balancing with the toe of your sliding foot. The standing leg bends and the hip drops until the front knee ends up in a 90-degree position, allowing your front thigh to be parallel to the ground. Return to the starting position by pushing the front foot into the floor, extending both the knee and hip, simultaneously sliding the foot with the towel underneath back toward the stationary front foot, and rise to a standing position.

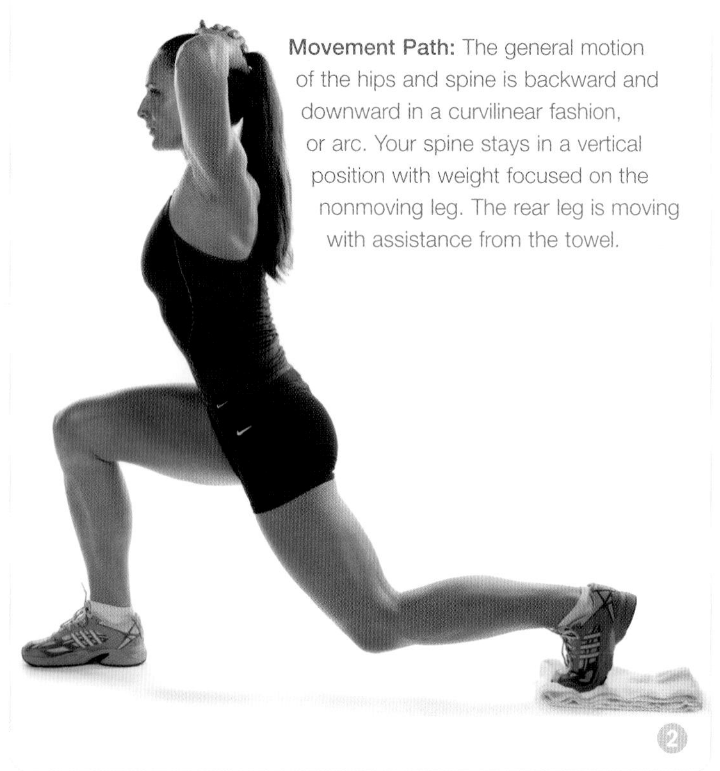

Movement Path: The general motion of the hips and spine is backward and downward in a curvilinear fashion, or arc. Your spine stays in a vertical position with weight focused on the nonmoving leg. The rear leg is moving with assistance from the towel.

2

LOOK FOR
- Body to be in center of balance
- Neutral spine position
- Towel sliding at a 45-degree angle across and behind the standing foot

AVOID
- Back extension—shoulders should be slightly in front of the hips.
- Raising the heel of the front foot (non-towel-sliding foot) off the ground
- Back foot being dragged forward
- Allowing the front knee to move forward and exceed the toe line
- Allowing the front knee to migrate inward toward the midline
- Keeping the back leg tense so that it remains straight

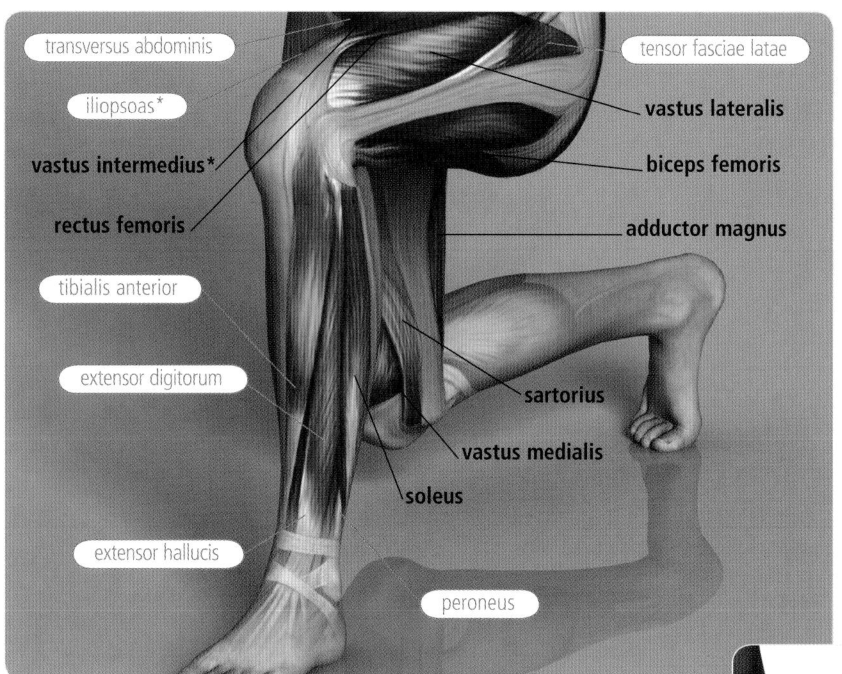

MUSCLES USED

- gluteus maximus
- vastus lateralis
- vastus medialis
- vastus intermedius
- rectus femoris
- biceps femoris
- adductor magnus
- iliopsoas
- erector spinae
- soleus
- anterior tibialis

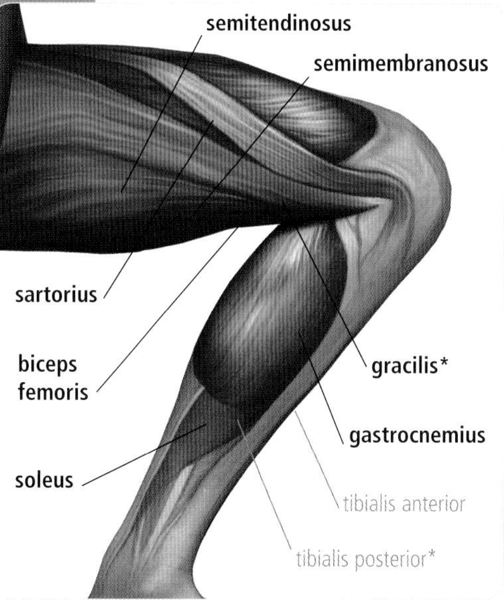

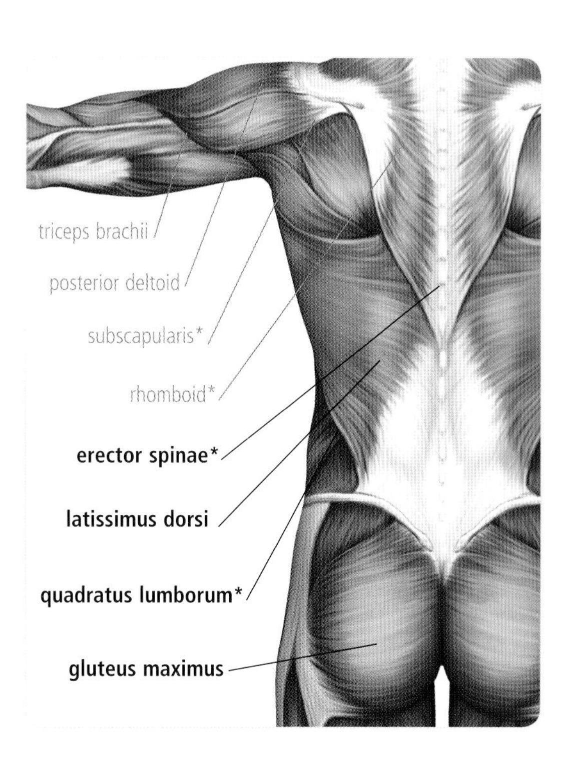

ANNOTATION KEY

Black text indicates active muscles

Gray text indicates stabilizing muscles

* indicates deep muscles

CROSS-BODY TOWEL SLIDE

1 **Starting Position:** With your hands placed behind your head, start with your feet close together, one foot centered on a small towel.

Action: Looking straight ahead, keep your head neutral and spine long. Now, slide the foot with the towel directly out to the side at a 45-degree angle. As you begin the movement, your chest should move forward and your hips backward. Retract your hips on the stationary leg while keeping your spine neutral. This should allow the upper thigh to be parallel to the ground. Stop at the bottom of the movement when the towel-sliding leg is fully extended. Return to the starting position by pushing into the ground with the standing foot and sliding the foot with the towel underneath back toward the stationary front foot, moving the hips forward and spine upward to vertical.

Movement Path: The general motion of the hips and pelvis is lateral downward and backward at a 45-degree angle. Your spine flexes slightly forward and arms extend, with weight focused on the nonmoving leg. The towel-sliding leg is moving with assistance from the towel. The towel foot bears little to no weight and is used primarily for balance. The stationary foot is the balance lever and prime mover.

2

LOOK FOR
- Body is in center of balance
- Neutral spine position
- Towel to slide at a 45-degree angle across and behind standing foot
- Shoulders should be slightly in front of the hips during back extension

AVOID
- Rotation of the hips
- Raising the heel of the front foot off the ground
- Dragging the back foot forward
- Allowing the front knee to move forward and exceed the toe line
- Allowing the front knee to migrate inward toward the midline
- Keeping the back leg tense so that it remains straight

STABILIZE BY
- Keeping the torso solid and chest up
- Keeping the hips and shoulders facing forward

CROSS-BODY TOWEL SLIDE • LUNGE

ANNOTATION KEY
Black text indicates active muscles
Gray text indicates stabilizing muscles
* indicates deep muscles

MUSCLES USED

- gluteus maximus
- vastus lateralis
- vastus medialis
- vastus intermedius
- rectus femoris
- biceps femoris
- adductor magnus
- iliopsoas
- erector spinae
- soleus
- anterior tibialis

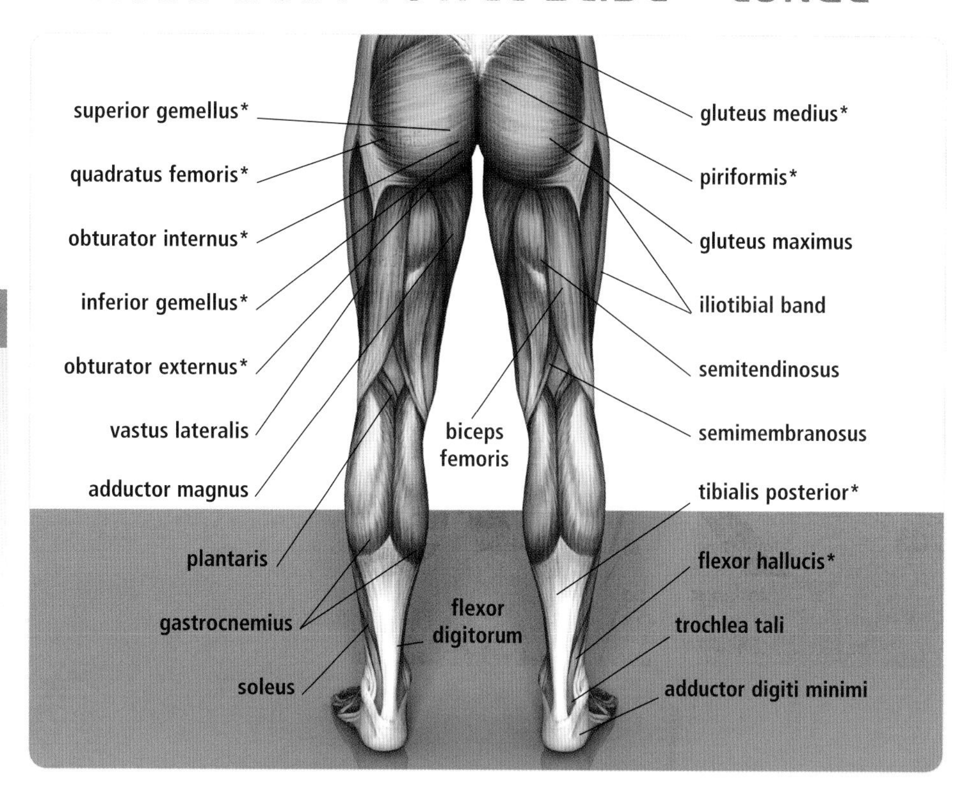

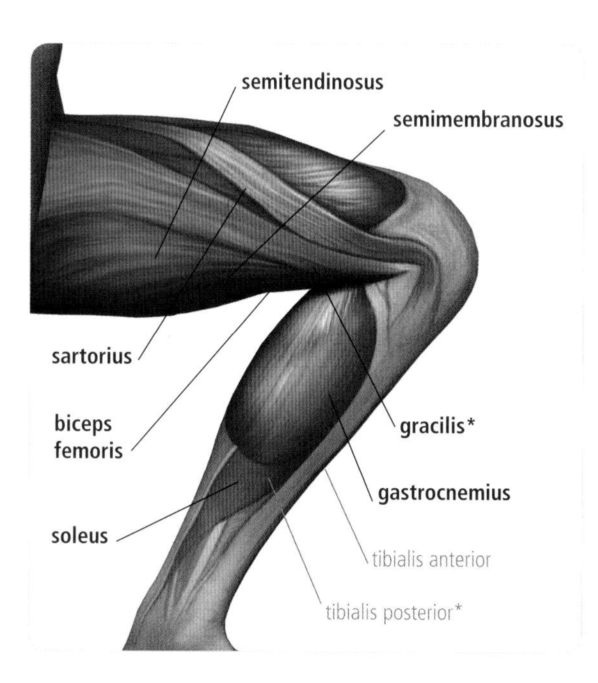

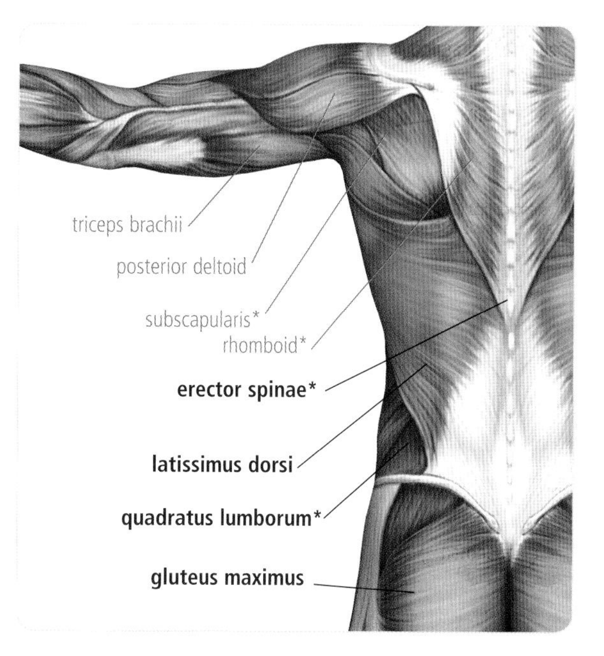

REVERSE BARBELL SLIDE

1

Starting Position: Grasp a bar directly above your head with hands wider than shoulder-width and your feet close together, one foot centered on a small towel, bearing little to no weight.

Action: Looking straight ahead, keep your head neutral and spine long. Now, slide the foot with the towel underneath directly behind you, so that you are balancing on the toe of your foot to create a 90-degree angle in your knee joint and a straight line from your spine through your bottom knee. The front knee should end up in a 90-degree position, allowing your front thigh to be parallel to the ground. Both the arms and bar remain directly above the head throughout the movement. Return to the starting position by pushing the front foot into the floor, extending both the knee and hip, simultaneously sliding the foot with the towel underneath back toward the stationary front foot and rise to a standing position.

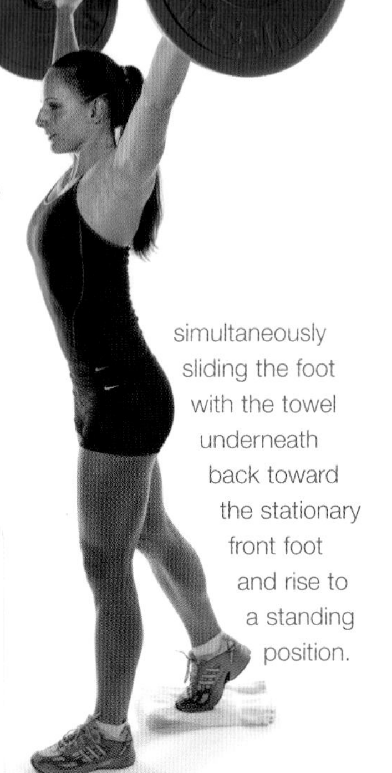

2

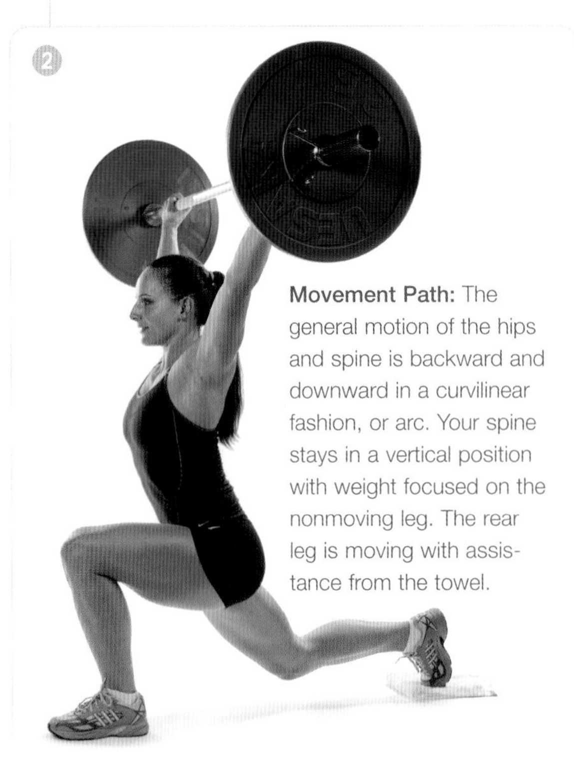

Movement Path: The general motion of the hips and spine is backward and downward in a curvilinear fashion, or arc. Your spine stays in a vertical position with weight focused on the nonmoving leg. The rear leg is moving with assistance from the towel.

LOOK FOR
- Bar to remain directly above head, arms extended
- Body is in center of balance
- Neutral spine position
- Towel sliding straight back with deceleration

AVOID
- Rotation of any kind
- Back extension—shoulders should be directly above the hips.
- Raising the heel of the front foot (non-towel-sliding foot) off the ground
- Back foot being dragged forward
- Allowing the front knee to move forward and exceed the toe line
- Allowing the front knee to migrate inward toward the midline
- Keeping the back leg tense so that it remains straight

STABILIZE BY
- Keeping the spine vertical, rib cage pulled up and in
- Keeping chest high and shoulders down
- Arms completely extended

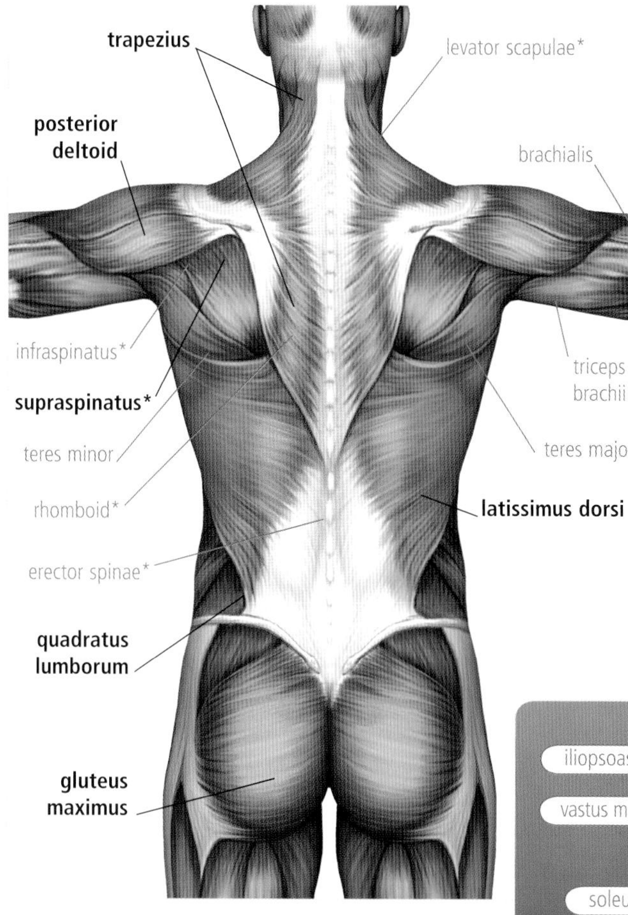

MUSCLES USED

- latissimus dorsi
- quadratus lumborum
- trapezius
- supraspinatus
- infraspinatus
- teres major
- teres minor
- gluteus maximus
- vastus lateralis
- vastus medialis
- vastus intermedius
- rectus femoris
- biceps femoris
- adductor magnus
- iliopsoas
- erector spinae
- soleus
- anterior tibialis

ANNOTATION KEY

Black text indicates active muscles

Gray text indicates stabilizing muscles

* indicates deep muscles

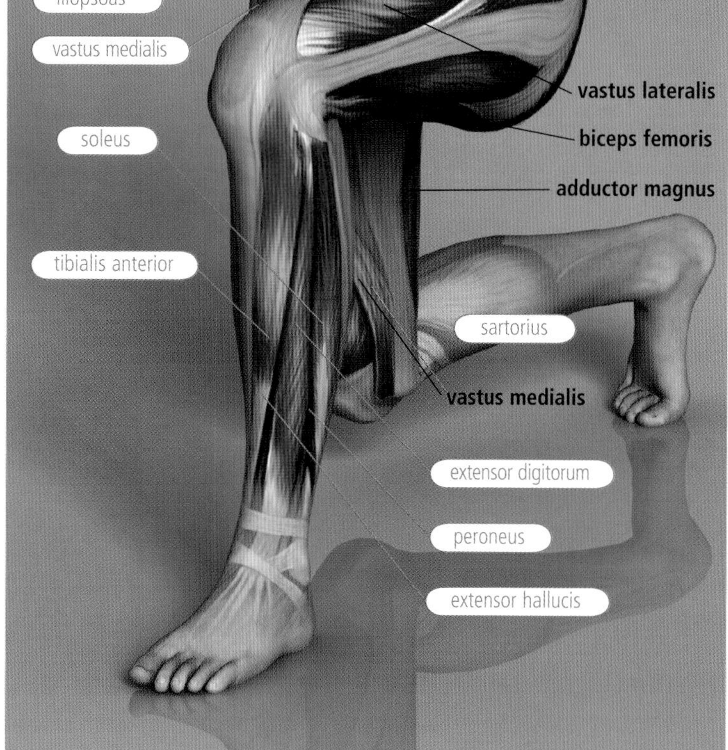

REVERSE WITH OVERHEAD KETTLEBELL

Starting Position: Stand with your feet close together and your hands on your hips. With palms facing each other and arms extended at chest height, grasp the kettlebell on the sides.

Action: Keeping your head up, your spine in a neutral position, and your hands in front of you, take a step forward, bending your front knee to a 90-degree angle and dropping your front thigh until it is parallel with the ground. Your back knee drops straight down behind you, so that you are balancing on the toe of your foot, to create a 90-degree angle in your knee joint and a straight line from your spine through your bottom knee. During the stepping-out process, simultaneously move the ball across your body 45 degrees to the side of the forward leg, keeping arms extended and level.

STABILIZE BY

- Keeping your chest high, stomach up, and spine neutral
- Evenly distributing your weight across your front foot, from front to back
- Keeping your back foot on the toe and your weight in the back of the stepping leg

Movement Path: A forward motion and a descending motion. Your spine stays in a vertical position and is translated forward and down by the step and the deceleration. Return to the starting position by pushing on your front foot and elevating with your back leg while bringing the ball back to starting position. Repeat with other leg.

LOOK FOR

- Body is in center of balance
- Neutral spine position

AVOID

- Back extension—shoulders should be slightly in front of the hips.
- Raising the heel of the front foot (non-towel-sliding foot) off the ground
- Back foot being dragged forward
- Allowing the front knee to move forward and exceed the toe line
- Allowing the front knee to migrate inward toward the midline
- Keeping the back leg tense so it remains straight

MODIFICATIONS

Less Difficult: Fold hands behind head. Use same action and movement path.

More Difficult: Rest a barbell across your shoulders. Maintain the same activation pattern and movement sequence, keeping the bar's weight balanced on your torso. Keep your shoulders down, with your hands wider than shoulder-width, your torso vertical and your chest and chin up.

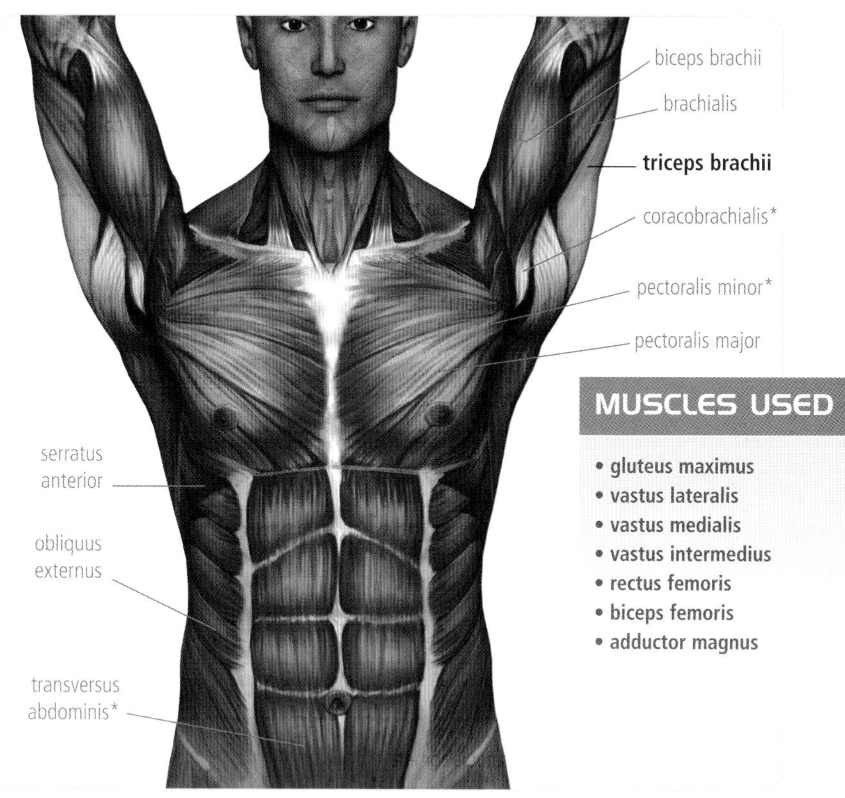

MUSCLES USED

- gluteus maximus
- vastus lateralis
- vastus medialis
- vastus intermedius
- rectus femoris
- biceps femoris
- adductor magnus

levator scapulae*
trapezius
triceps brachii
posterior deltoid
infraspinatus*
teres major
rhomboid*
erector spinae*
quadratus lumborum*
gluteus maximus

ANNOTATION KEY

Black text indicates active muscles

Gray text indicates stabilizing muscles

* indicates deep muscles

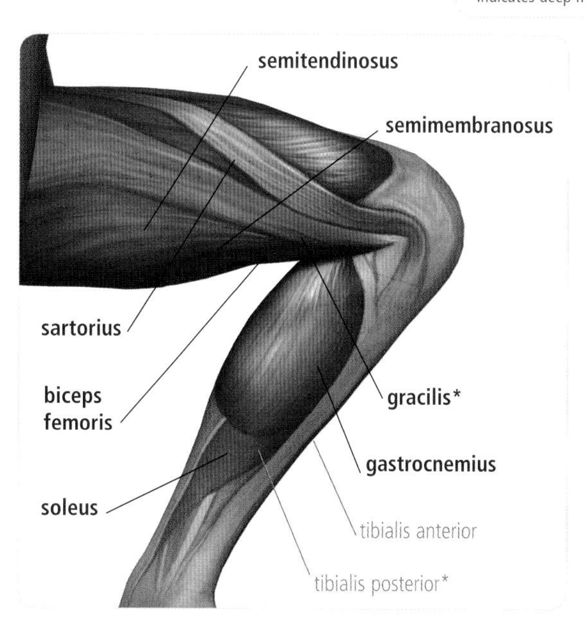

UP TO BOX

STABILIZE BY
- Keeping your upper back muscles and shoulders down and back
- Not allowing your momentum to bring forward either the weights or your torso
- Keeping you hip, shoulder, and ankle in a line from the bottom weight

Starting Position: Stand vertically with your feet directly below your hips and your hands either on your hips or clasped behind your head, elbows pointing outward.

Action: Step forward, placing one foot on a step in front of you, dropping the front thigh and hip so that both the raised knee and hip are close to a 90-degree angle. Make sure that your body is vertical, your chest is up, and your front knee is directly over your foot. Your raised knee should not exceed the toe line, and your foot should be flat on the surface of the step. Back knee and hip drop directly downward, spine remains erect. Keeping your back leg bent, push through your top leg, extending your knee and hips simultaneously to drive your body upward and backward. Do not allow your back leg to push off the floor.

LOOK FOR
- A slight forward translation and directly upward movement of your spine

AVOID
- Straightening your back knee
- Allowing your front knee to slip forward beyond the toe line or any part of your front foot to lift off the step
- Moving your knee either laterally or medially; keep it directly over the stepping foot

Movement Path: A forward and slightly downward movement. Your head should begin above the moving foot and end directly between both feet. Allow your arms to simply stabilize the weight, keeping shoulders back. Ascend in the same fashion.

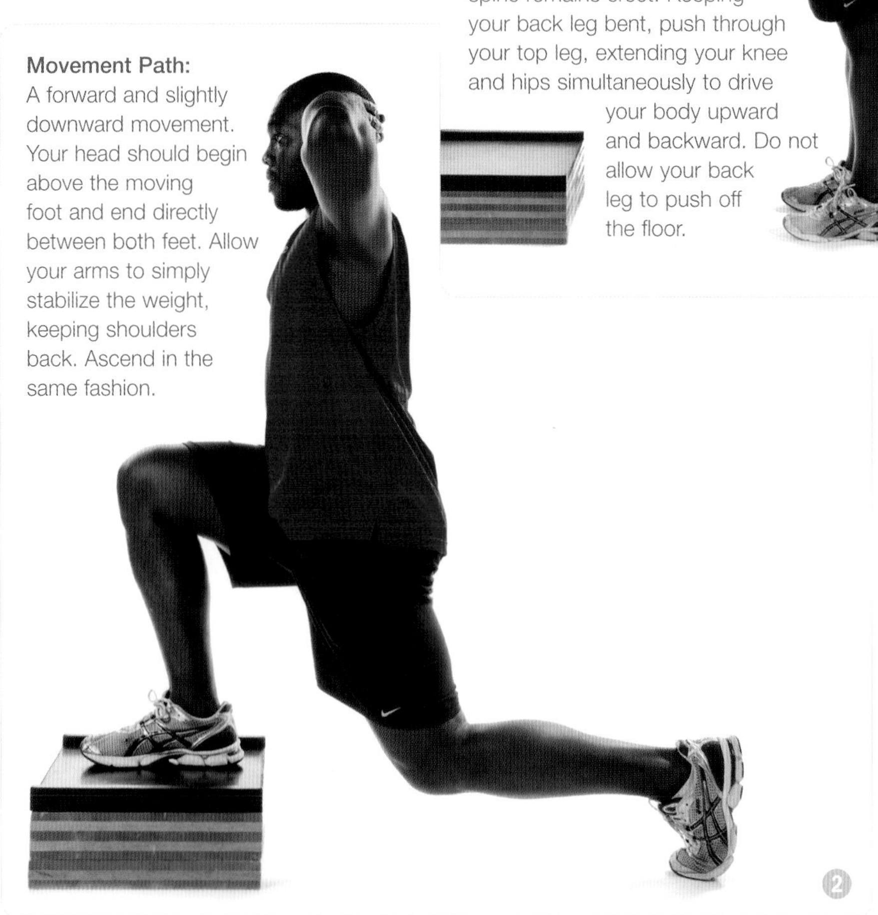

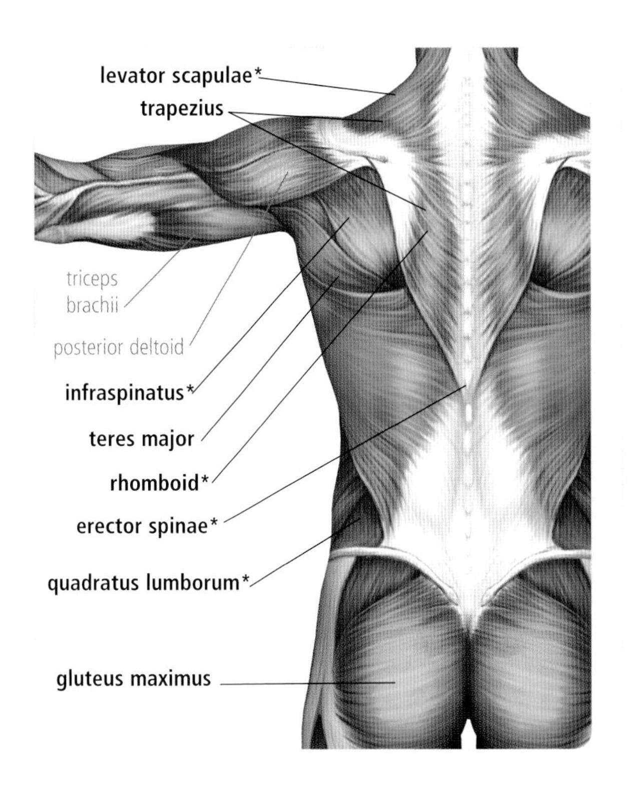

MODIFICATION

More Difficult: Holding a barbell directly above your head, shoulders down, elbows extending, repeat same action and movement path.

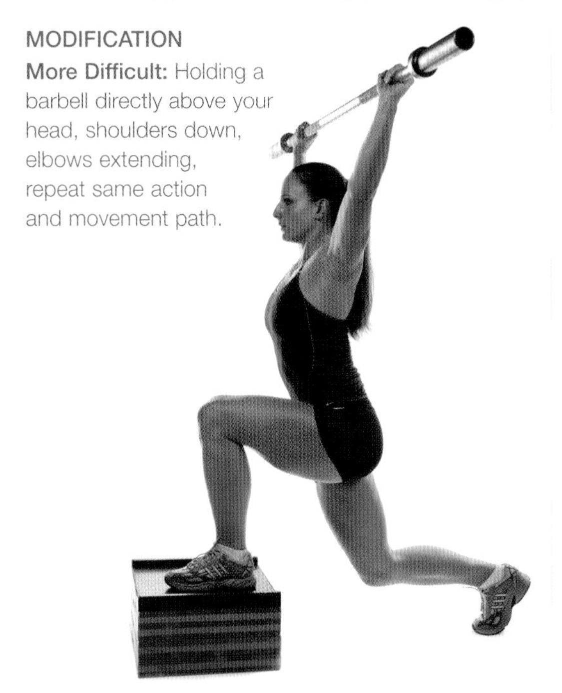

MUSCLES USED

- rectus femoris
- sartorius
- biceps femoris
- semitendinosus
- semimembranosus
- soleus
- tibialis posterior
- tibialis anterior
- adductor magnus

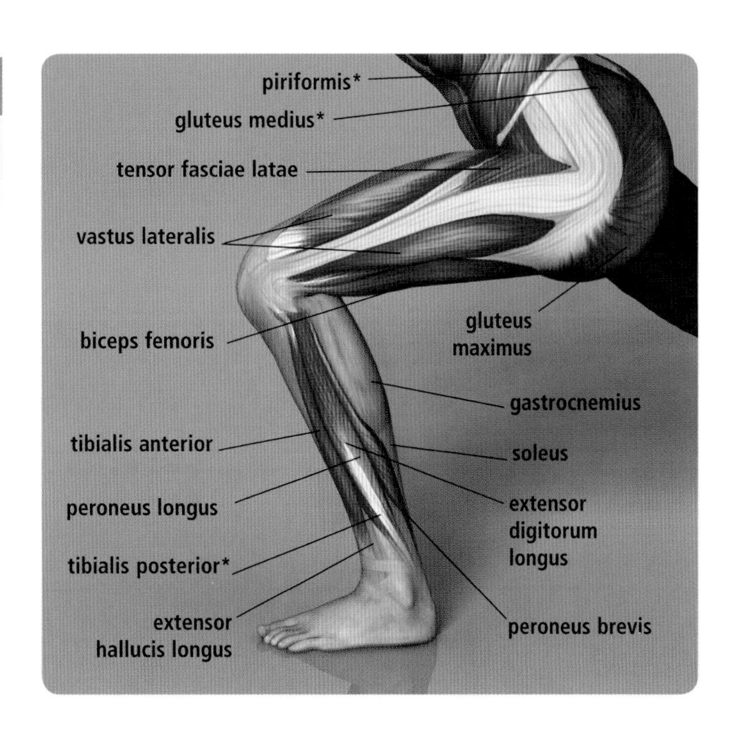

ANNOTATION KEY

Black text indicates active muscles

Gray text indicates stabilizing muscles

* indicates deep muscles

OFF BOX

LUNGE

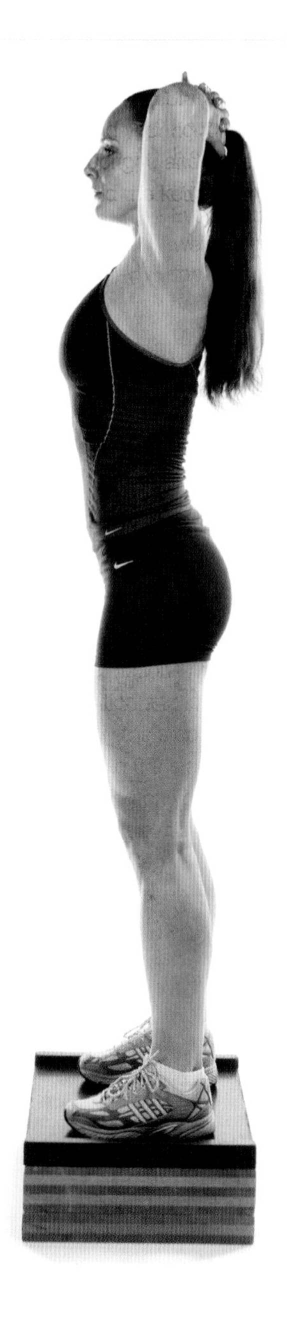

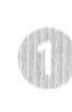

Starting Position: Begin by standing in a vertical position on a block, feet together, hands clasped behind head, chest erect, and head high.

Action: Step directly forward off the block, bending your knee and allowing your torso to ride forward. Torso remains erect as the front foot contacts the ground. Drop the torso and hips directly down by bending both the front and back knee until the front thigh is parallel to the ground and back knee comes almost to the ground.

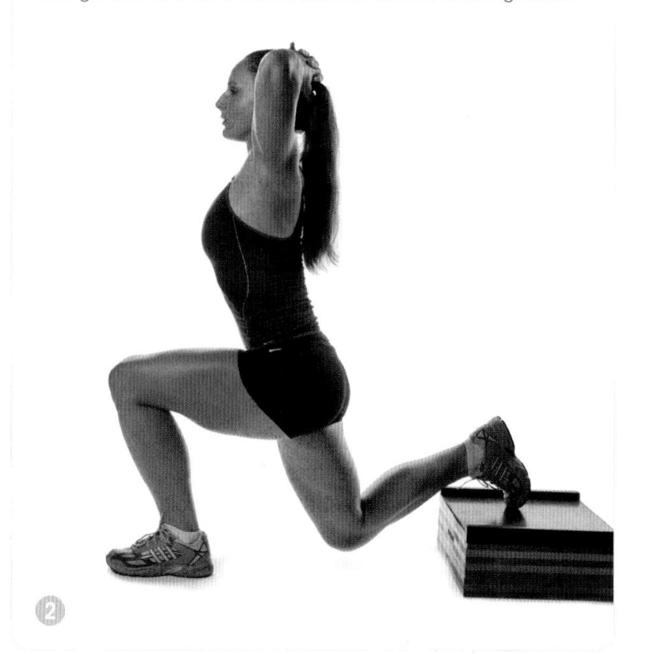

LOOK FOR
- Your head to remain directly above your hip
- Your knee and hips to move simultaneously

AVOID
- Extending your knee beyond your toe line
- Any rotation in your hips or torso
- Any deviation of standing knee from above the weight-bearing foot

STABILIZE BY
- Keeping your spinal muscles active, your shoulders retracted and depressed, the opposite leg involved, and your opposite foot relaxed

OFF BOX • LUNGE

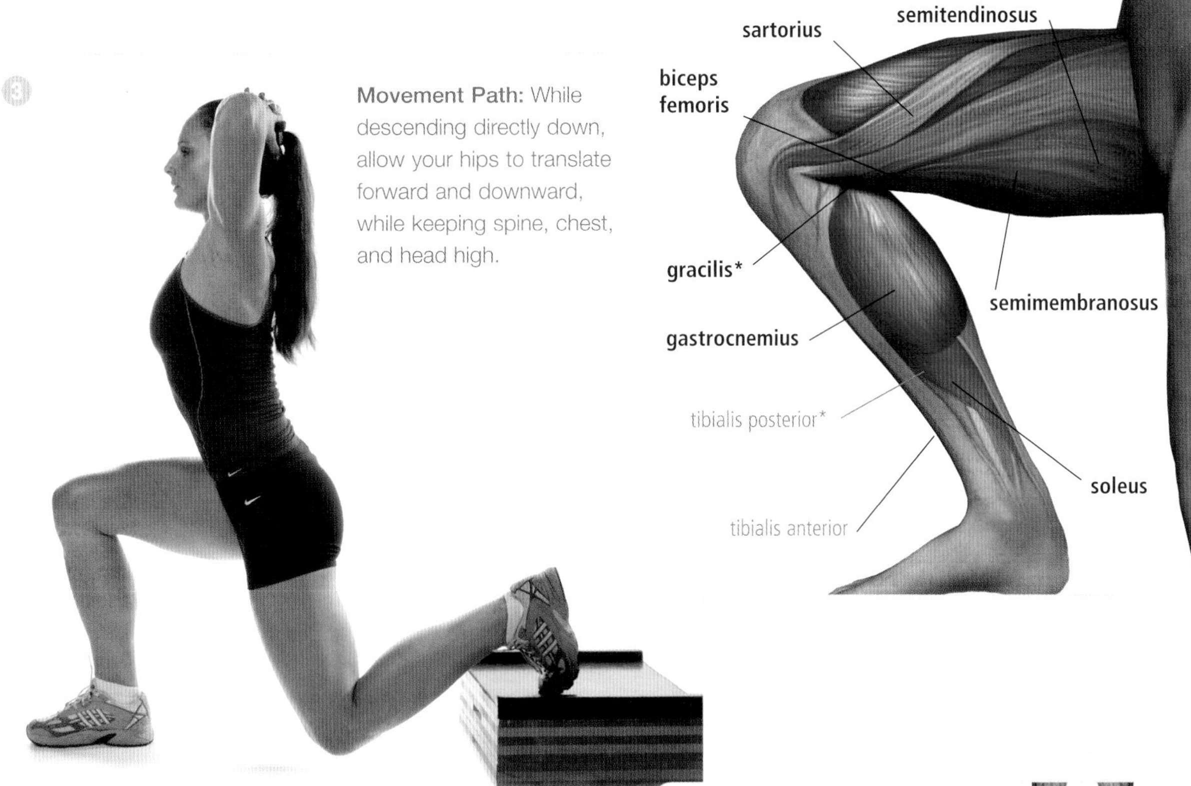

Movement Path: While descending directly down, allow your hips to translate forward and downward, while keeping spine, chest, and head high.

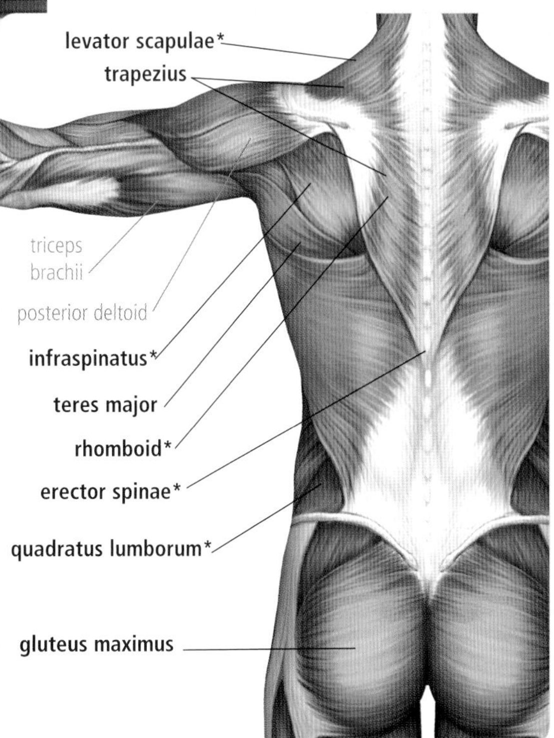

MUSCLES USED

- vastus lateralis
- vastus medialis
- vastus intermedius
- rectus femoris
- sartorius
- semitendinosus
- semimembranosus
- gluteus maximus
- erector spinae
- quadratus lumborum
- anterior deltoid
- transverses abdominis
- rhomboids
- adductor magnus
- tensor fasciae latae
- gluteus medius

ANNOTATION KEY

Black text indicates active muscles

Gray text indicates stabilizing muscles

* indicates deep muscles

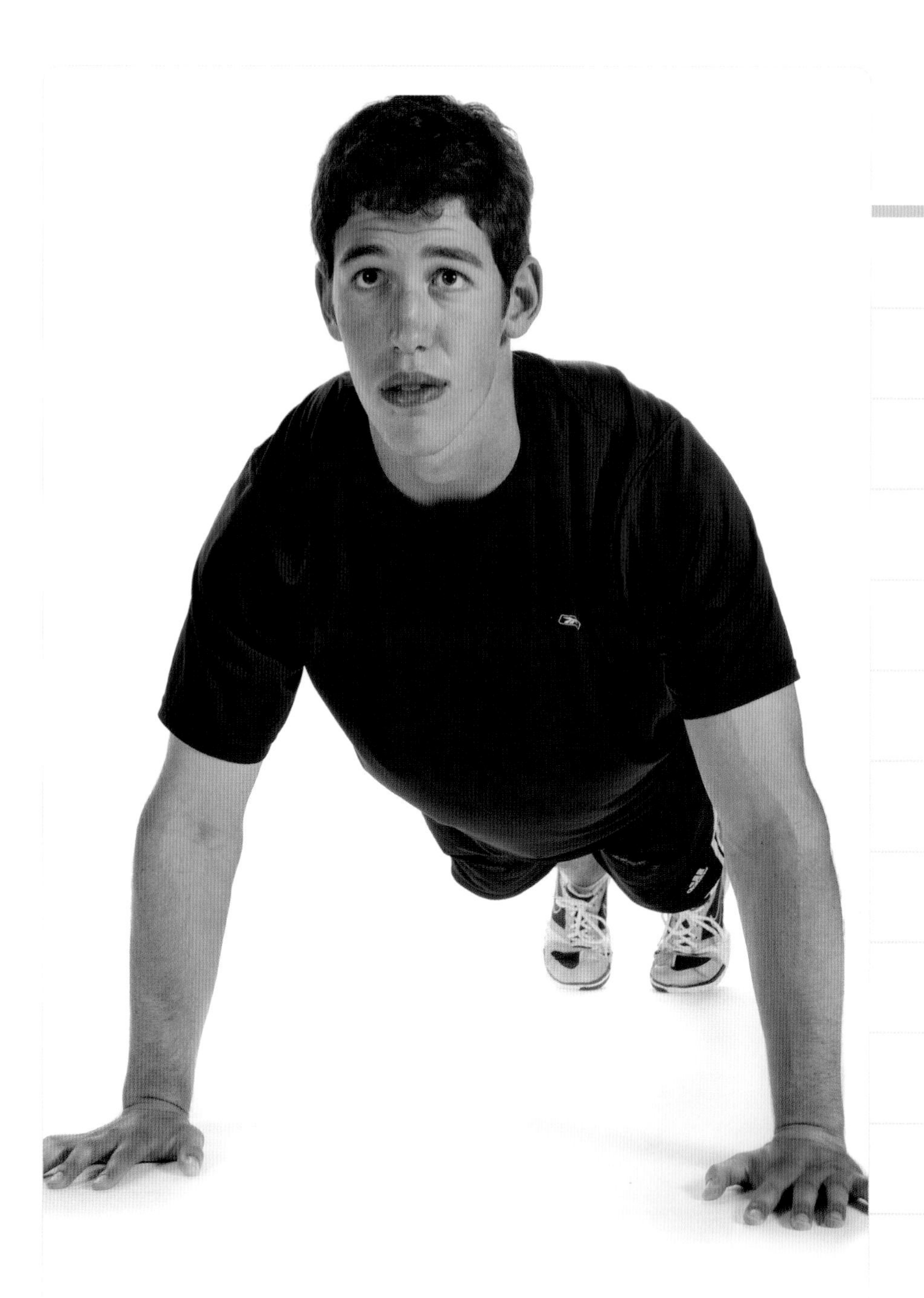

PUSH-UP

The classic. The mighty push-up has been around for thousands of years (as an exercise) and for very good reason. It has the reputation of being a very simple exercise, but, if done correctly, it can contribute to almost every part of the body in both meaningful and beneficial ways.

At La Palestra we use the push-up as a diagnostic tool during our evaluations to measure not only chest and arm endurance but also shoulder stability, abdominal and low-back strength, hip stability, and leg endurance.

Joints involved are the shoulder, elbow, and wrist. The primary muscles are the chest, shoulder, and triceps.

The primary benefits of this exercise are shoulder, back, and hip stability; upper-body strength and endurance; and abdominal endurance.

BASIC

PUSH-UP

Starting Position: Lie flat on the ground, face down. Place your hands slightly outside of your shoulders and your fingertips parallel to your collarbone. Make sure that your elbows are at 45-degree angles to your torso. Place both feet on your tiptoes.

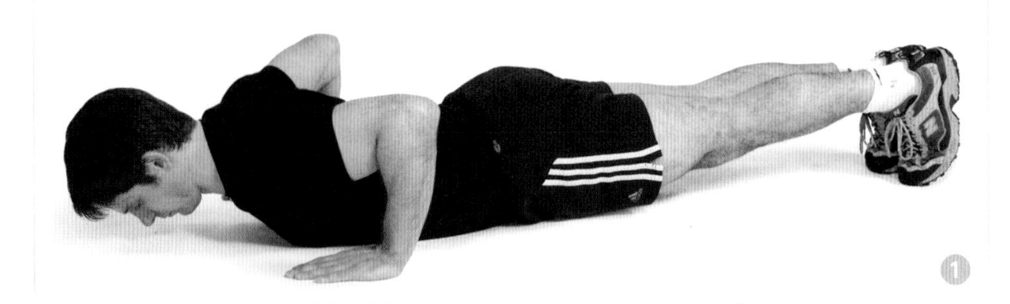

LOOK FOR

- A single plane of movement, i.e., a straight line from head to ankle

AVOID

- Segmental elevation, i.e., your shoulders rising before your hips or vice versa
- Elevating your shoulders toward your ears
- Moving your head forward

Action: Raise your legs and hips off the ground. Your lower back should arch slightly. Extend your arms, pushing into the ground. To return, lower your body in a single plane by bending your arms.

Movement Path: The plane of your body rotates upward in an arc. Use your feet as a lever.

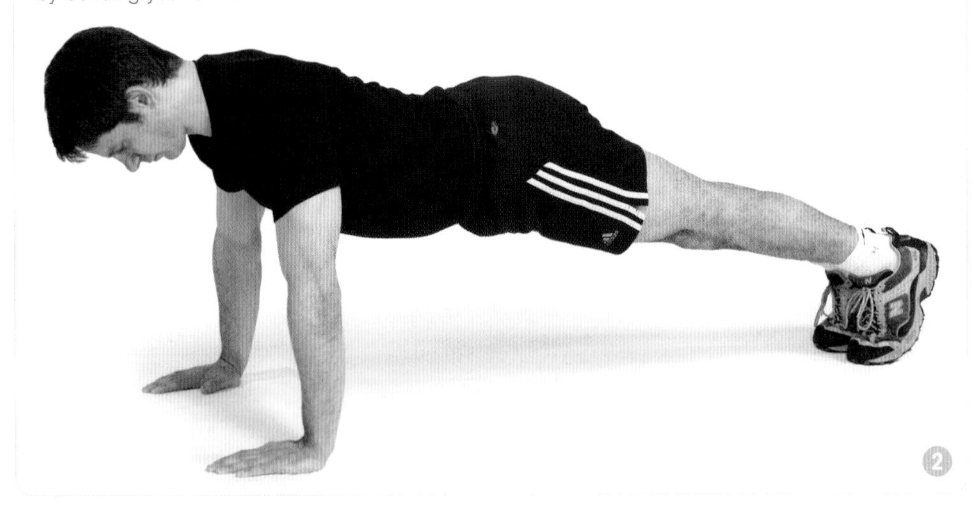

STABILIZE BY

- Keeping your knees locked
- Fixing your ankles in a stable position
- Keeping your hips, abdominal muscles, and lower back rigid

BASIC • PUSH-UP

MUSCLES USED

ANNOTATION KEY

Black text indicates active muscles

Gray text indicates stabilizing muscles

* indicates deep muscles

- **anterior deltoid**
- **coracobrachialis**
- **pectoralis major**
- **pectoralis minor**
- **triceps brachii**

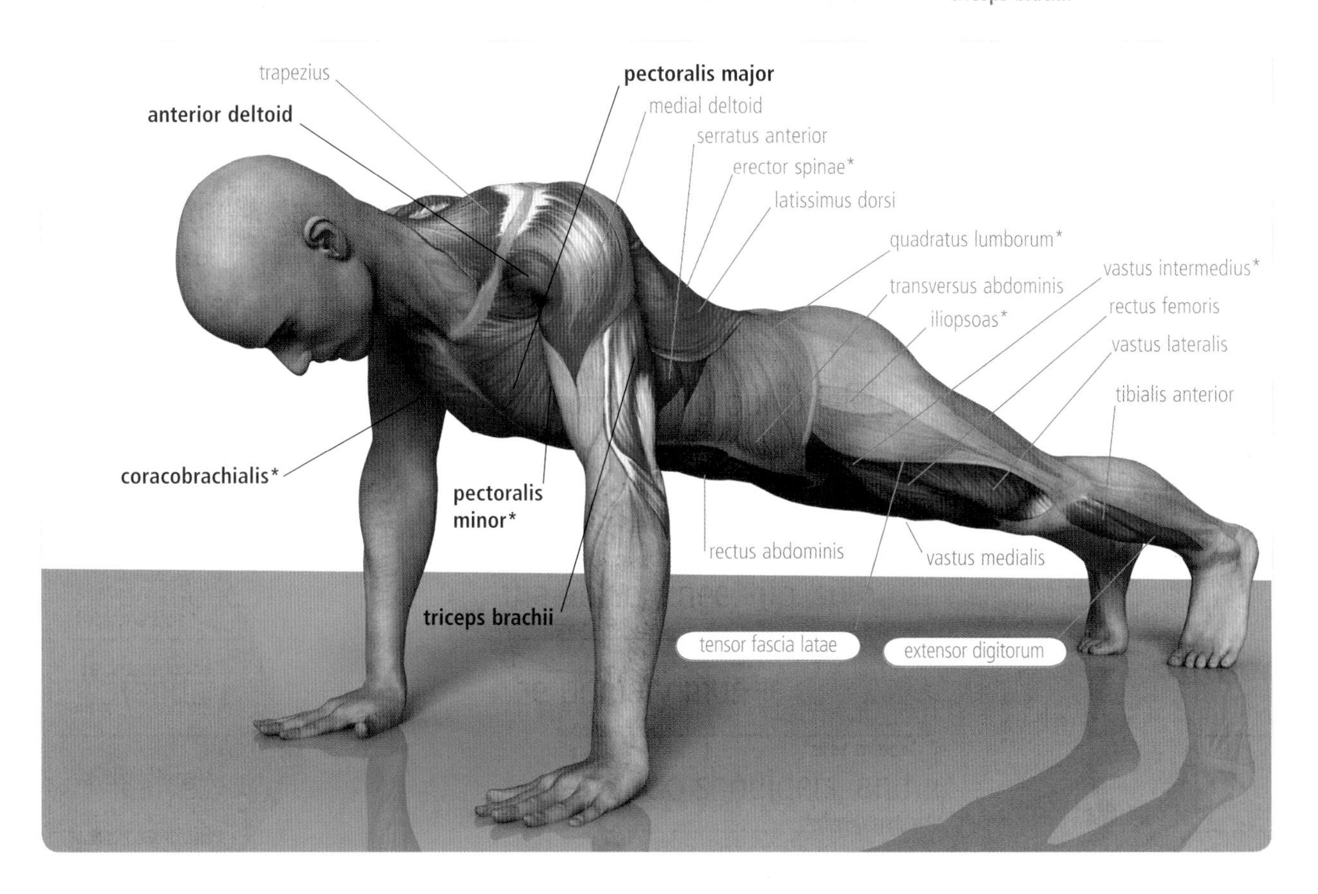

MODIFICATIONS

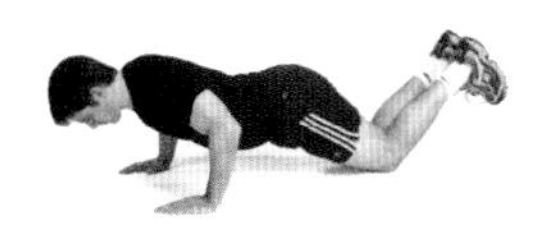

Less Difficult: Shorten the lever by bending your knees to the floor. Maintain the same action and movement path.

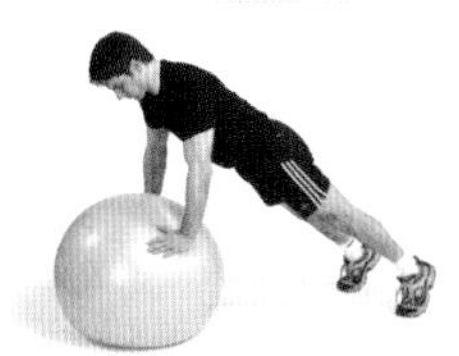

More difficult: Raise the angle of elevation to 45 degrees by placing your hands on a physio ball.

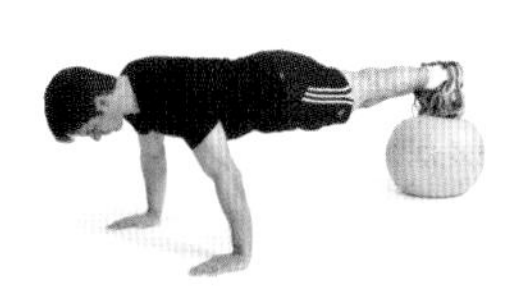

More difficult: Place your feet on a Swiss ball.

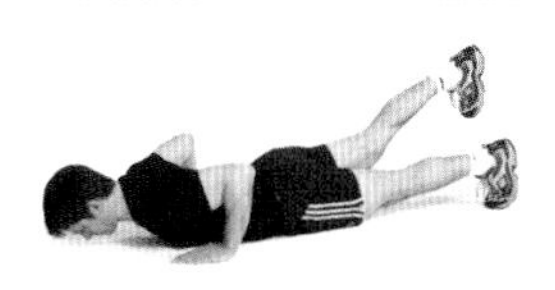

More difficult: Raise one leg and maintain the same activation pattern and movement sequence.

PUSH-UP & ROLL-OUT

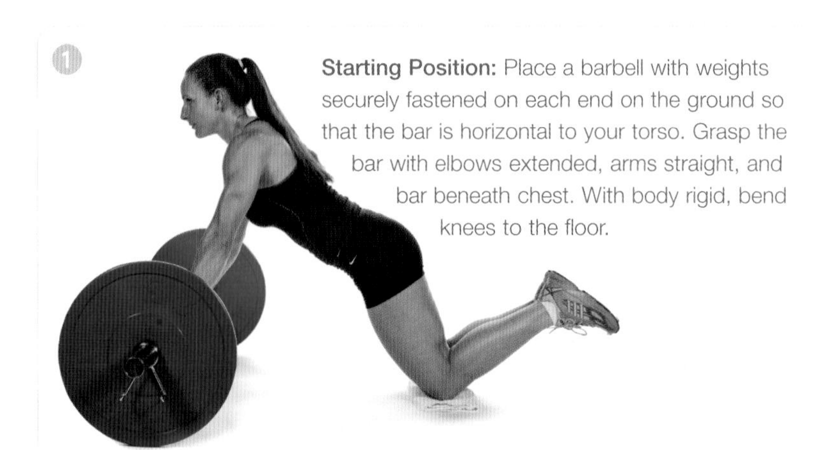

Starting Position: Place a barbell with weights securely fastened on each end on the ground so that the bar is horizontal to your torso. Grasp the bar with elbows extended, arms straight, and bar beneath chest. With body rigid, bend knees to the floor.

Action: Keeping your elbows at 45-degree angles to your torso, use your knees as a fulcrum and let your body drop until your chest touches the bar. Extend elbows and push up and away until arms are fully extended. Pause. Then, putting pressure on the heel of the hand, push on the bar, rolling it forward with arms remaining extended. Pause briefly, and pull back on bar, returning it to starting position.

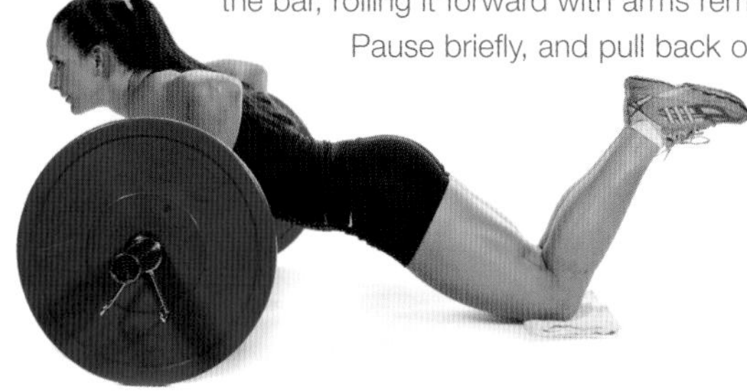

Movement Path: First, lower your body in a single plane by bending your arms. Your hips and shoulders should move simultaneously upward. Use your feet as a lever. Then, elevate arms and allow torso to drop.

LOOK FOR

- Spine remains motionless throughout both movements of the arms and shoulders
- Spine to remain solid
- Shoulders to remain down
- Bar to not move during push-up phase

AVOID

- A segmental elevation, i.e., your shoulders rising before your hips or vice versa
- Elevating your shoulders toward your ears
- Moving your head forward
- Bar to roll forward or backward unevenly

STABILIZE BY

- Keeping your knees locked
- Fixing your ankles in a stable position
- Keeping your hips, abdominal muscles, and lower back rigid

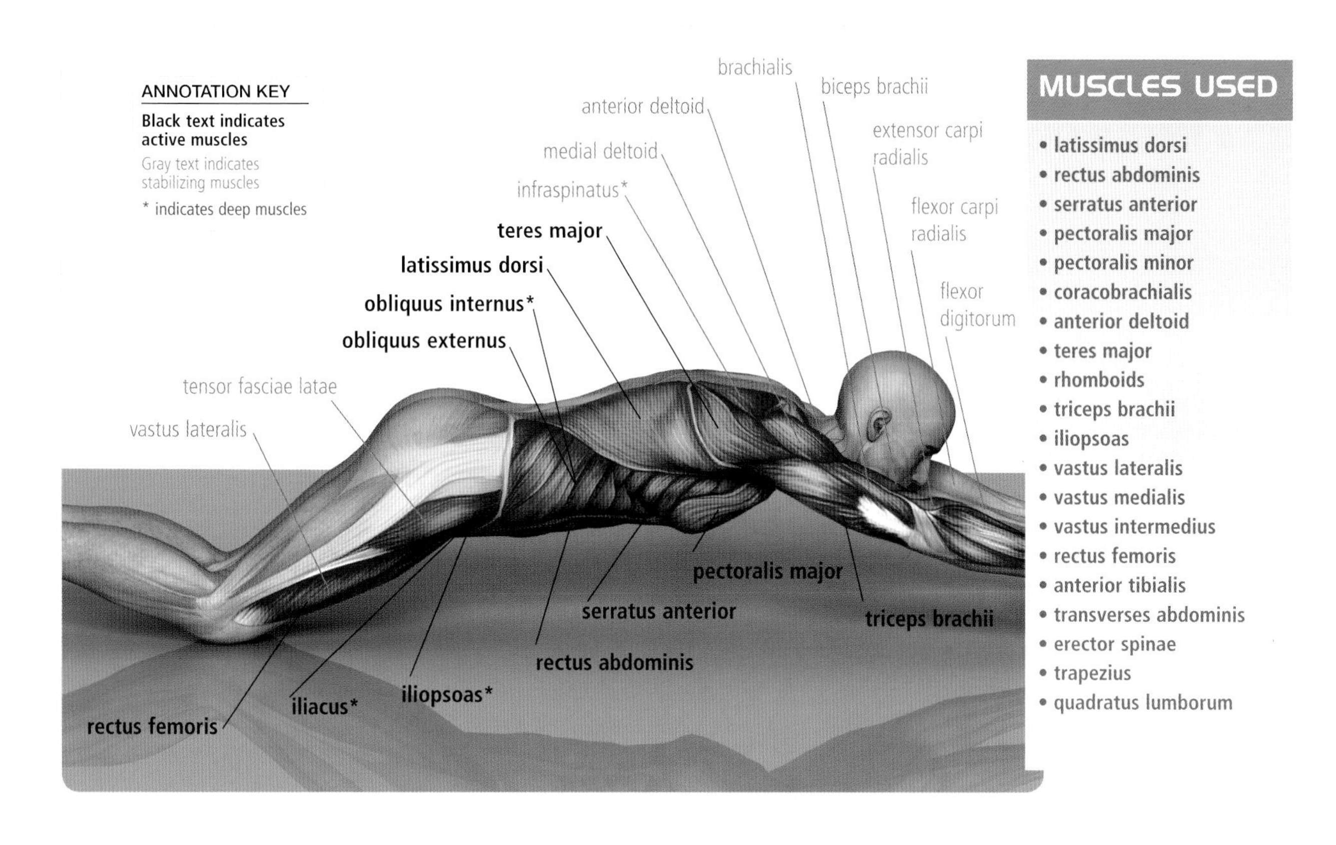

MUSCLES USED

- latissimus dorsi
- rectus abdominis
- serratus anterior
- pectoralis major
- pectoralis minor
- coracobrachialis
- anterior deltoid
- teres major
- rhomboids
- triceps brachii
- iliopsoas
- vastus lateralis
- vastus medialis
- vastus intermedius
- rectus femoris
- anterior tibialis
- transverses abdominis
- erector spinae
- trapezius
- quadratus lumborum

MODIFICATIONS

More Difficult: Extend legs so that body is rigid. Maintain same action and movement path.

OTHER MODIFICATIONS

More Difficult: Place feet on Swiss ball. Maintain same action and movement path.

More Difficult: Raise one leg and maintain same action and movement path.

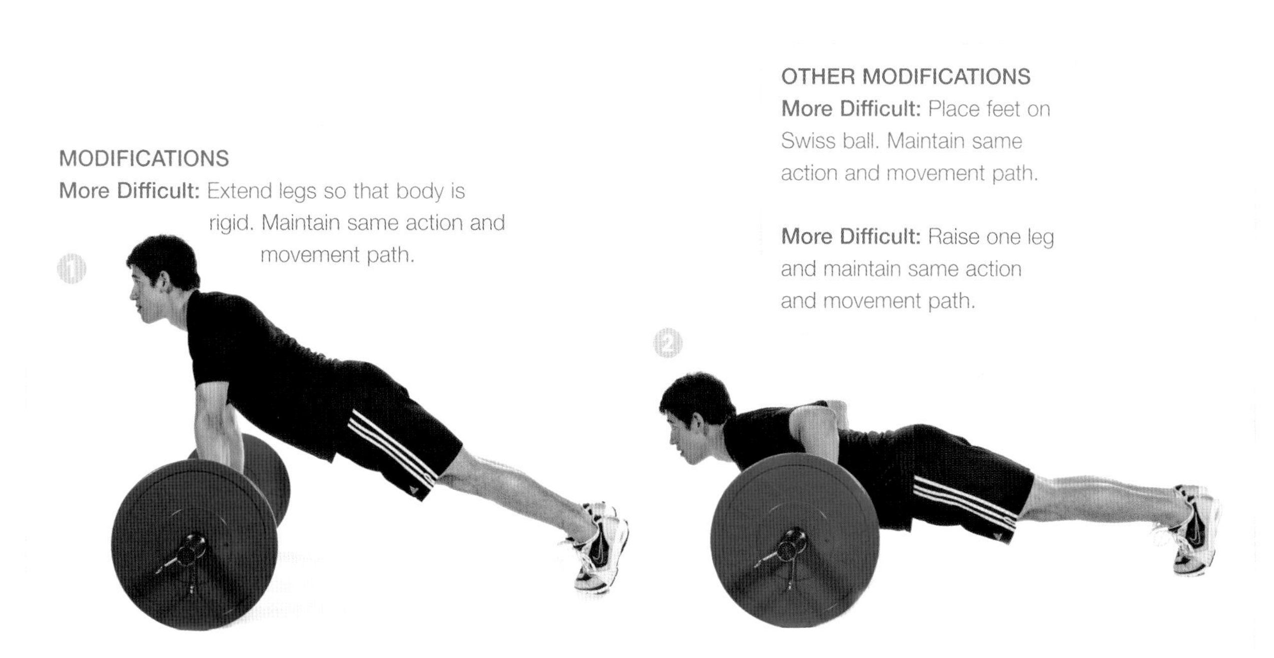

ON PHYSIO BALL & BLOCKS

1

Starting Position: With hands wider than shoulder-width and fingertips parallel to collar-bone, place hands on blocks (or bench) and place feet with ankles fixed at 90-degree angles, toes down on physio ball so that body is horizontal.

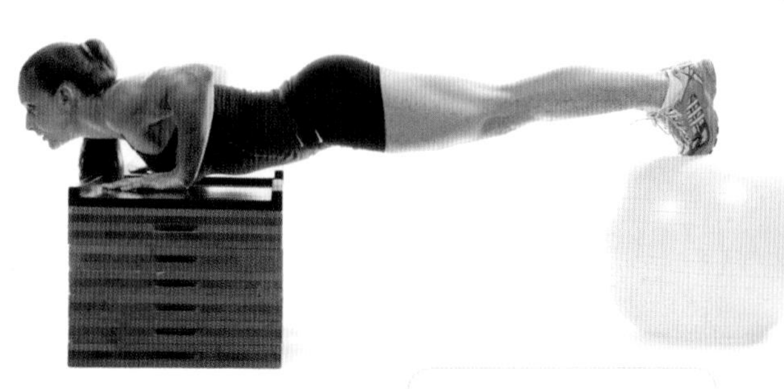

STABILIZE BY
- Keeping your knees locked
- Fixing your ankles in a stable position
- Keeping your hips, abdominal muscles, and lower back rigid

2

Action: Lower your entire body by allowing the elbows to bend until your torso has dropped into a position where the chest is at the level of your hands. Return by extending the elbows and pushing into the blocks, elevating entire body simultaneously.

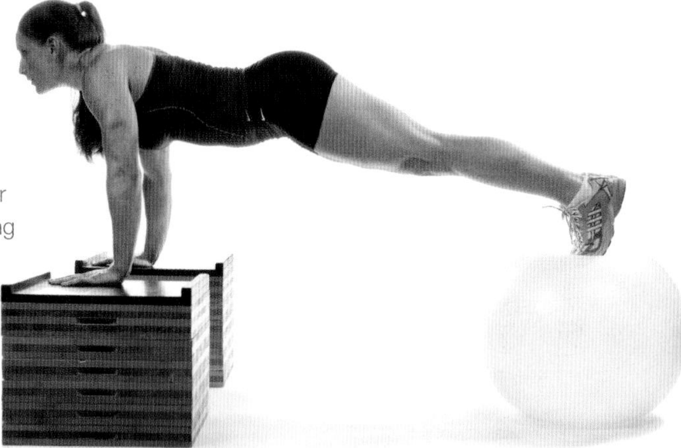

LOOK FOR
- A single plane of movement, i.e., a straight line from head to ankle

AVOID
- A segmental elevation, i.e., your shoulders rising before your hips or vice versa
- Elevating your shoulders toward your ears
- Moving your head forward
- Allowing the ankles to change position
- Allowing the ball or body to migrate laterally

3 **Movement Path:** The plane of your body rotates upward in an arc. Use your feet as a lever.

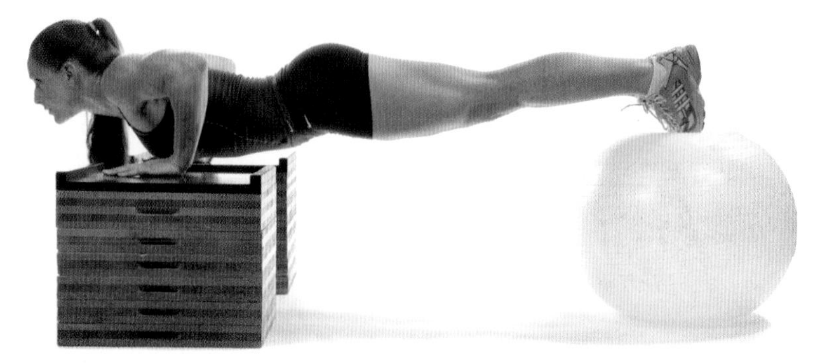

MODIFICATIONS

More Difficult: Keeping toes of one foot on physio ball, elevate other leg. Follow same action and movement path.

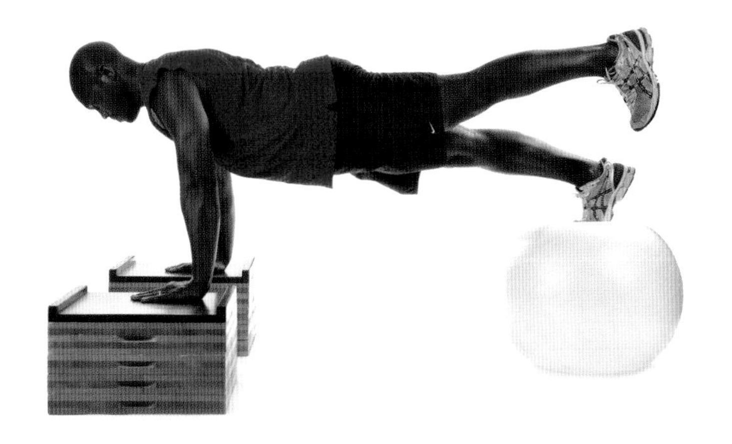

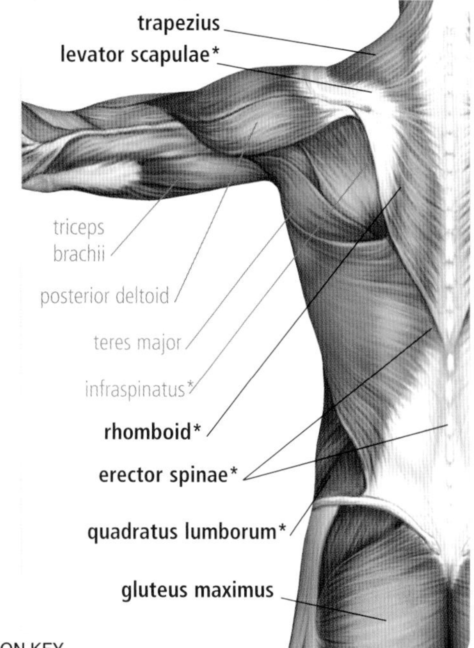

ANNOTATION KEY

Black text indicates active muscles

Gray text indicates stabilizing muscles

* indicates deep muscles

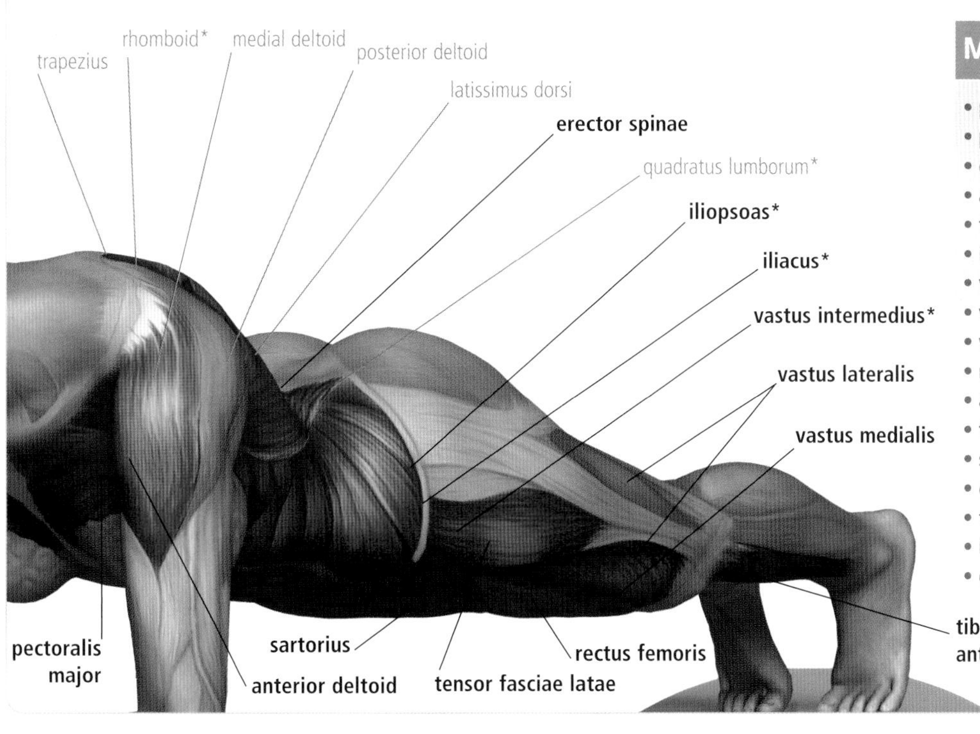

MUSCLES USED

- pectoralis major
- pectoralis minor
- coracobrachialis
- anterior deltoid
- triceps brachii
- iliopsoas
- vastus lateralis
- vastus medialis
- vastus intermedius
- rectus femoris
- anterior tibialis
- transversus abdominis
- serratus anterior
- erector spinae
- trapezius
- latissimus dorsi
- quadratus lumborum

PUSH-UP

ON DUMBBELLS WITH ROTATION

1

Starting Position: Lie flat on the floor with your hands slightly wider than shoulder width, grasping dumbbells, so that the dumbbell handles are parallel to your spine. Point your elbows directly at the ceiling. Your feet should be slightly wider than shoulder width and your spine should be neutral.

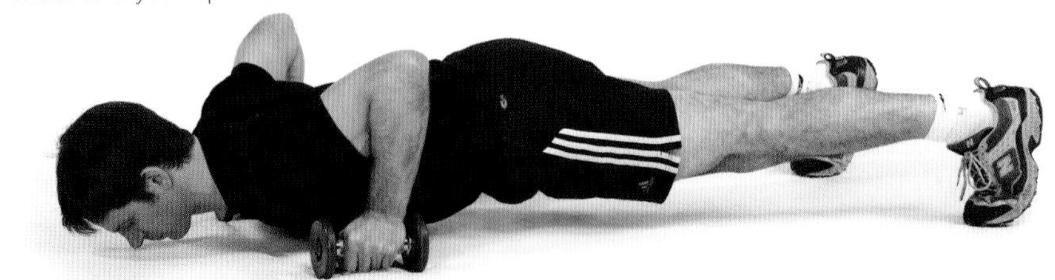

2

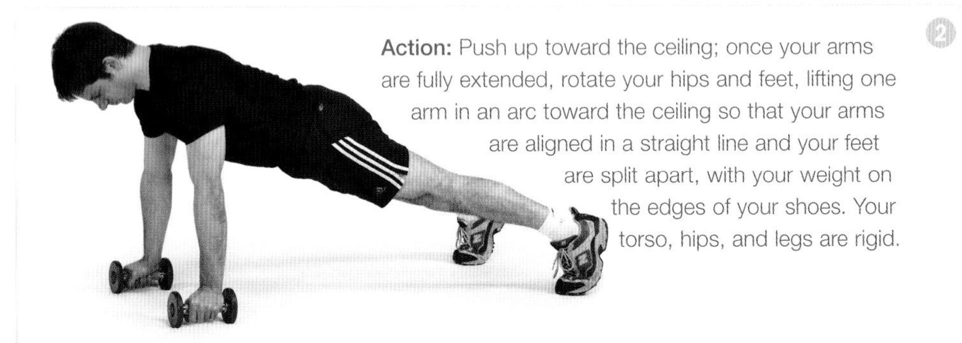

Action: Push up toward the ceiling; once your arms are fully extended, rotate your hips and feet, lifting one arm in an arc toward the ceiling so that your arms are aligned in a straight line and your feet are split apart, with your weight on the edges of your shoes. Your torso, hips, and legs are rigid.

LOOK FOR
- Your shoulders to remain depressed
- Your neck to remain long
- Your hips to remain elevated
- Your shoulders, hips, and feet to remain in the same plane from the floor

AVOID
- Bending your knees, dropping your hips, or excessive rotation in shoulder and hip

3

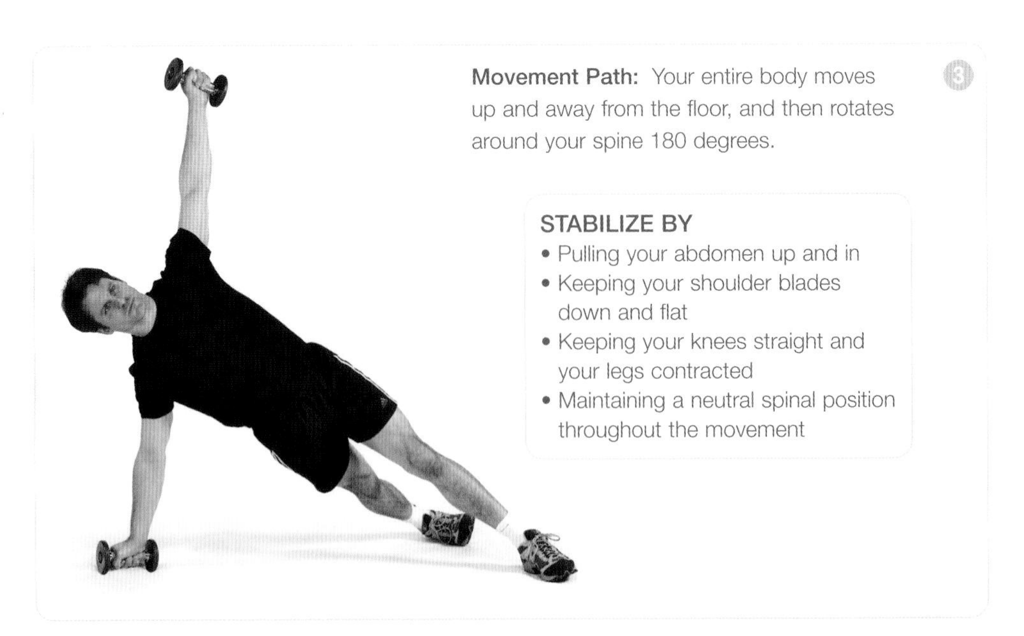

Movement Path: Your entire body moves up and away from the floor, and then rotates around your spine 180 degrees.

STABILIZE BY
- Pulling your abdomen up and in
- Keeping your shoulder blades down and flat
- Keeping your knees straight and your legs contracted
- Maintaining a neutral spinal position throughout the movement

ON DUMBELLS WITH ROTATION • PUSH-UP

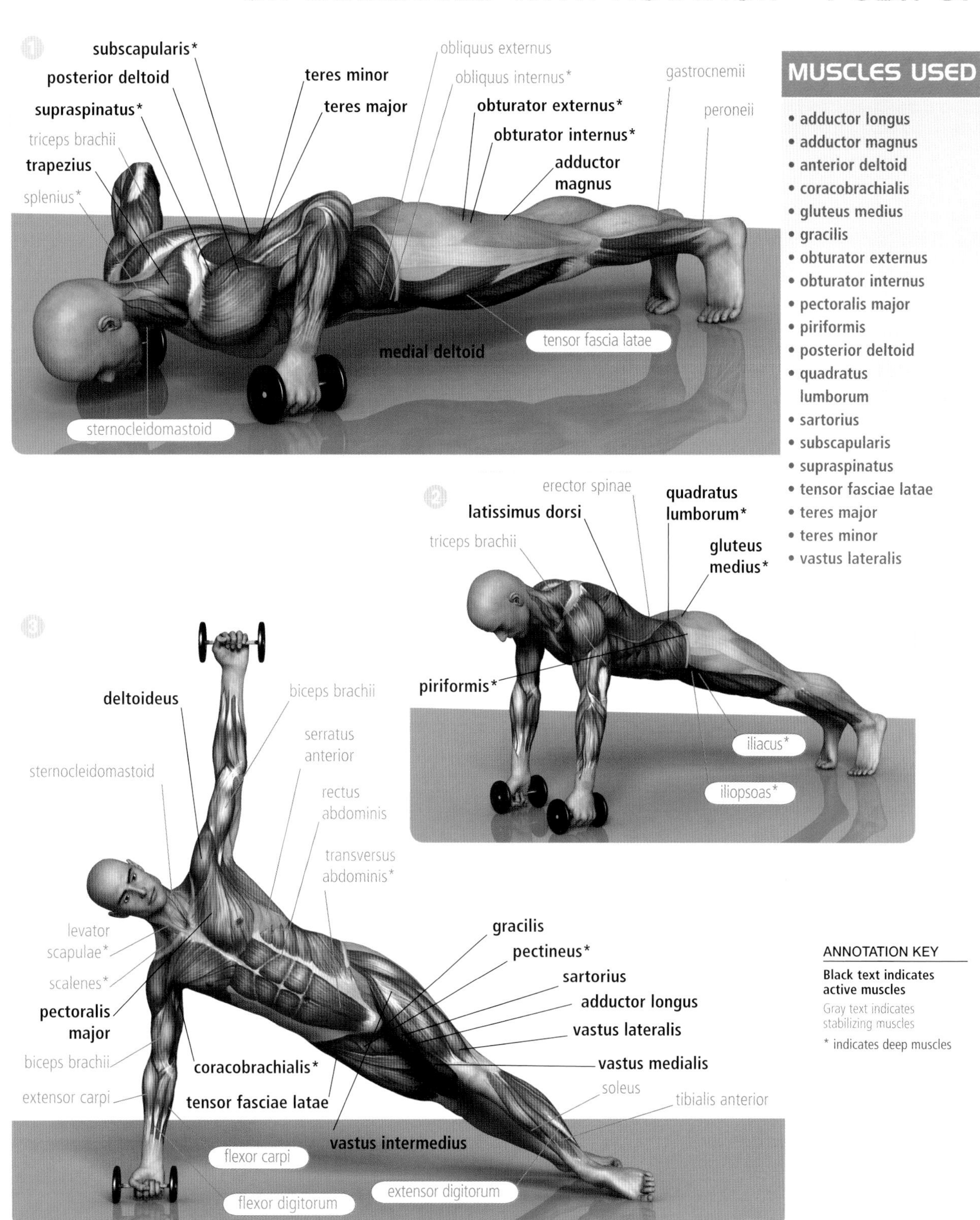

MUSCLES USED

- adductor longus
- adductor magnus
- anterior deltoid
- coracobrachialis
- gluteus medius
- gracilis
- obturator externus
- obturator internus
- pectoralis major
- piriformis
- posterior deltoid
- quadratus lumborum
- sartorius
- subscapularis
- supraspinatus
- tensor fasciae latae
- teres major
- teres minor
- vastus lateralis

ANNOTATION KEY

Black text indicates active muscles

Gray text indicates stabilizing muscles

* indicates deep muscles

TOWEL FLY

1

Starting Position: With fully extended arms, start from the top of the push-up position, with your hands wider than shoulder-width and placed on a towel so that the towel is taut between your hands and directly under your chest.

Action: Move your hands together while keeping your torso rigid and your arms extended. Return by spreading your hands to the starting position.

LOOK FOR

- Your arms to remain directly below your chest and perpendicular to your torso

AVOID

- Dropping your head forward or bending or extending your elbows
- Any change in your spinal position
- Elevating or widening your shoulder blades

STABILIZE BY

- Keeping your hips up and your knees and ankles locked
- Keeping your shoulders retracted and depressed throughout the movement

2

Movement Path: As your hands slide together, your torso (spine), hips, and legs elevate, using your toes as a lever.

Your hand movements should be smooth and simultaneous.

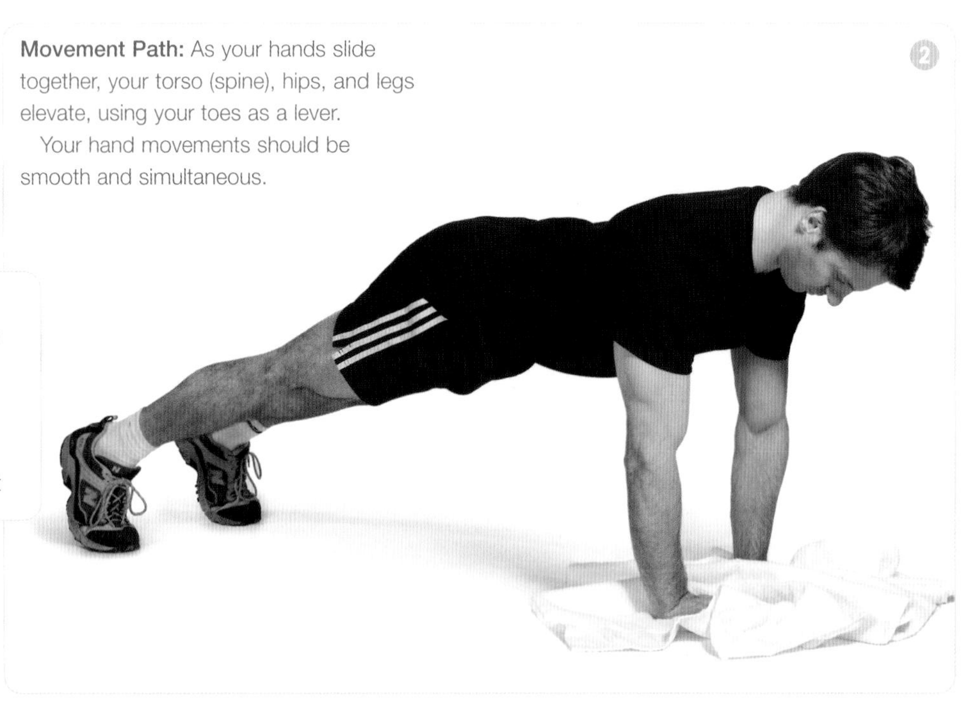

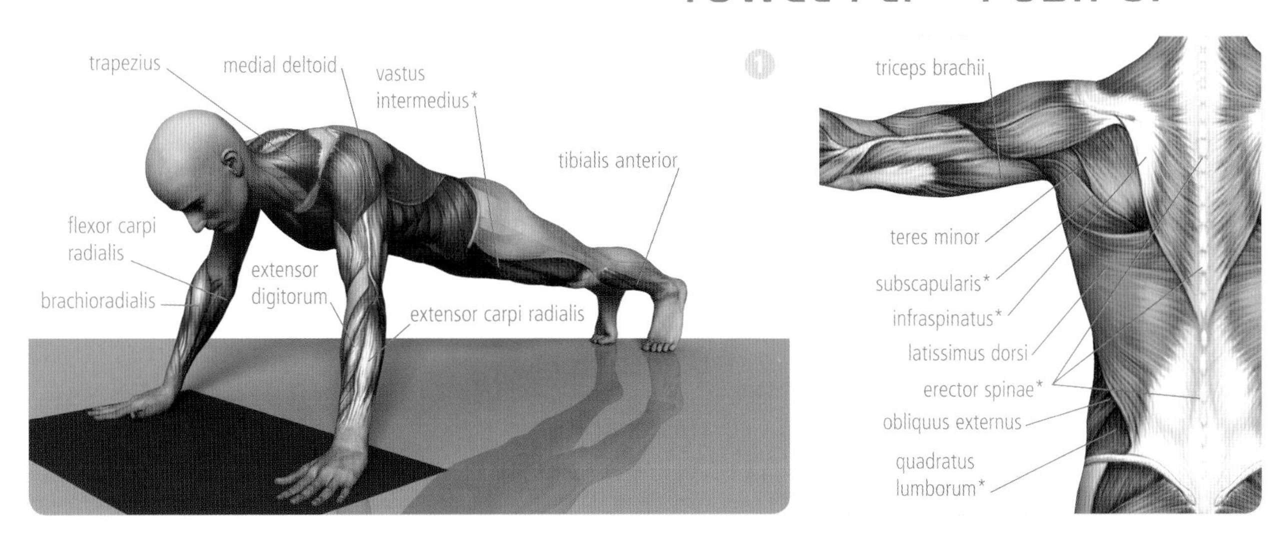

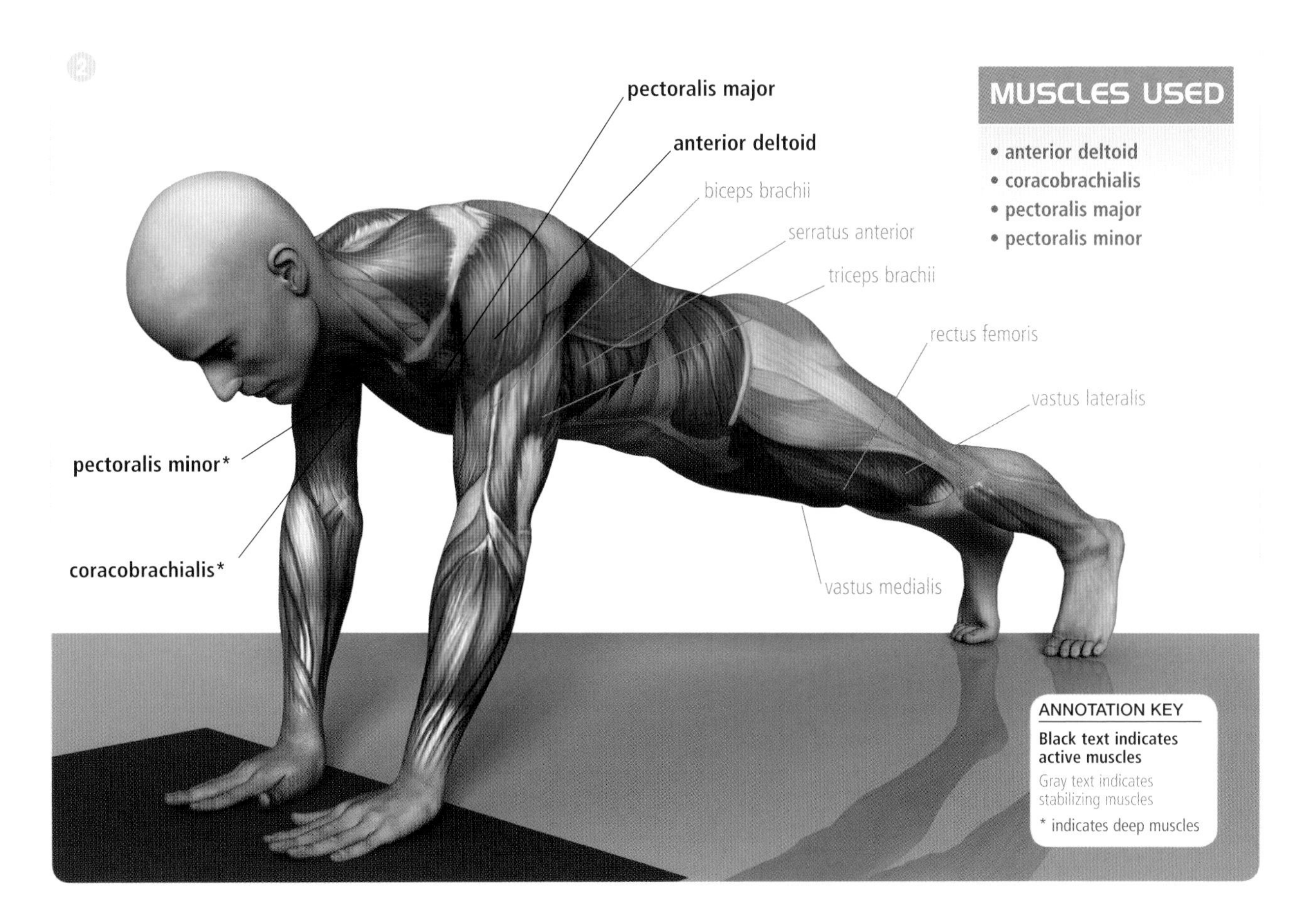

MUSCLES USED

- **anterior deltoid**
- **coracobrachialis**
- **pectoralis major**
- **pectoralis minor**

ANNOTATION KEY

Black text indicates active muscles

Gray text indicates stabilizing muscles

* indicates deep muscles

PIKE & PRESS

Starting Position: Place hands on blocks (or a bench), and place feet with ankles fixed at 90-degree angles on a physio ball, toes down, so that body is horizontal. Hands are wider than shoulder-width, and fingertips are parallel to collarbone. Feet are placed on ball with top of foot (shoelaces) contacting the ball, and toes are pointed.

LOOK FOR
- A single plane of movement, i.e., a straight line from head to ankle

AVOID
- A segmental elevation, i.e., your shoulders rising before your hips or vice versa
- Elevating your shoulders toward your ears
- Moving your head forward
- Allowing the ankles to change position
- Allowing the ball or body to migrate laterally

Action: Lower your entire body by allowing the elbows to bend until your torso has dropped into a position where the chest is at the level of your hands. Return by extending the elbows and pushing into the blocks, elevating entire body simultaneously.

From top position, pull ball forward by flexing foot and drawing the toes and hips upward so that the torso is bent at the hips. Toes are on top of the ball and both feet are at 90-degree angles. Upper body and head are facing downward. Keeping torso in that position, bend elbows and drop spine (head-first) between hands. Return by pushing hands into blocks until elbows are fully extended. Then, drop hips and extend toes until body returns to horizontal.

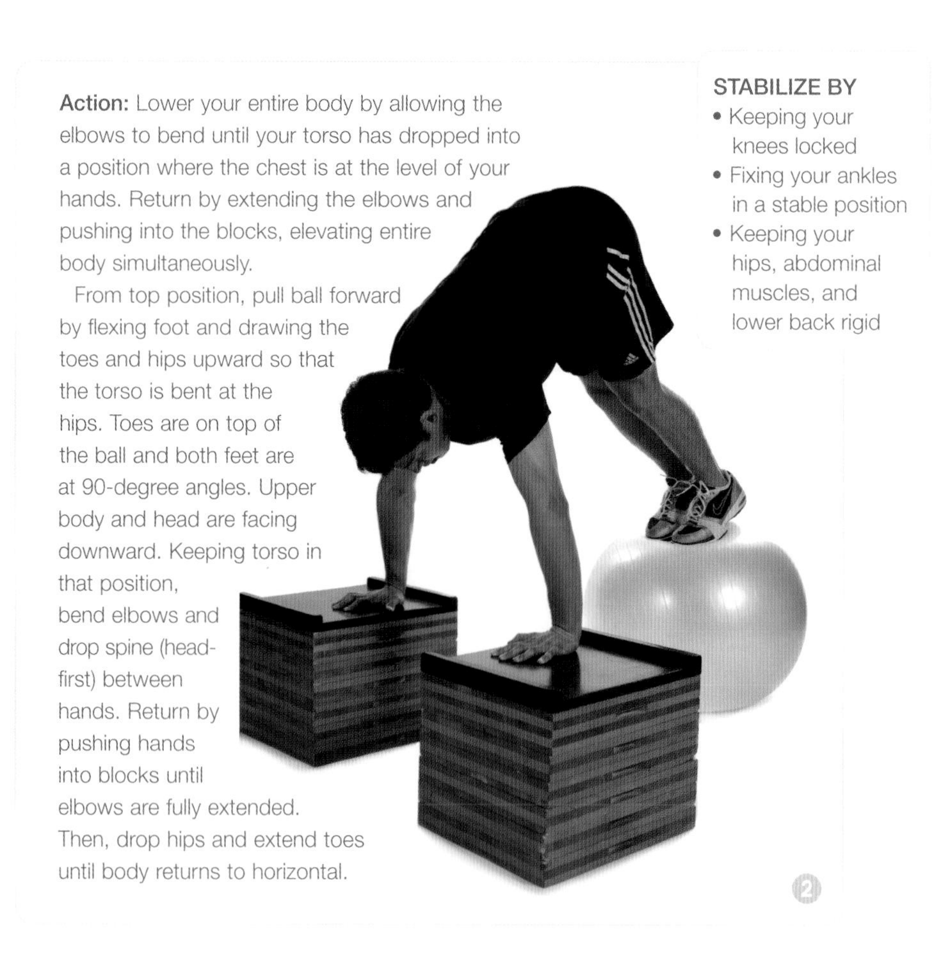

STABILIZE BY
- Keeping your knees locked
- Fixing your ankles in a stable position
- Keeping your hips, abdominal muscles, and lower back rigid

3

Movement Path: The plane of your body rotates upward in an arc. Use your feet as a lever.

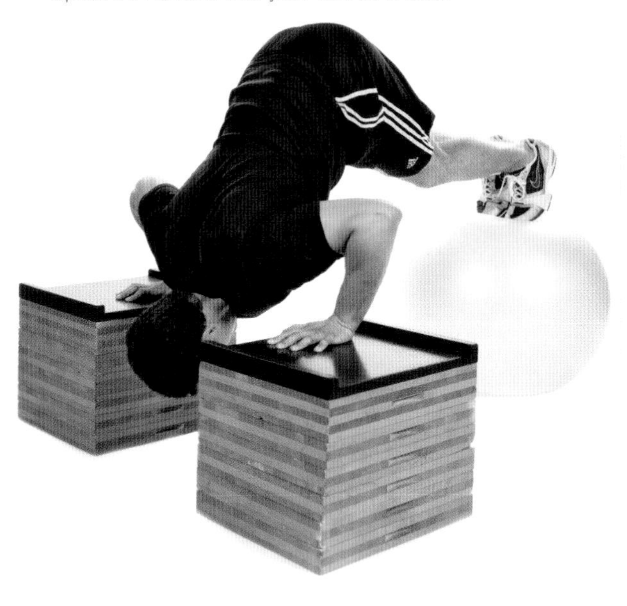

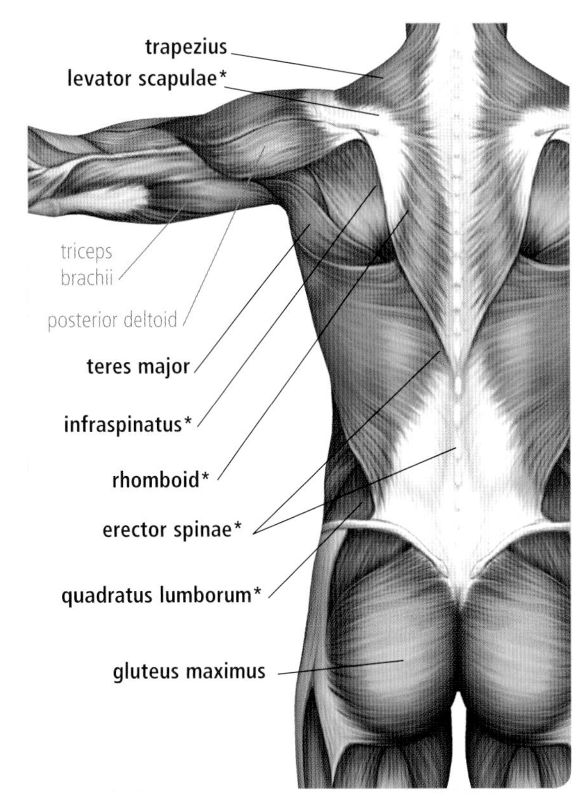

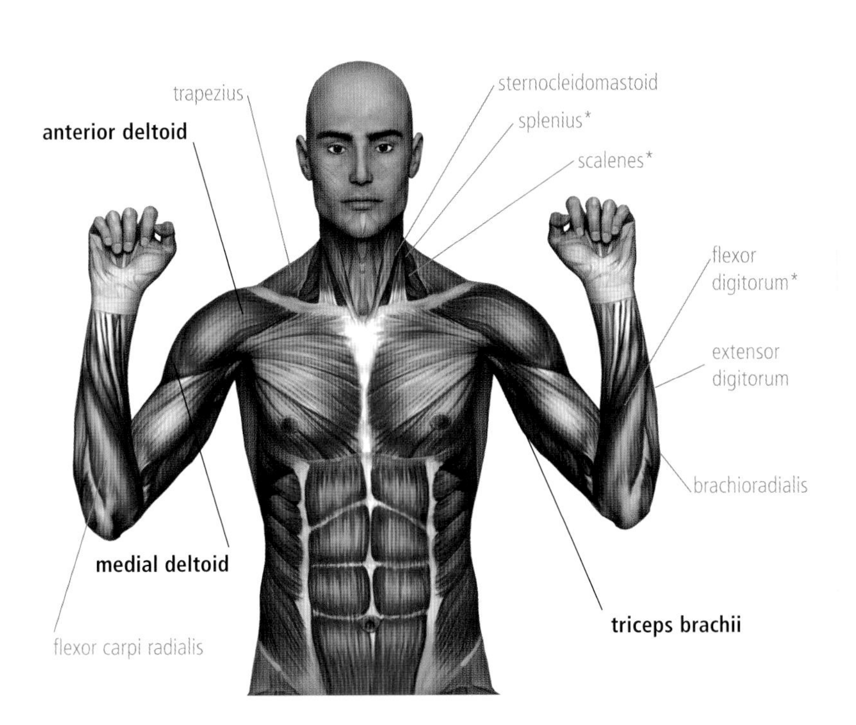

MUSCLES USED

- pectoralis major
- pectoralis minor
- coracobrachialis
- anterior deltoid
- triceps brachii
- iliopsoas
- vastus lateralis
- vastus medialis
- vastus intermedius
- rectus femoris
- anterior tibialis
- transversus abdominis
- serratus anterior
- erector spinae
- trapezius
- latissimus dorsi
- quadratus lumborum

ANNOTATION KEY

Black text indicates active muscles

Gray text indicates stabilizing muscles

* indicates deep muscles

LOWER-BODY ROTATION

1. **Starting Position:** With hand position same as in a push-up, rotate the lower body with either feet split and bottom foot forward, or one foot on top of the other.

LOOK FOR
- Fingertips to remain parallel
- Hips to remain in position throughout movement
- Feet to remain rigid and contact the ground only with the edges

AVOID
- Shoulders to elevate toward the ears
- Ankles to drop and contact the ground

2. **Action:** Raise your legs and hips off the ground. Your lower back should arch slightly. Extend your arms, pushing into the ground. To return, lower your body in a single plane by bending your arms. Repeat on opposite side.

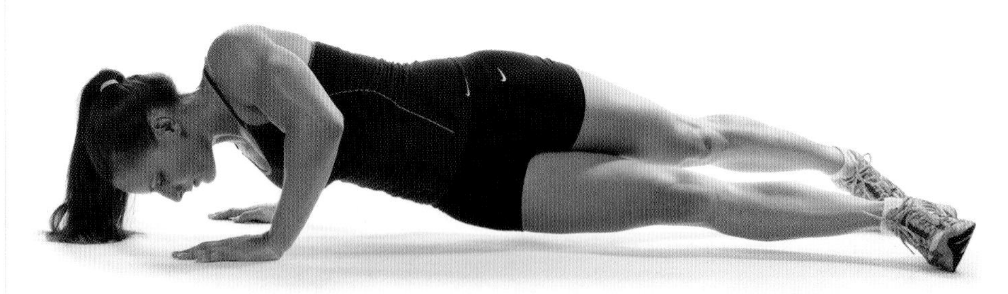

Movement Path: The plane of your body rotates upward in an arc. Use your feet as a lever.

STABILIZE BY
- Keeping your knees locked
- Fixing your ankles in a stable position
- Keeping your hips, abdominal muscles, and lower back rigid

ANNOTATION KEY

Black text indicates active muscles

Gray text indicates stabilizing muscles

* indicates deep muscles

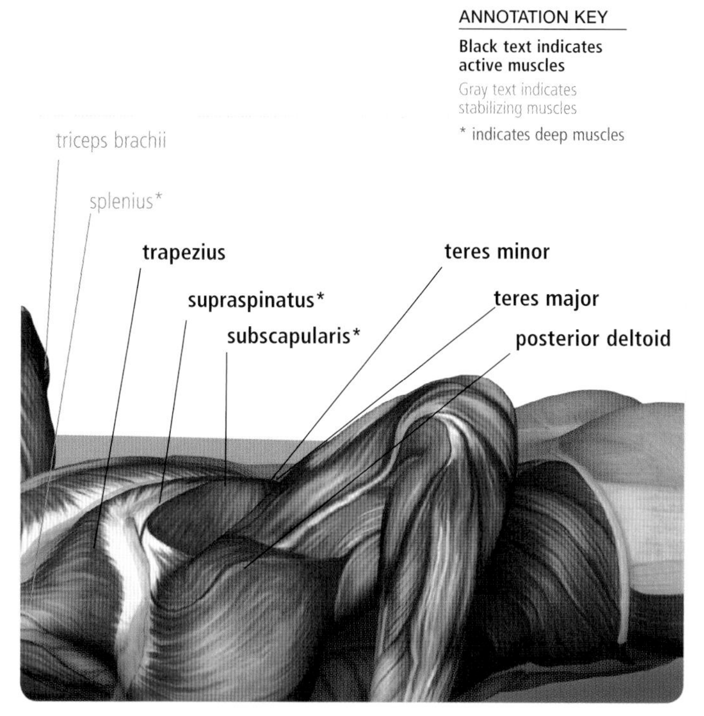

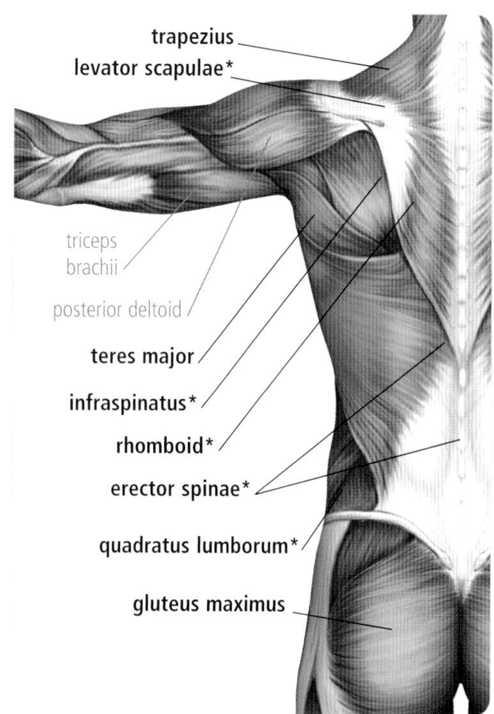

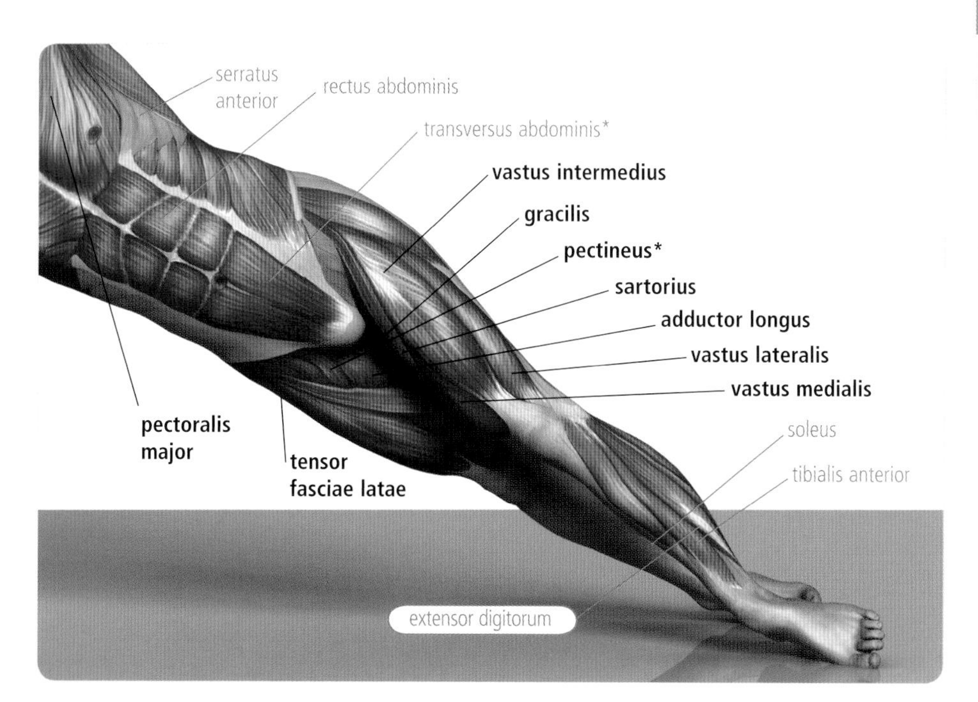

MUSCLES USED

- pectoralis major
- pectoralis minor
- coracobrachialis
- anterior deltoid
- triceps brachii
- iliopsoas
- vastus lateralis
- vastus medialis
- vastus intermedius
- rectus femoris
- anterior tibialis
- transversus abdominis
- serratus anterior
- erector spinae
- trapezius
- latissimus dorsi
- quadratus lumborum

CLAP PUSH-UP

1 **Starting Position:** Lie flat on the ground, face down. Place your hands slightly outside of your shoulders and your fingertips parallel to your collarbone. Make sure that your elbows are at 45-degree angles to your torso. Place both feet on tiptoes.

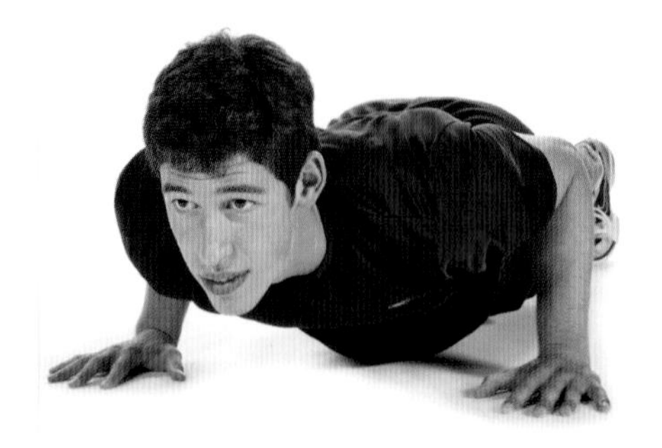

2

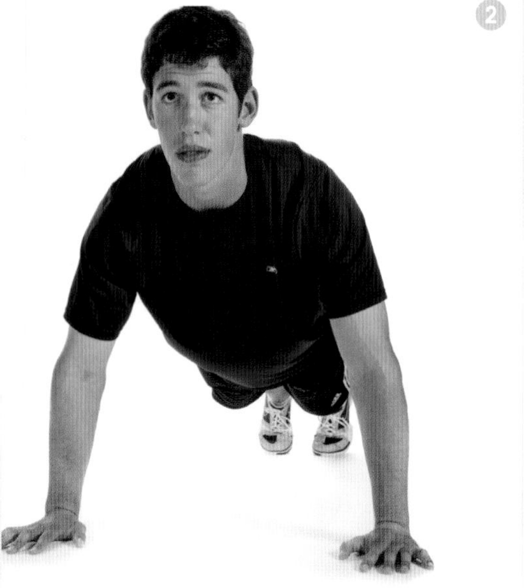

3

Action: Keeping body rigid, forcefully and quickly push hands into the ground so that enough momentum is generated for the hands to come off the ground. Just as the body reaches its highest point remove hands and clap them directly underneath the chest, immediately returning them to original position and allowing the body to return toward start position, decelerating as it descends to a position just above the floor. Quickly repeat.

LOOK FOR

- Body to remain rigid
- Hands to return to original position
- Continuous movement

AVOID

- Stopping at the bottom of the movement
- Allowing hand position to vary substantially

STABILIZE BY

- Keeping your knees locked
- Fixing your ankles in a stable position
- Keeping your hips, abdominal muscles, and lower back rigid

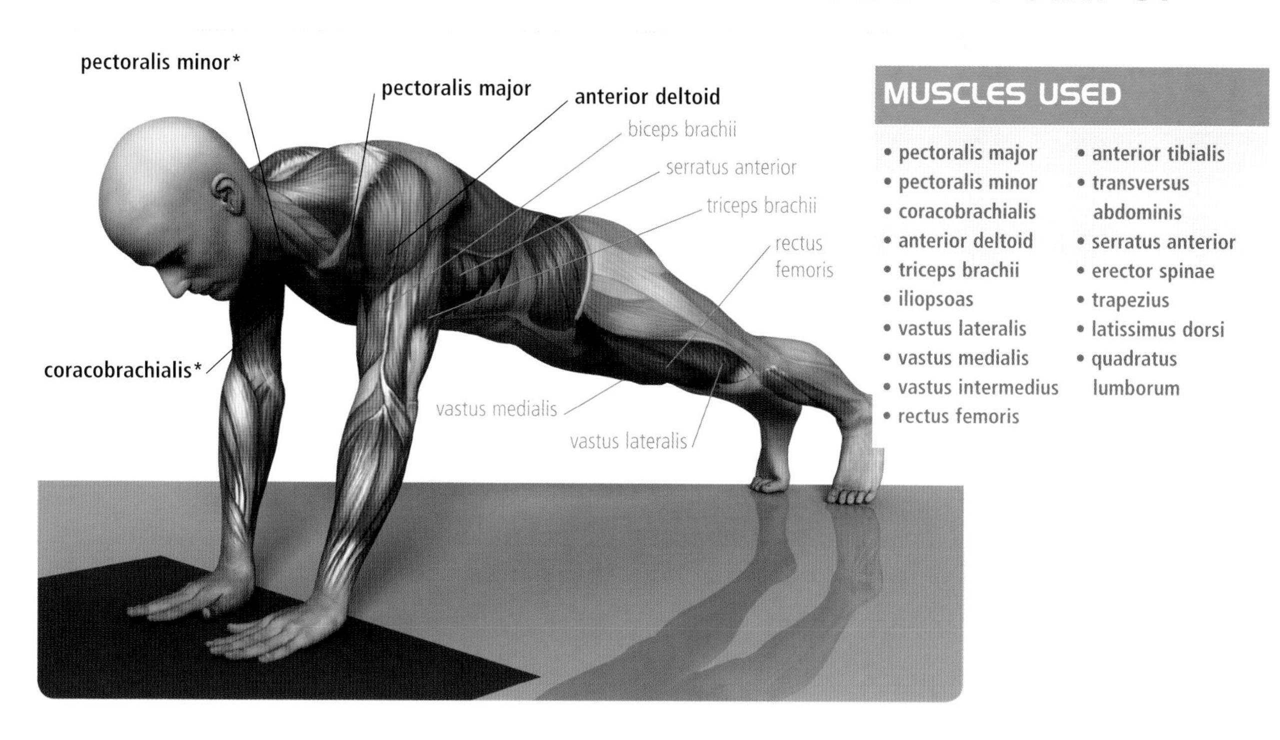

MUSCLES USED

- pectoralis major
- pectoralis minor
- coracobrachialis
- anterior deltoid
- triceps brachii
- iliopsoas
- vastus lateralis
- vastus medialis
- vastus intermedius
- rectus femoris
- anterior tibialis
- transversus abdominis
- serratus anterior
- erector spinae
- trapezius
- latissimus dorsi
- quadratus lumborum

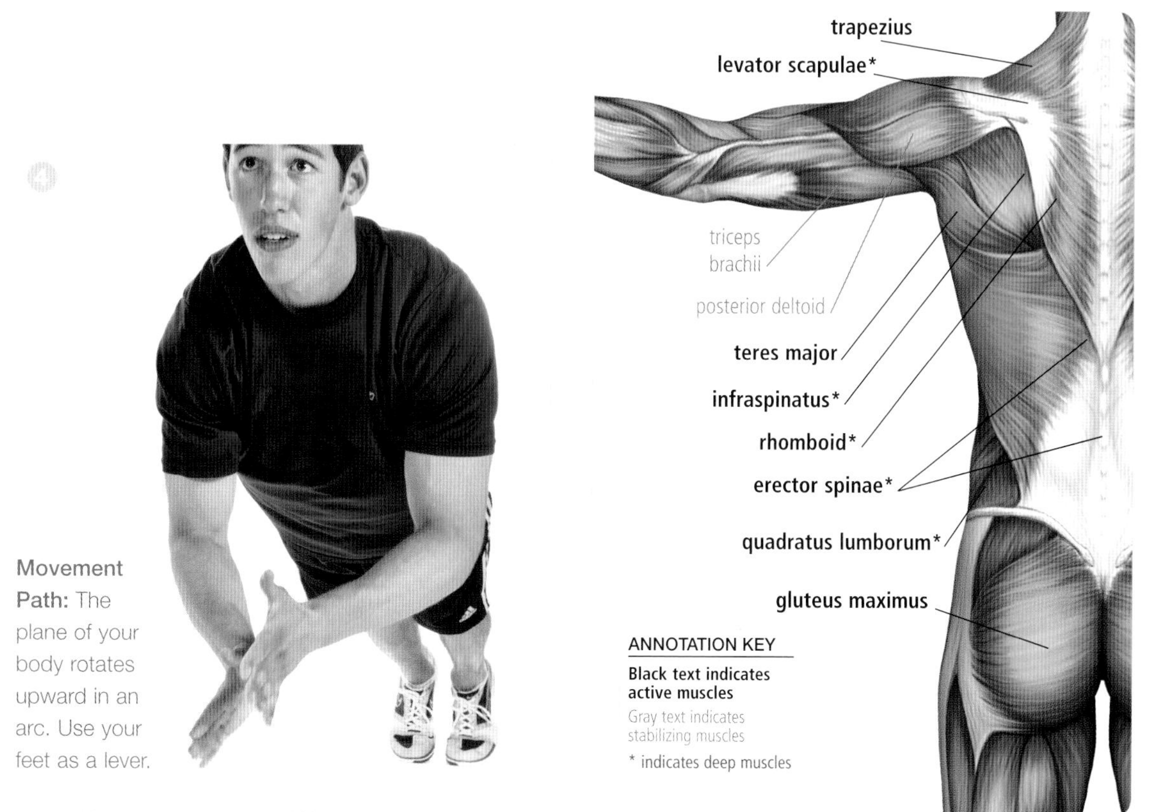

Movement Path: The plane of your body rotates upward in an arc. Use your feet as a lever.

ANNOTATION KEY

Black text indicates active muscles

Gray text indicates stabilizing muscles

* indicates deep muscles

ON KETTLEBELLS

PUSH-UP

1

Starting Position: Grasp handles of kettlebells set on ground slightly wider than shoulder-width and parallel to your collarbone. Make sure that your elbows are at 45-degree angles to your torso. Place both feet on tiptoes.

Action: Raise your legs and hips off the ground. Your lower back should arch slightly. Extend your arms, pushing into the ground. To return, lower your body in a single plane by bending your arms.

LOOK FOR
- A single plane of movement, i.e., a straight line from head to ankle

AVOID
- A segmental elevation, i.e., your shoulders rising before your hips or vice versa
- Elevating your shoulders toward your ears
- Moving your head forward

STABILIZE BY
- Keeping your knees locked
- Fixing your ankles in a stable position
- Keeping your hips, abdominal muscles, and lower back rigid

Movement Path: The plane of your body rotates upward in an arc. Use your feet as a lever.

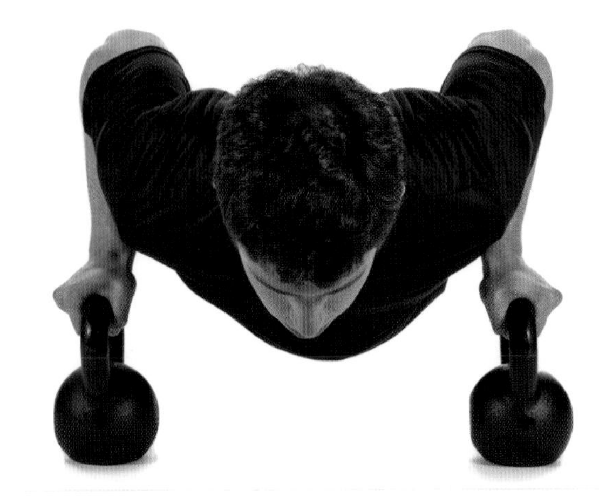

2

MODIFICATION

More Difficult: Place one hand on a medicine ball, the other on the floor. Follow same action and movement path.

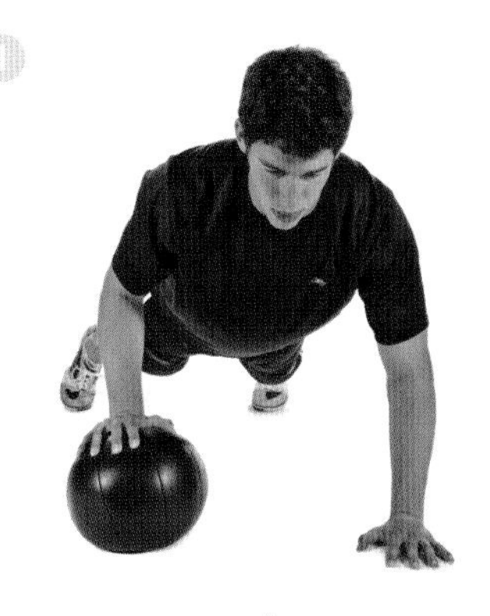

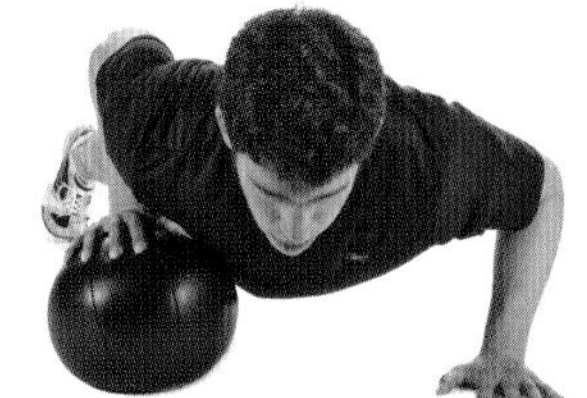

MUSCLES USED

- pectoralis major
- pectoralis minor
- coracobrachialis
- anterior deltoid
- triceps brachii
- iliopsoas
- vastus lateralis
- vastus medialis
- vastus intermedius
- rectus femoris
- tibialis anterior
- transversus abdominis
- serratus anterior
- erector spinae
- trapezius
- latissimus dorsi
- quadratus lumborum

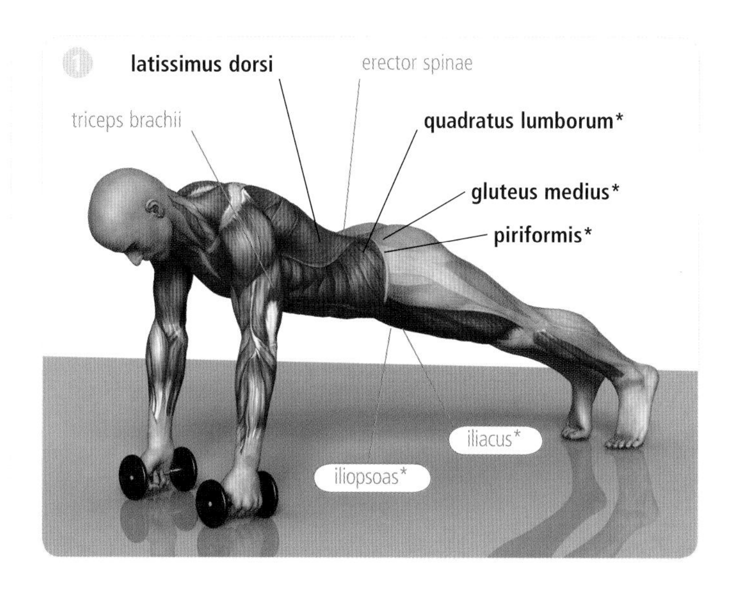

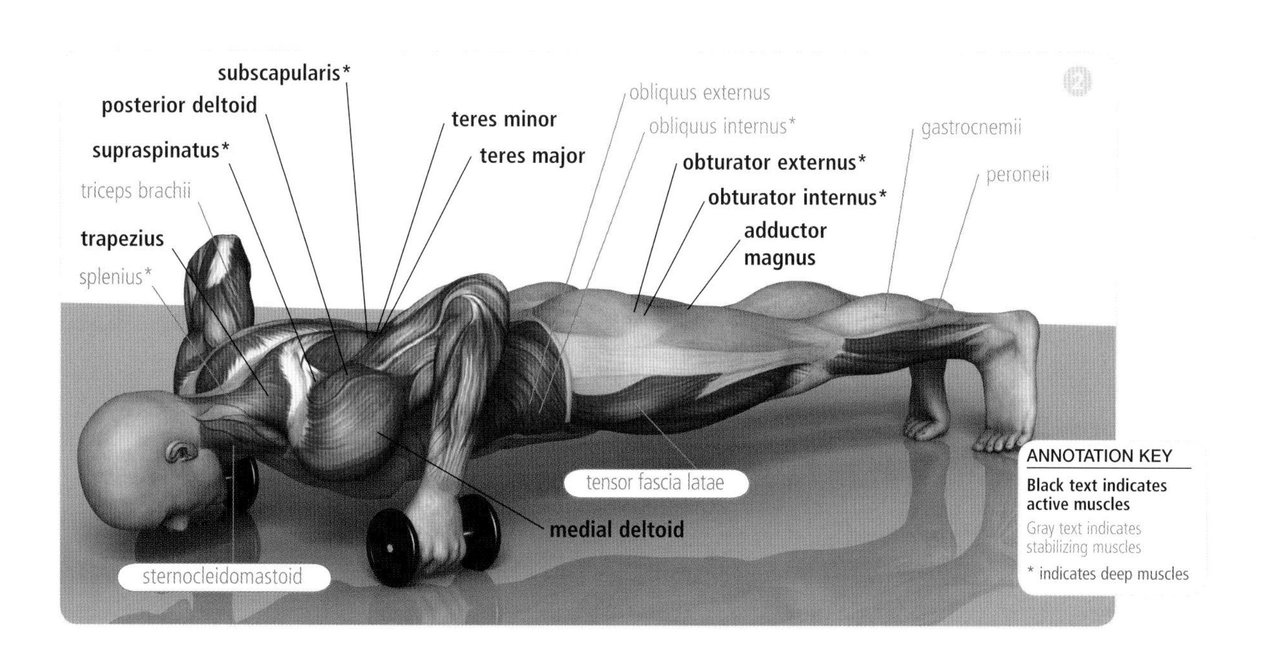

HAND WALKOVER

1 **Starting Position:** Begin with one hand on floor and one elevated on a box.

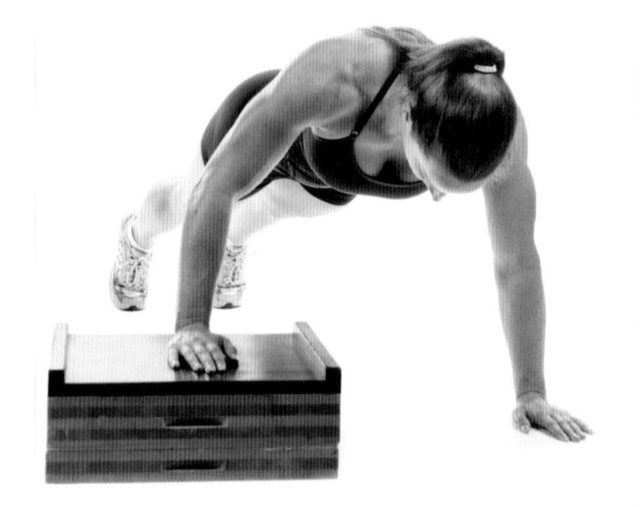

STABILIZE BY
- Keeping torso rigid
- Keeping legs straight and feet firm but relaxed

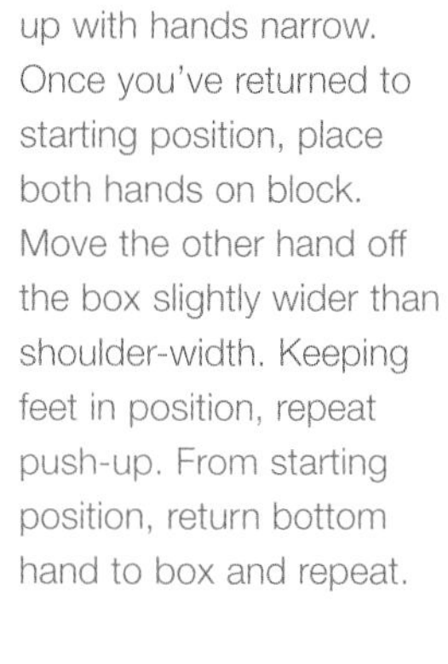

Action: Perform a push-up with hands narrow. Once you've returned to starting position, place both hands on block. Move the other hand off the box slightly wider than shoulder-width. Keeping feet in position, repeat push-up. From starting position, return bottom hand to box and repeat.

LOOK FOR
- Shoulders to remain horizontal
- Rib cage and chest up
- Elbow of elevated hand to be slightly bent, while other is completely straight at top position

AVOID
- Dropping one shoulder
- Any sagging or extending of the hips
- Bending knees

2

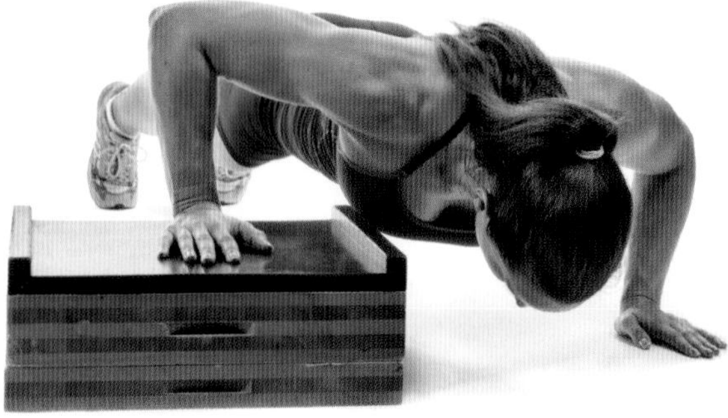

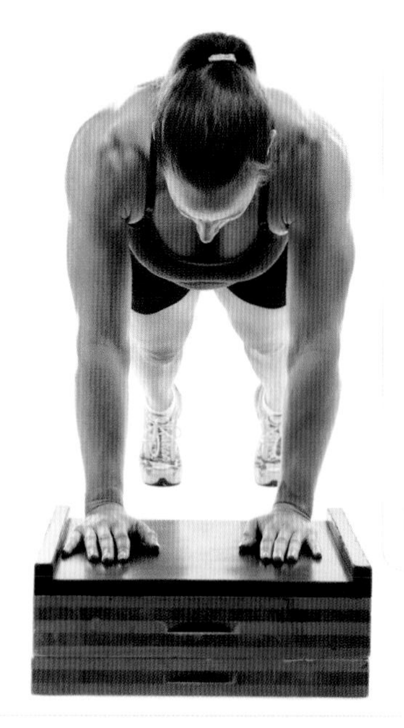

3

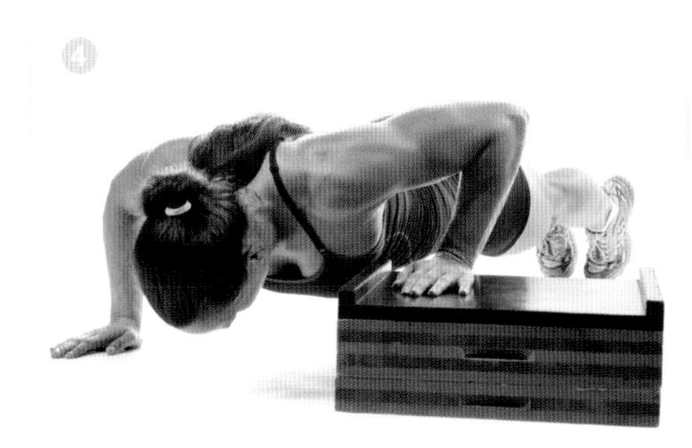

Movement Path: The spine moves in a horizontal plane in an arc with the feet as a fulcrum, torso descending directly toward the floor and returning.

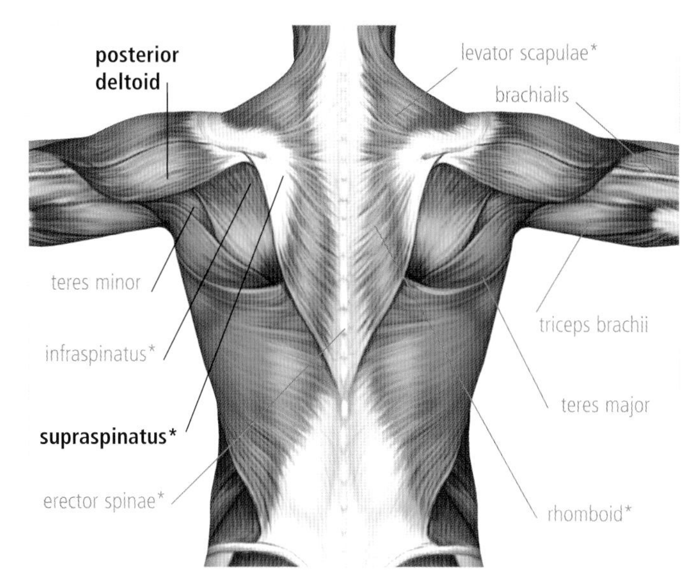

MUSCLES USED

- pectoralis major
- pectoralis minor
- coracobrachialis
- anterior deltoid
- triceps brachii
- iliopsoas
- vastus lateralis
- vastus medialis
- vastus intermedius
- rectus femoris
- anterior tibialis
- transversus abdominis
- serratus anterior
- erector spinae
- trapezius
- latissimus dorsi
- quadratus lumborum

ANNOTATION KEY

Black text indicates active muscles

Gray text indicates stabilizing muscles

* indicates deep muscles

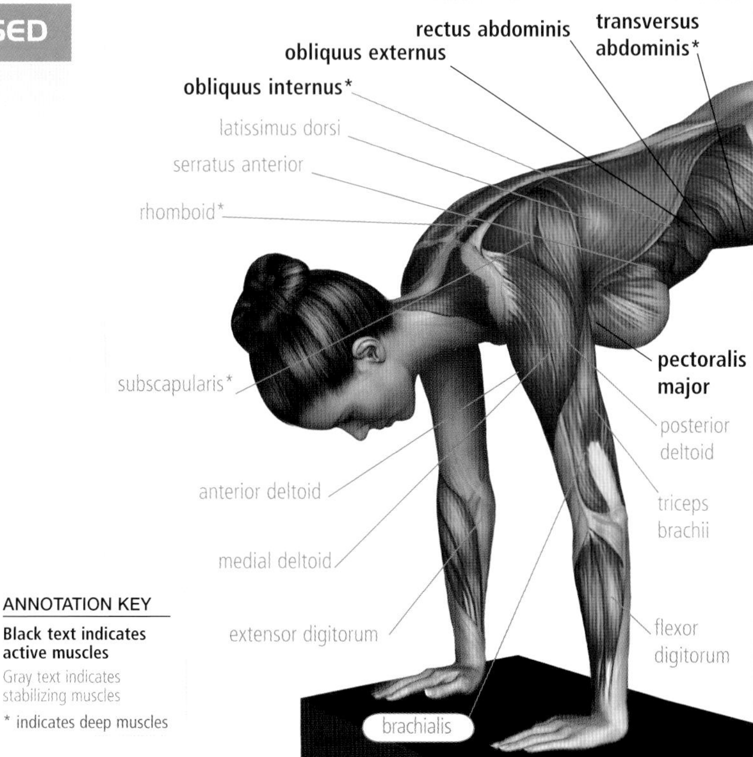

HANDS ON RINGS

1

Starting Position: With body rigid, grasp rings slightly wider than shoulder-width apart with a palms-down grip, so that rings are parallel and directly above the chest.

Action: Allow the entire body to descend chest-first in a controlled manner by allowing elbows to bend and using toes as a fulcrum. While descending, move hands apart laterally, until chest is directly between the hands at ring level, and elbows are bent to 90 degrees. Return by extending arms, pushing toward the floor until elbows are straightened.

LOOK FOR
- A single plane of movement, i.e., a straight line from head to ankle

AVOID
- Segmental elevation, i.e., your shoulders rising before your hips or vice versa.
- Elevating your shoulders toward your ears
- Moving your head forward

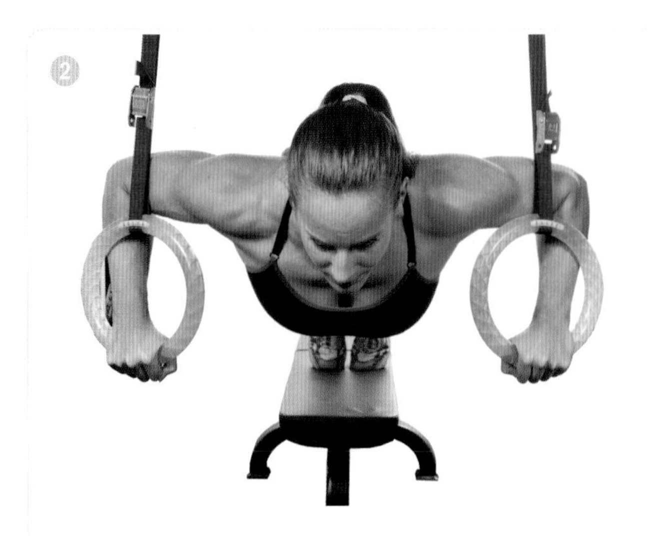

2

Movement Path: Torso moves directly downward, and hands move outward on the descent and inward on the ascent.

STABILIZE BY
- Keeping your knees locked
- Fixing your ankles in a stable position
- Keeping your hips, abdominal muscles, and lower back rigid

HANDS ON RINGS • PUSH-UP

MUSCLES USED

- pectoralis major
- pectoralis minor
- coracobrachialis
- anterior deltoid
- triceps brachii
- iliopsoas
- vastus lateralis
- vastus medialis
- vastus intermedius
- rectus femoris
- anterior tibialis
- transversus abdominis
- serratus anterior
- erector spinae
- trapezius
- latissimus dorsi
- quadratus lumborum

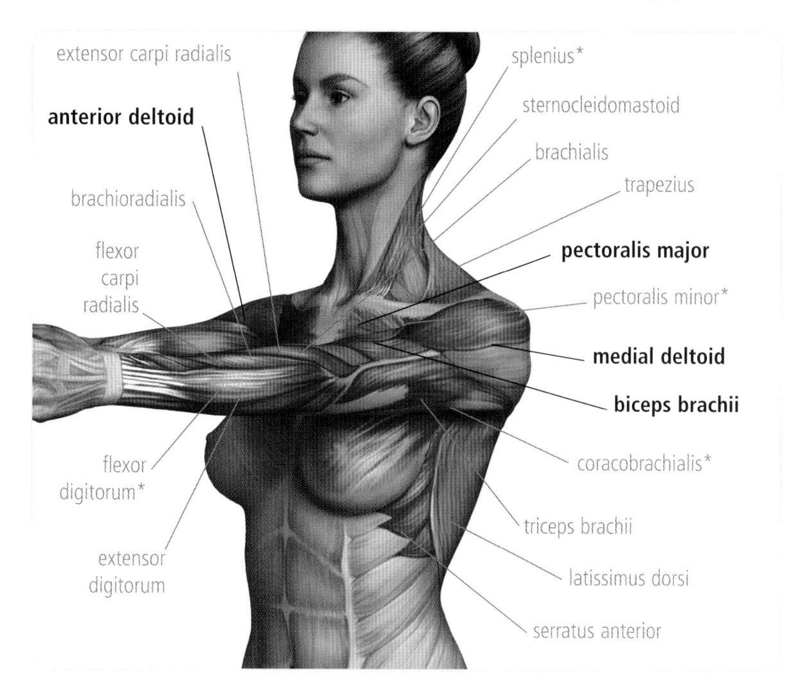

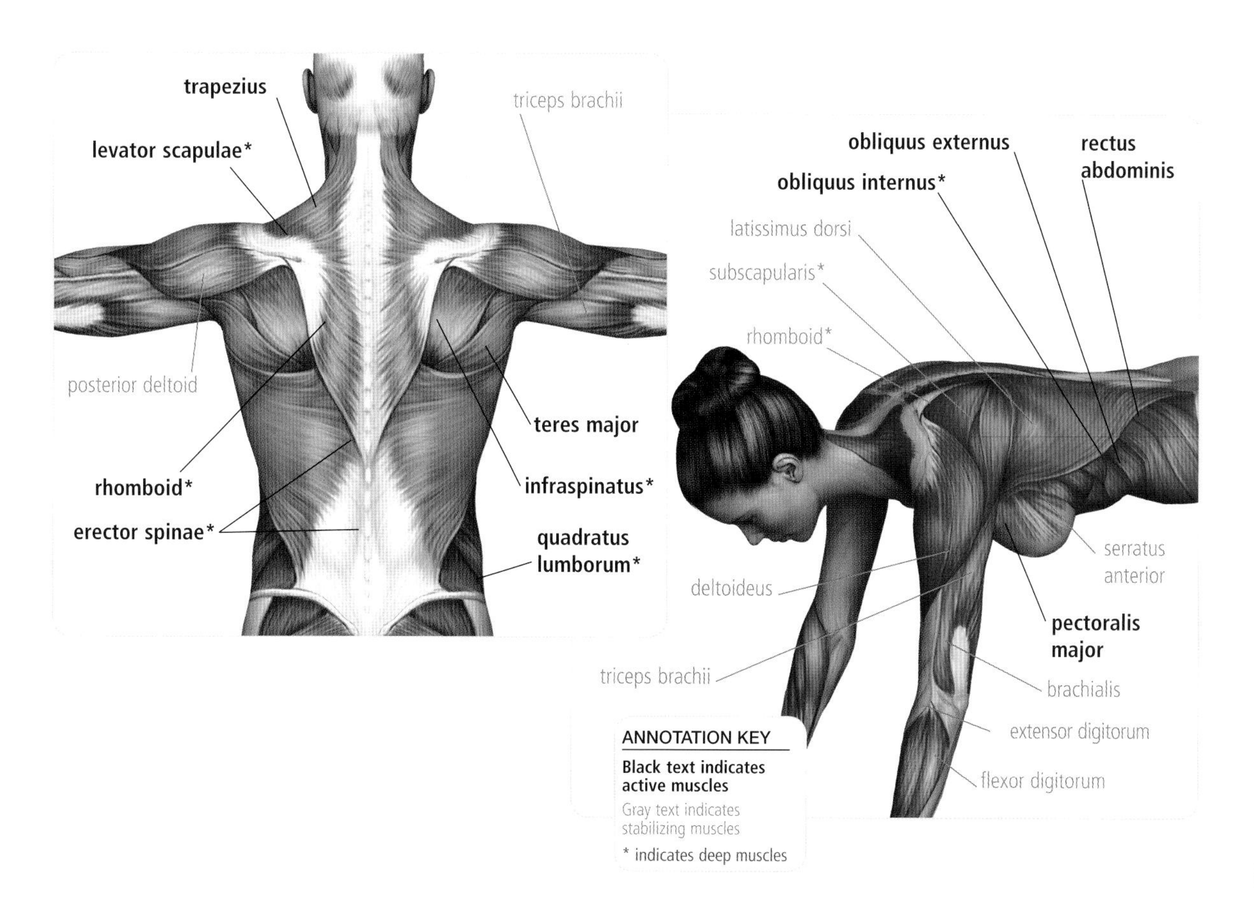

ANNOTATION KEY

Black text indicates active muscles

Gray text indicates stabilizing muscles

* indicates deep muscles

SINGLE-ARM FORWARD SLIDE

1 **Starting Position:** On a smooth flat surface (preferably wood) assume a push-up position with legs straight and each hand placed on a small individual towel. Hands are directly beneath shoulders.

LOOK FOR
- Smooth transitions
- All parts to move at once

AVOID
- Touching the ground with the torso
- Bending knees
- Allowing body to rotate

2 **Action:** Bend one elbow and simultaneously slide the other hand upward, keeping that elbow straight to cause your torso to descend. Return by pushing into the floor with the bent arm and pulling downward with the overhead, straightened one, until torso returns to original position. Alternate arms.

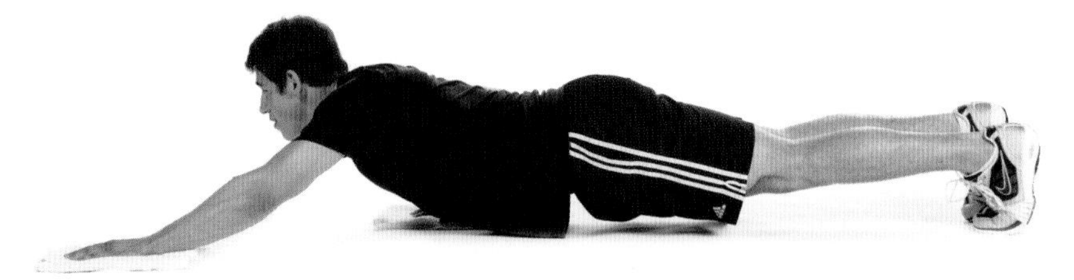

3 **Movement Path:** Spine moves directly downward. One arm moves upward.

STABILIZE BY
- Keeping tension on both hands
- Keeping legs straight and hips even

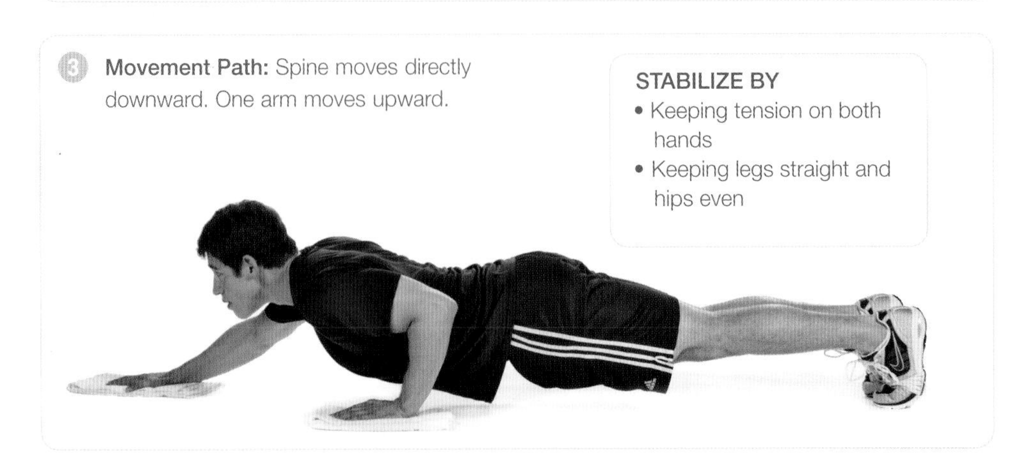

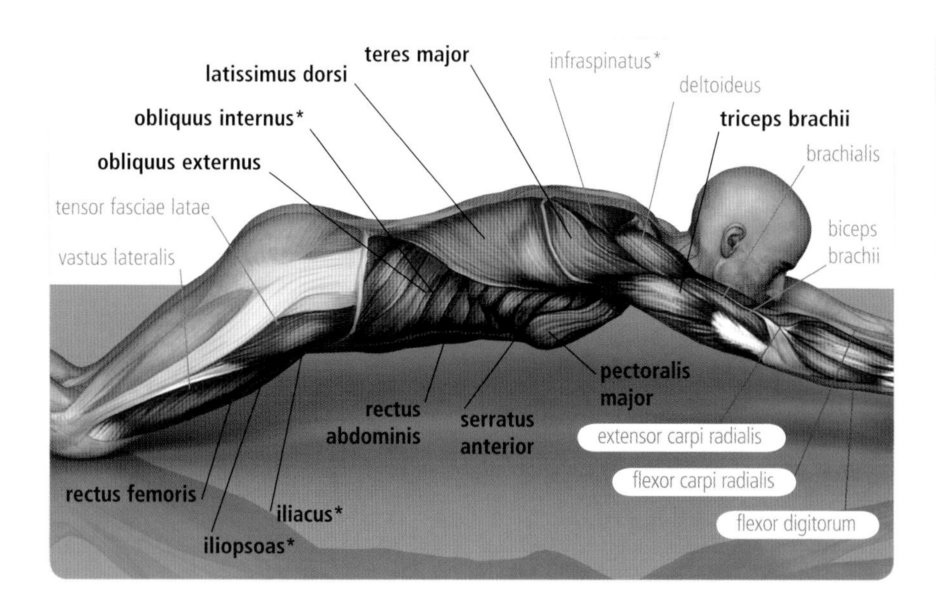

MUSCLES USED

- pectoralis major
- pectoralis minor
- coracobrachialis
- anterior deltoid
- triceps brachii
- iliopsoas
- vastus lateralis
- vastus medialis
- vastus intermedius
- rectus femoris
- anterior tibialis
- transversus abdominis
- serratus anterior
- erector spinae
- trapezius
- latissimus dorsi
- quadratus lumborum

ANNOTATION KEY
Black text indicates active muscles
Gray text indicates stabilizing muscles
* indicates deep muscles

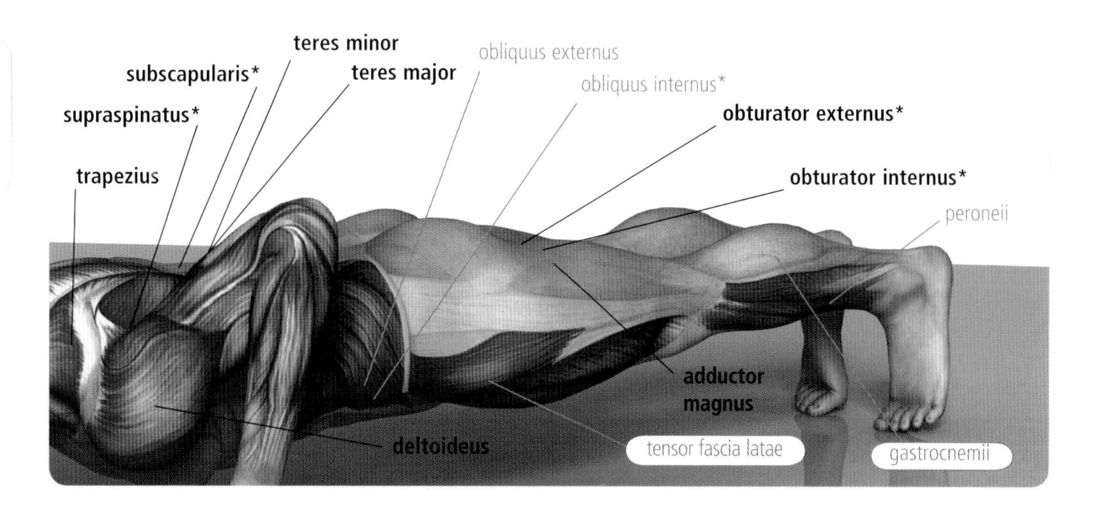

MODIFICATIONS

Less Difficult: Assume a push-up position with knees bent. Follow same action and movement path.

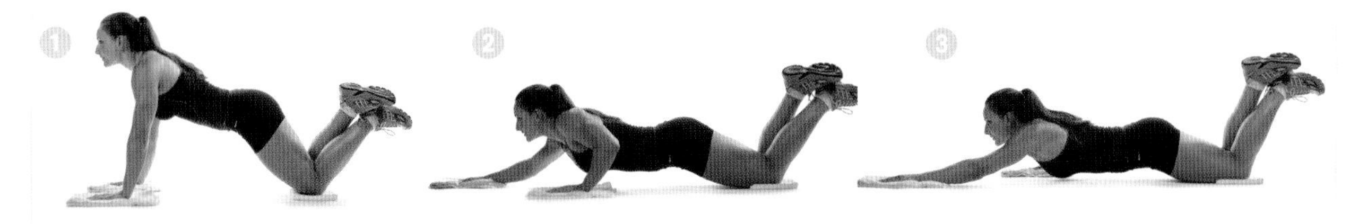

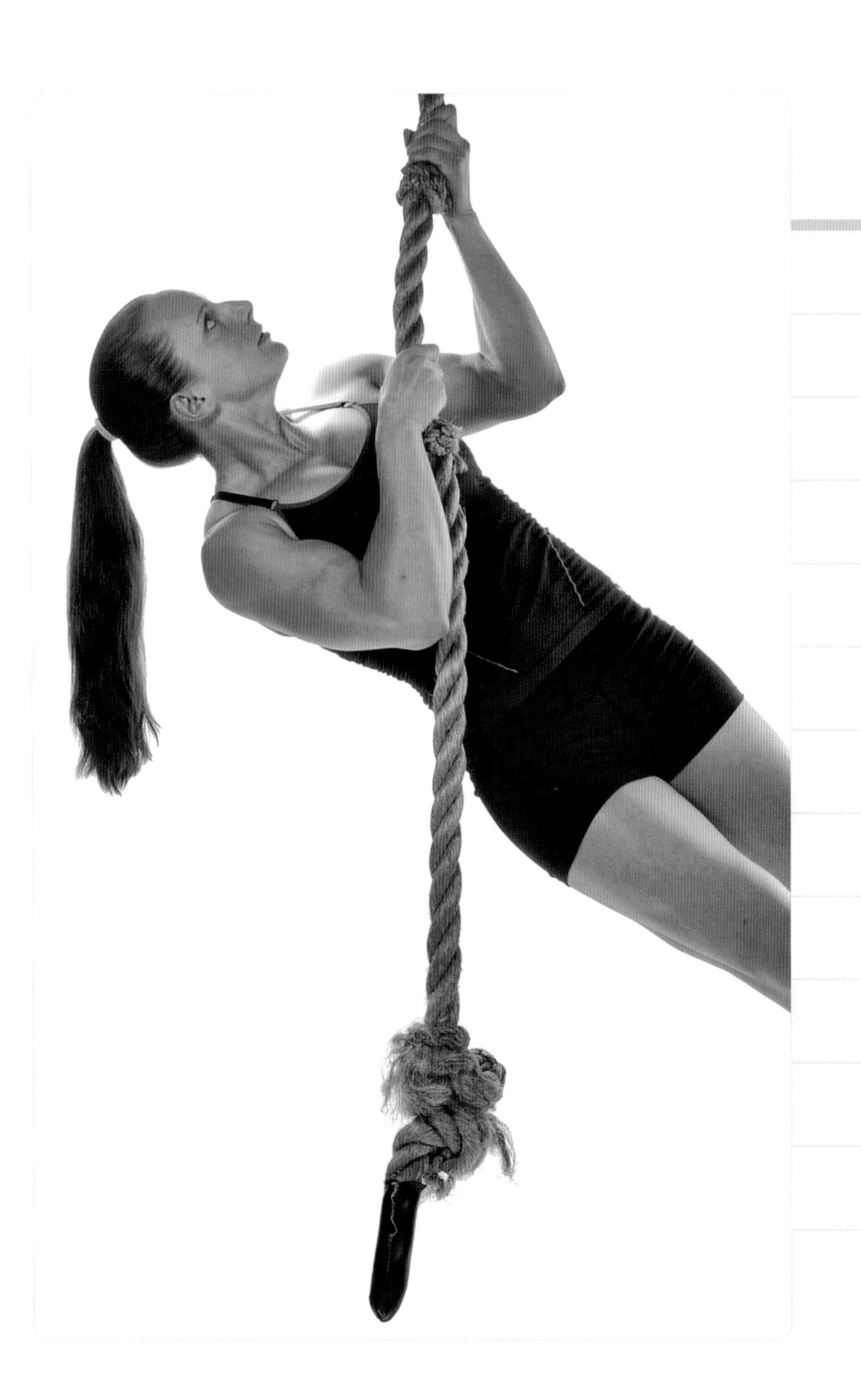

CHIN-UP

Like its other half, (the push-up), the chin-up has also been around as an exercise for thousands of years. These two are the yin and yang of the upper body's function: push and pull. The chin-up is perhaps the most intimidating of all exercises because there is only you and the bar, and either you can pull yourself up to it or you cannot. Gravity is relentless, and no matter how strong you are, when you begin to fail (and you will) there is no way to cheat it: when you're done, you're done. As an upper-body conditioning exercise it is rivaled by only its partner the push-up (and perhaps the dip) as an absolute necessity for anyone at any level.

Joints involved are the shoulder, elbow, and wrist. Muscles are back, shoulders, and biceps.

The primary benefits derived from chin-ups are upper-body pulling strength and endurance, shoulder stability, grip strength, and posture.

CHIN-UP

Starting Position: Gripping the bar with your palms in (facing your body), hang with your knees bent only very slightly. Keep your head in a neutral alignment. Your hands should be shoulder-width apart.

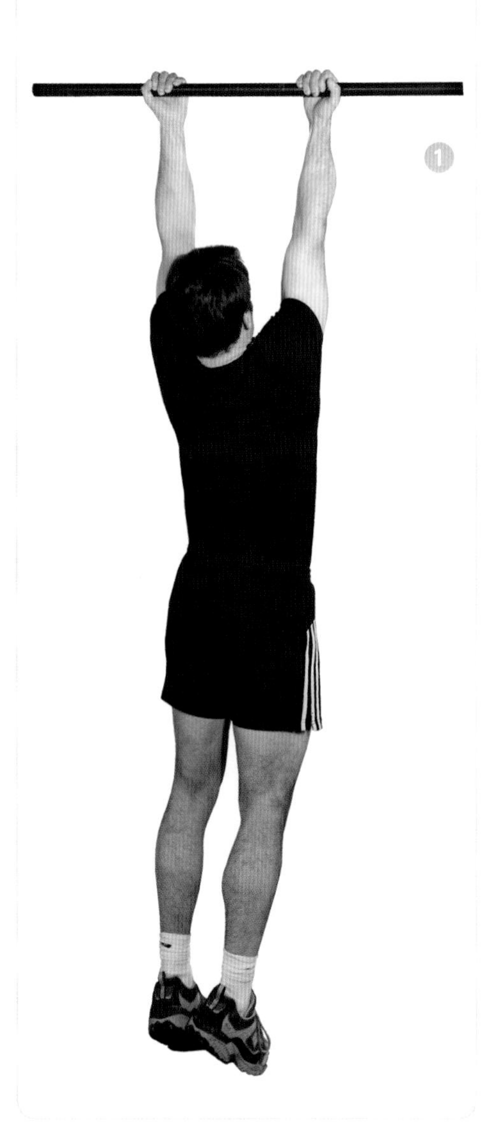

Action: Pull your body up vertically until your upper chest is aligned with the bar: this is the end of the concentric phase. Lower your body back down to the starting position with your elbows fully extended (the end of the eccentric phase).

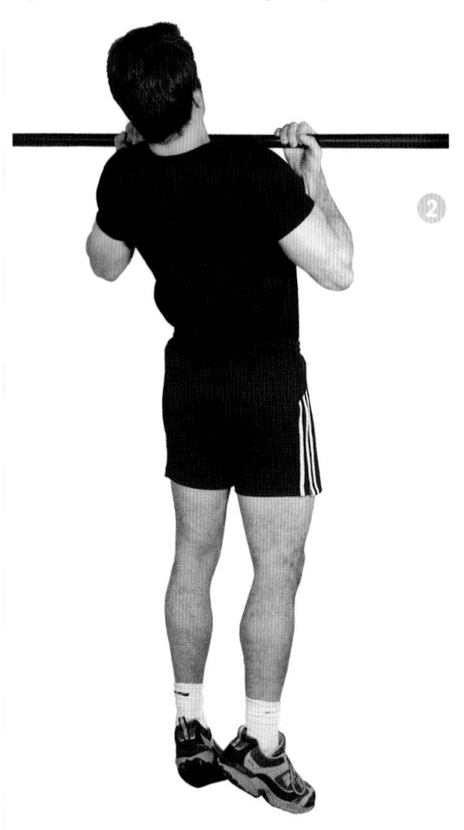

Movement Path: Your body moves vertically up. Your upper body tilts back slightly to allow your chin to smoothly pass the bar line.

STABILIZE BY
- Retracting your scapula
- Keeping your core tight to prevent swinging

LOOK FOR
- Your arms to return to a full extension
- You shoulder blades to draw together and downward at the beginning of the movement

AVOID
- Swinging, jerking, chin "pecking," or hyper-extension of elbows

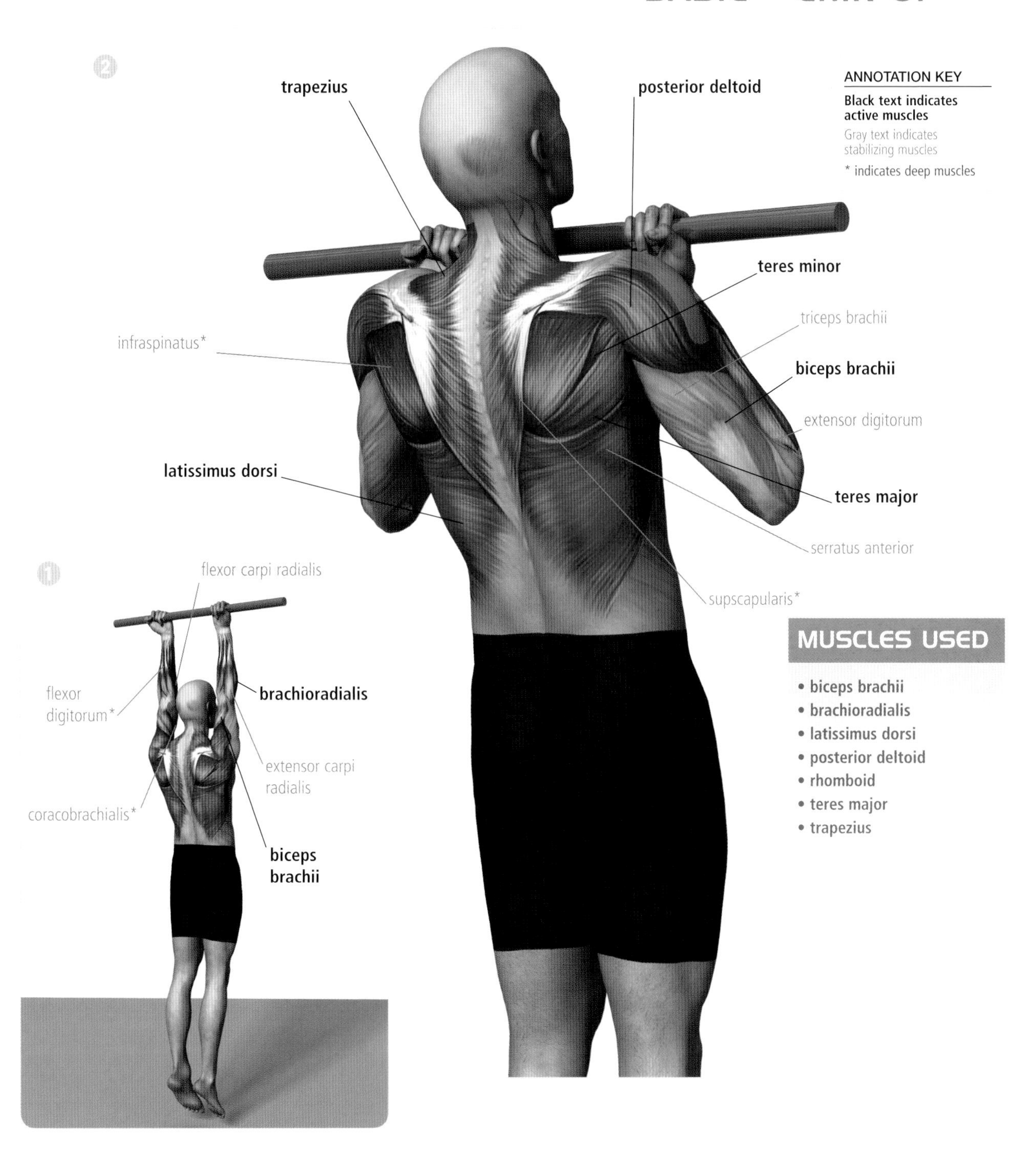

ANNOTATION KEY

Black text indicates active muscles

Gray text indicates stabilizing muscles

* indicates deep muscles

MUSCLES USED

- biceps brachii
- brachioradialis
- latissimus dorsi
- posterior deltoid
- rhomboid
- teres major
- trapezius

PULL-UP GRIP

Starting Position: Gripping the bar with your palms out (facing away from your body), hang with your knees bent and your ankles crossed. Keep your head in a neutral alignment. Your hands should be shoulder-width apart.

Action: Pull your body up vertically until your upper chest is aligned with the bar: this is the end of the concentric phase. Lower your body back down to the starting position with your elbows fully extended (the end of the eccentric phase).

Movement Path: Your body moves vertically up. Your upper body tilts back slightly to allow your chin to smoothly pass the bar line.

LOOK FOR
- Your arms to return to a full extension
- Your shoulder blades to draw together and downward at the beginning of the movement

AVOID
- Swinging, jerking, chin "pecking," or hyper-extension of elbows

STABILIZE BY
- Retracting your scapula
- Keeping your core tight to prevent swinging

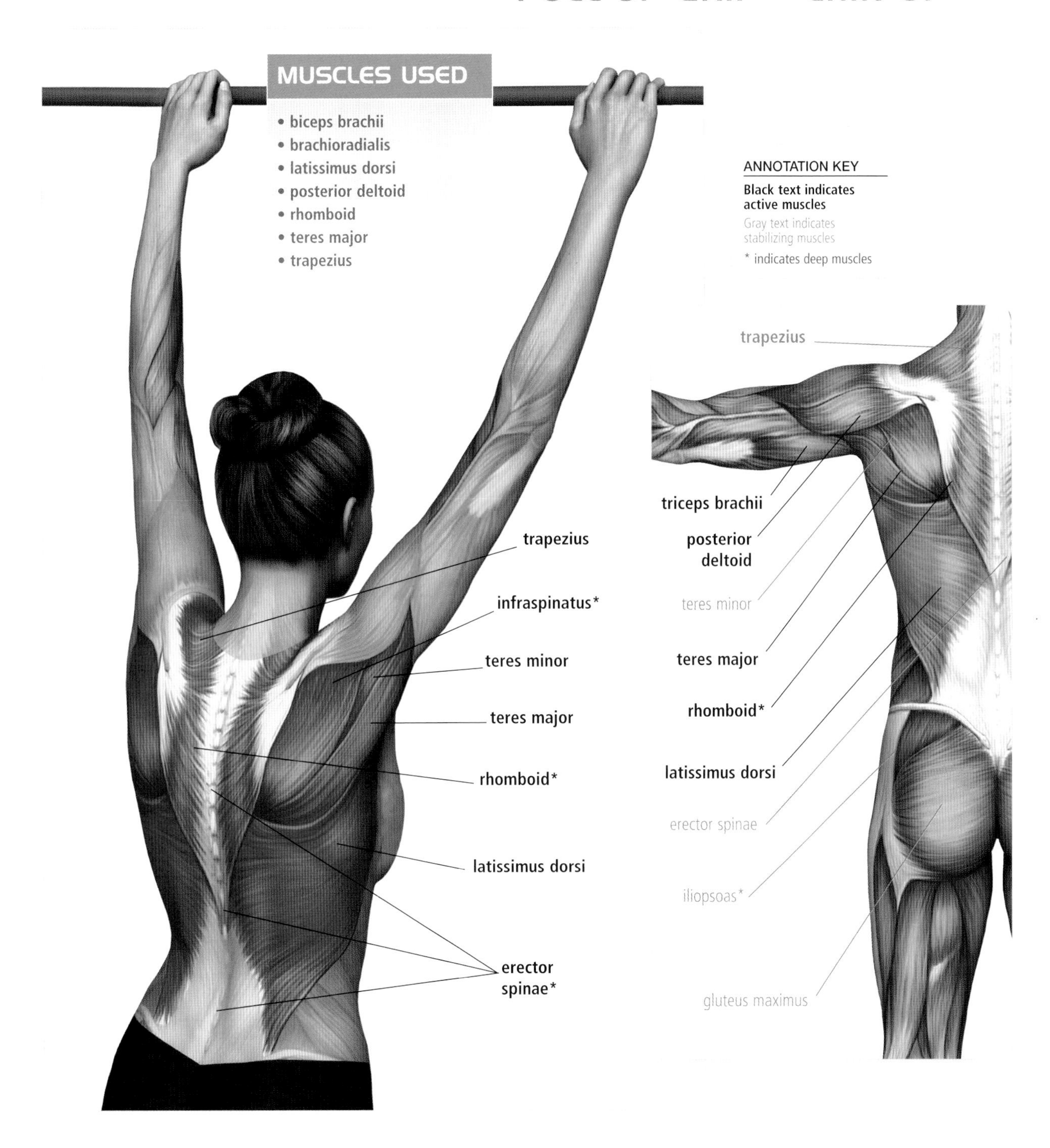
MUSCLES USED
• biceps brachii
• brachioradialis
• latissimus dorsi
• posterior deltoid
• rhomboid
• teres major
• trapezius
ANNOTATION KEY
Black text indicates active muscles
Gray text indicates stabilizing muscles
* indicates deep muscles
trapezius
infraspinatus*
teres minor
teres major
rhomboid*
latissimus dorsi
erector spinae*
trapezius
triceps brachii
posterior deltoid
teres minor
teres major
rhomboid*
latissimus dorsi
erector spinae
iliopsoas*
gluteus maximus

45° BODY ROW

Starting Position: Hang from a bar with your body in a flat plane. The line of your body should be at a 45-degree angle to the floor. Grasp the bar with both arms in supine or prone grips. Your elbows should be at 90-degree angles.

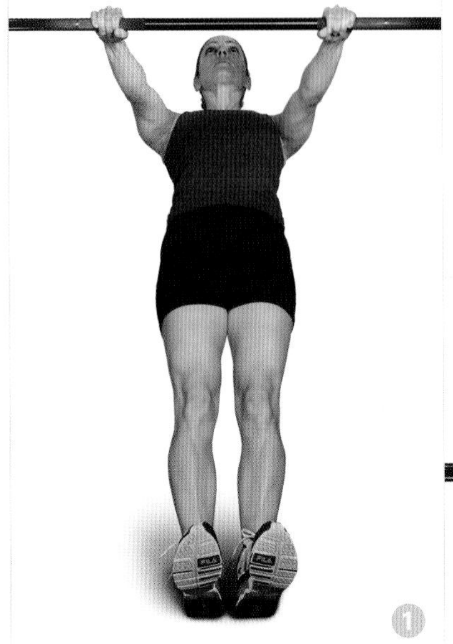

STABILIZE BY
- Fixing your shoulders in one position
- Locking your knees
- Keeping your ankles in a fixed position
- Keeping your hips, abdominal muscles, and lower back rigid

LOOK FOR
- A single plane of movement, maintaining a straight line from your head to your ankles

AVOID
- A segmental elevation, such as your shoulders rising before hips or vice versa
- Elevating your shoulders toward your ears
- Moving your head forward

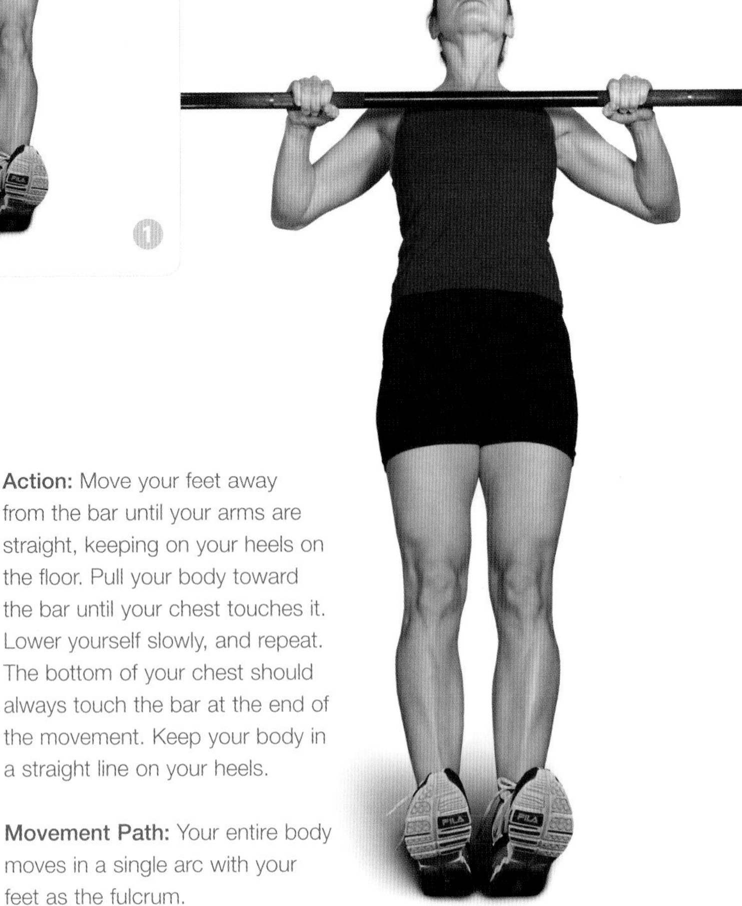

Action: Move your feet away from the bar until your arms are straight, keeping on your heels on the floor. Pull your body toward the bar until your chest touches it. Lower yourself slowly, and repeat. The bottom of your chest should always touch the bar at the end of the movement. Keep your body in a straight line on your heels.

Movement Path: Your entire body moves in a single arc with your feet as the fulcrum.

45° BODY ROW • CHIN-UP

MUSCLES USED

- biceps brachii
- brachialis
- brachioradialis
- infraspinatus
- latissimus dorsi
- rhomboid
- teres major
- teres minor
- trapezius

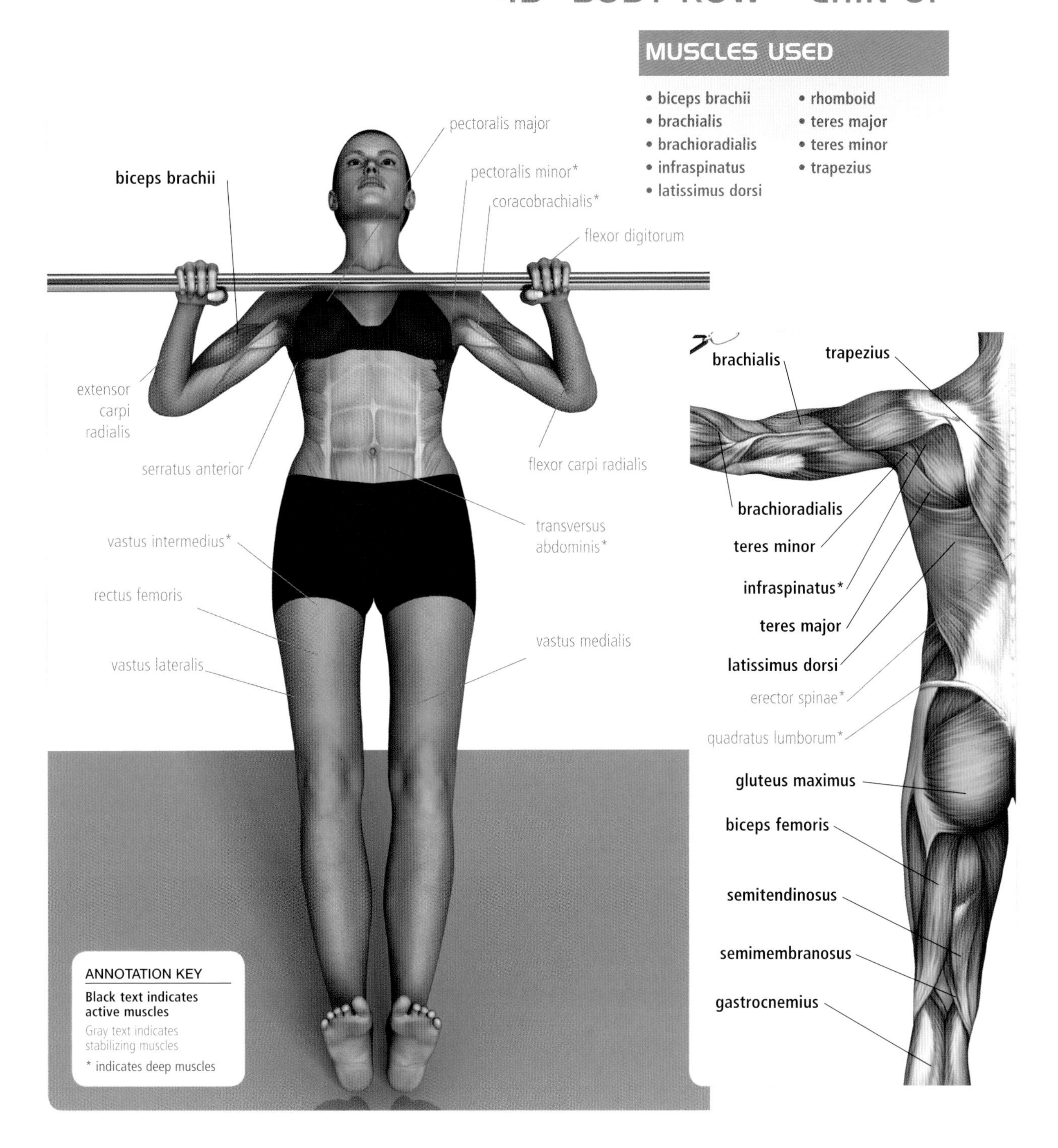

HORIZONTAL BODY ROW

Starting Position: Hang from a bar with your body in a flat plane. Elevate your feet so that your body is parallel to the ground. Grasp the bar with both arms in supine or prone grips. Your elbows should be at 90-degree angles.

Action: Keeping your weight on your heels, pull your body toward the bar until your chest touches it. Lower yourself slowly, and repeat. The bottom of your chest should always touch the bar at the end of the movement. Keep your body in a straight line on your heels.

LOOK FOR
- A single plane of movement, maintaining a straight line from your head to your ankles

AVOID
- A segmental elevation, such as your shoulders rising before hips or vice versa
- Elevating your shoulders toward your ears
- Moving your head forward

STABILIZE BY
- Fixing your shoulders in one position
- Locking your knees
- Keeping your ankles in a fixed position
- Keeping your hips, abdominal muscles, and lower back rigid

Movement Path: Your entire body moves in a single arc with your feet as the fulcrum.

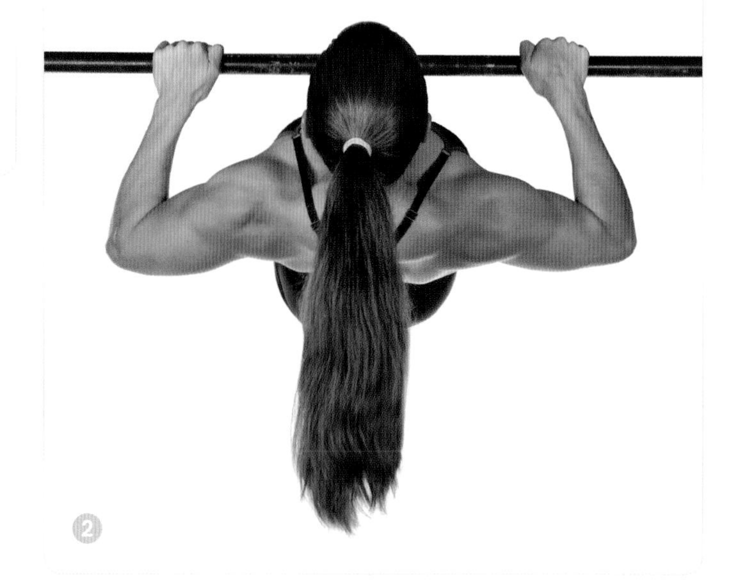

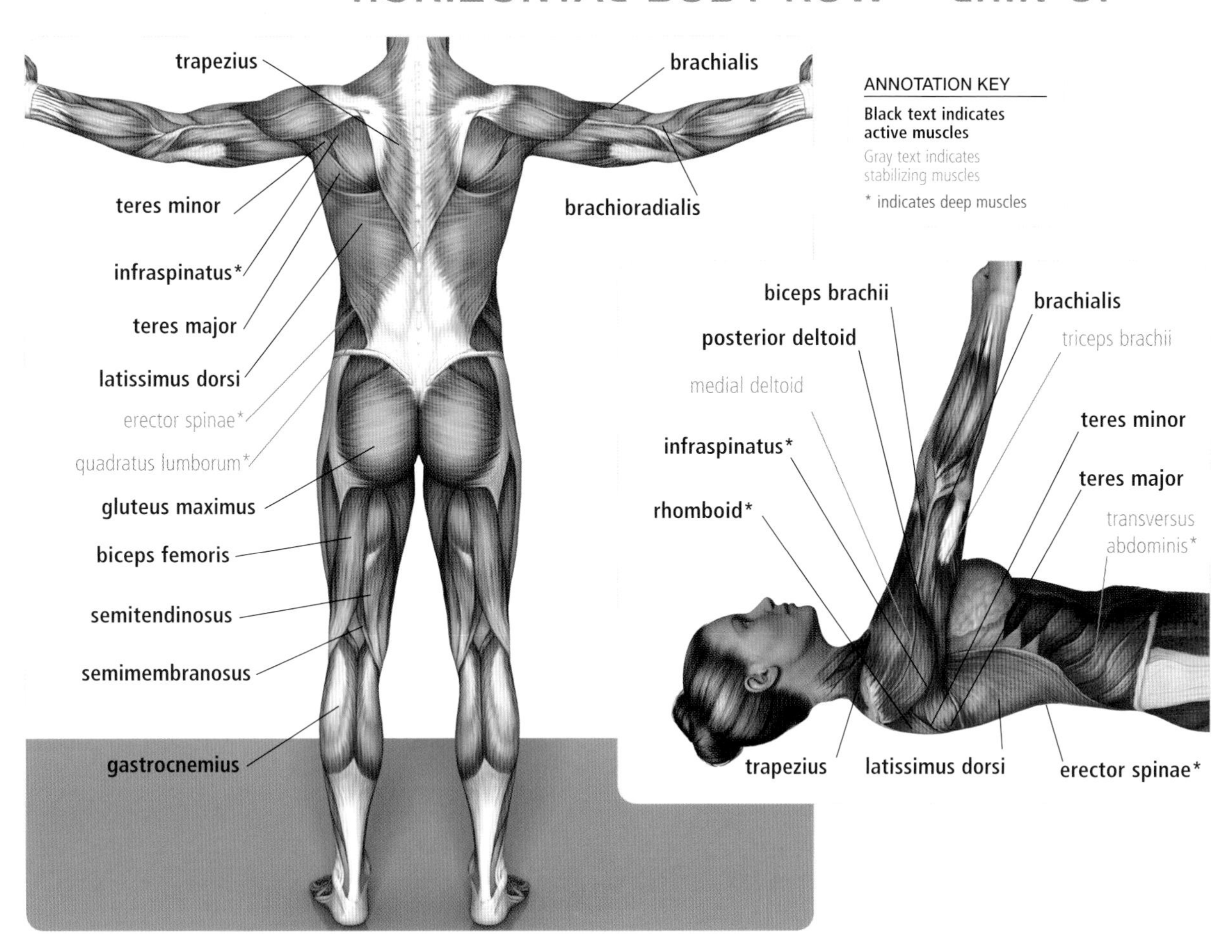

ANNOTATION KEY

Black text indicates active muscles

Gray text indicates stabilizing muscles

* indicates deep muscles

MUSCLES USED

- biceps brachii
- brachialis
- brachioradialis
- infraspinatus
- latissimus dorsi
- rhomboid
- teres major
- teres minor
- trapezius

MODIFICATIONS

More difficult: Put both of your feet on a Swiss ball.

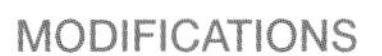

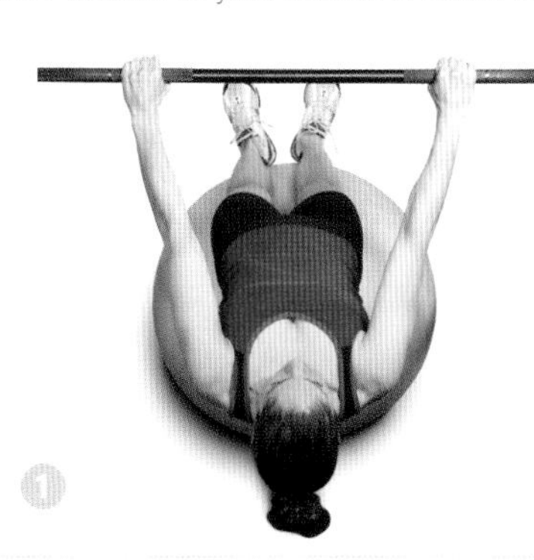

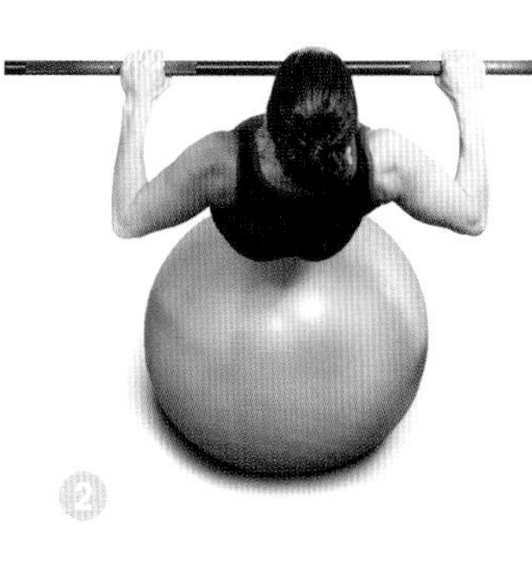

LATERAL ROPE PULL

1

Starting Position: Elevate feet on bench. Lean at an approximately 30-degree angle from the ground, with feet rigid and weight on the edges of the shoes. With the rope at chest height, grasp it across your body with an alternating grip, top hand farthest away, bottom hand closest to you. The body is completely rigid.

Action: Keeping body rigid, pull down and across body keeping the rope adjacent to chest throughout movement.

LOOK FOR
- Feet to work as a fulcrum
- Rope to remain adjacent to chest

AVOID
- Dropping your hips
- Allowing the body to rotate

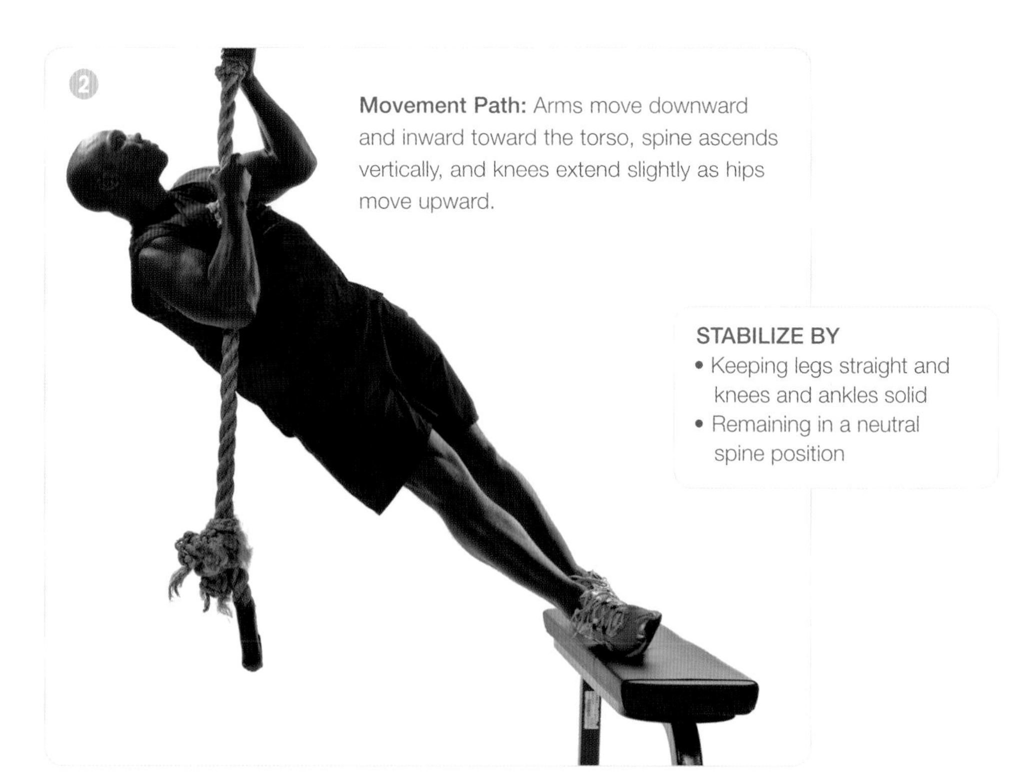

2

Movement Path: Arms move downward and inward toward the torso, spine ascends vertically, and knees extend slightly as hips move upward.

STABILIZE BY
- Keeping legs straight and knees and ankles solid
- Remaining in a neutral spine position

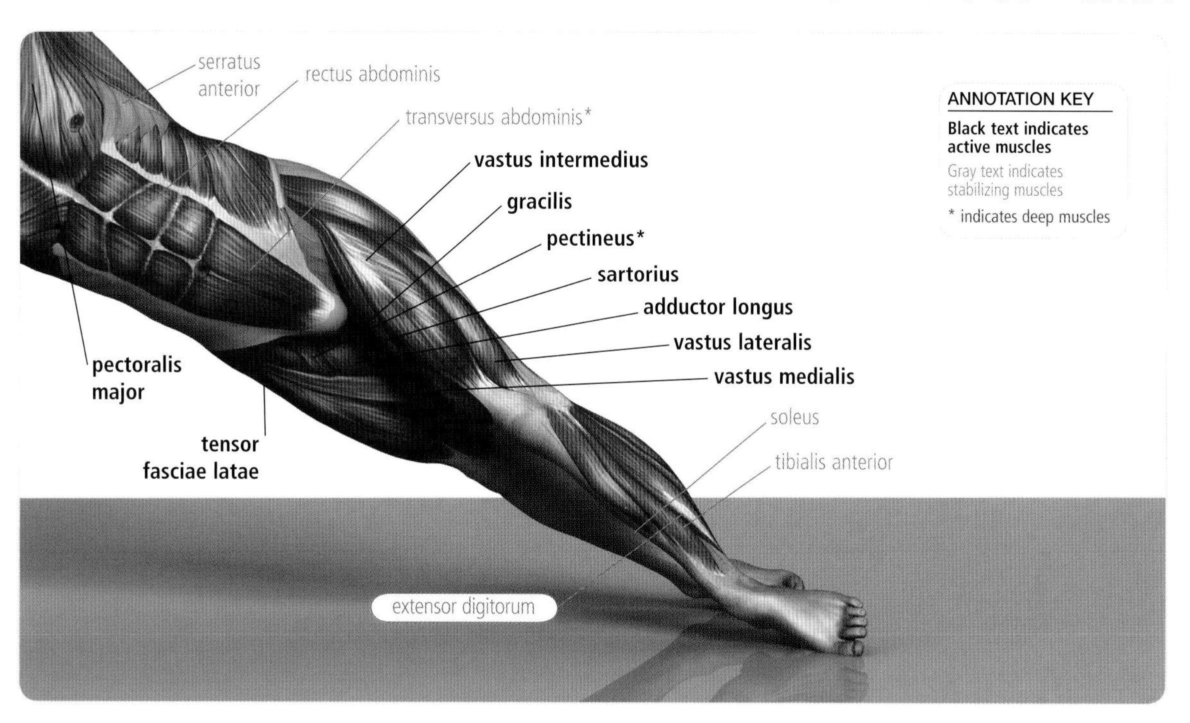

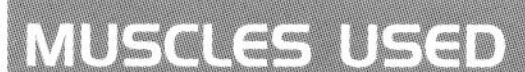

MUSCLES USED

- serratus anterior
- external oblique
- rectus abdominis
- posterior deltoid
- teres major
- teres minor
- supraspinatus
- infraspinatus
- subscapularis
- triceps brachii
- pectoralis major
- pectoralis minor
- latissimus dorsi
- transversus abdominis
- gluteus medius
- piriformis
- obturator externus
- obturator internus
- iliopsoas
- gluteus maximus
- pectineus
- vastus lateralis
- vastus medialis
- vastus intermedius
- rectus femoris
- biceps femoris
- semitendinosus
- semimembranosus
- tensor fasciae latae
- adductor longus
- adductor magnus
- gracilis
- quadratus lumborum
- erector spinae

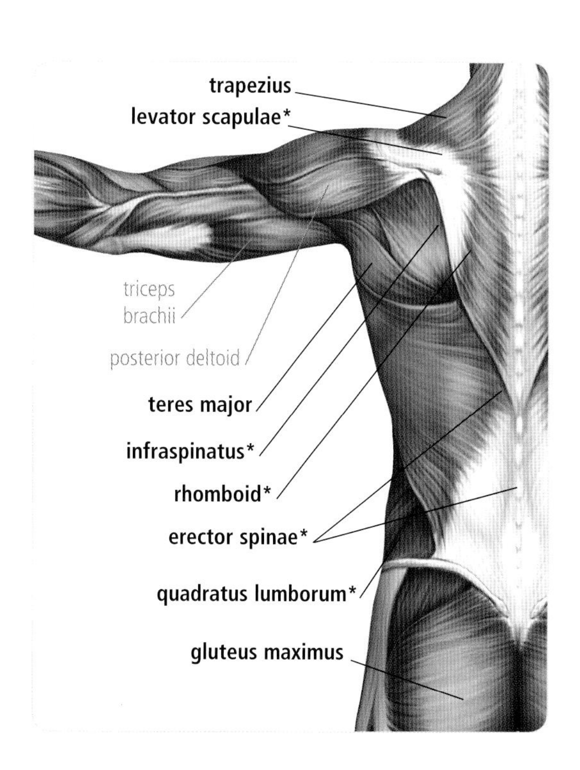

PULL-DOWN NEUTRAL GRIP

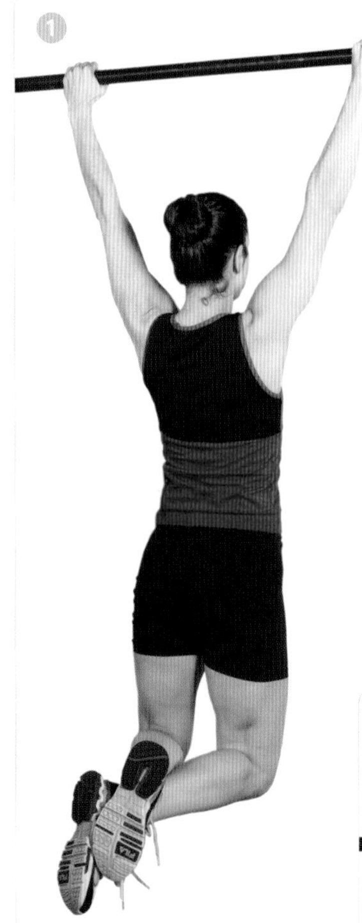

Starting Position: Gripping the bar with your palms out (facing away from your body), hang with your knees bent and your ankles crossed. Keep your head in a neutral alignment. Your hands should be shoulder-width apart.

Action: Pull your body up vertically until your upper chest is aligned with the bar: this is the end of the concentric phase. Lower your body back down to the starting position with your elbows fully extended (the end of the eccentric phase).

LOOK FOR
- Your arms to return to a full extension
- You shoulder blades to draw together and downward at the beginning of the movement

AVOID
- Swinging, jerking, chin "pecking," or hyper-extension of elbows

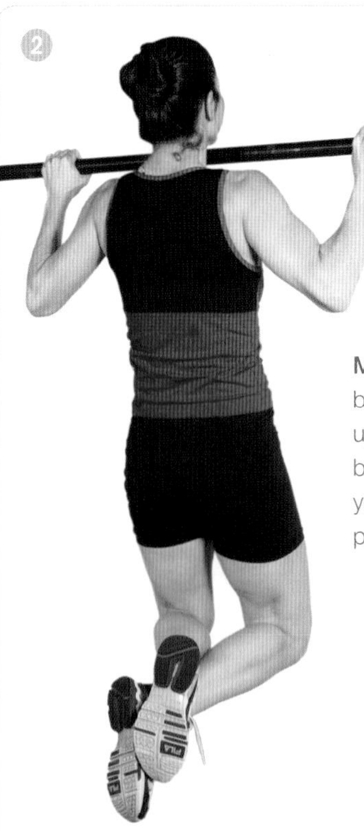

Movement Path: Your body moves vertically up. Your upper body tilts back slightly to allow your chin to smoothly pass the bar line.

STABILIZE BY
- Retracting your scapula
- Keeping your core tight to prevent swinging

PULL-DOWN NEUTRAL GRIP • CHIN-UP

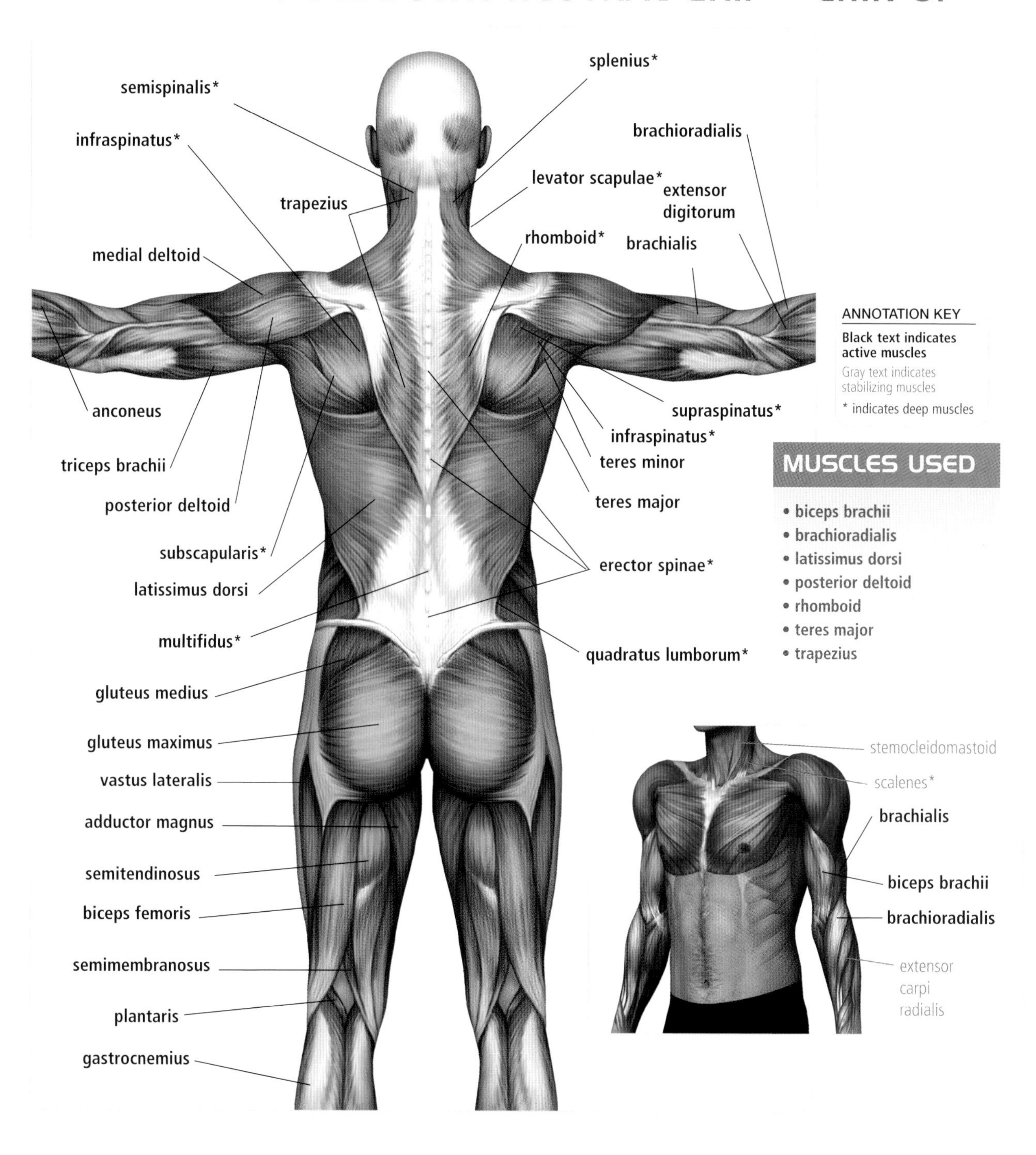

STAND-PULL

Starting Position: In standing position, grasp a bar at collarbone height with palms slightly wider than shoulder-width apart and palms facing away from you. The tops of your shoes should be directly beneath your hands, distributing your weight so that if you were to let go of the bar you would fall backward.

Action: Drop your hips down and backward, bending knees, extending the arms, and keeping spine in a vertical and neutral position until arms are fully extended. Return by simultaneously pulling downward with the elbows and the arms and extending the knees and hips again, keeping the spine vertical and neutral.

Movement Path: Spine travels downward and backward, arms extend upward and forward, hips retract and drop, upper legs move upward toward the torso. Lower legs remain stationary.

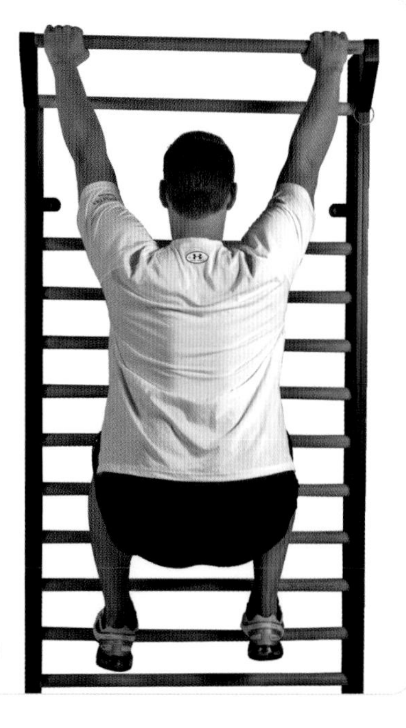

LOOK FOR
- Simultaneous movement of all parts
- Head and spine to remain vertical throughout movement
- Chest to be pulled up and to the bar
- Elbows to remain adjacent to the torso at top position

AVOID
- Allowing the torso to drop forward
- Pulling the elbows backward on the pull-up phase

STABILIZE BY
- Keeping the feet flat and weight evenly distributed
- Keeping the spine solid, rib cage and head up

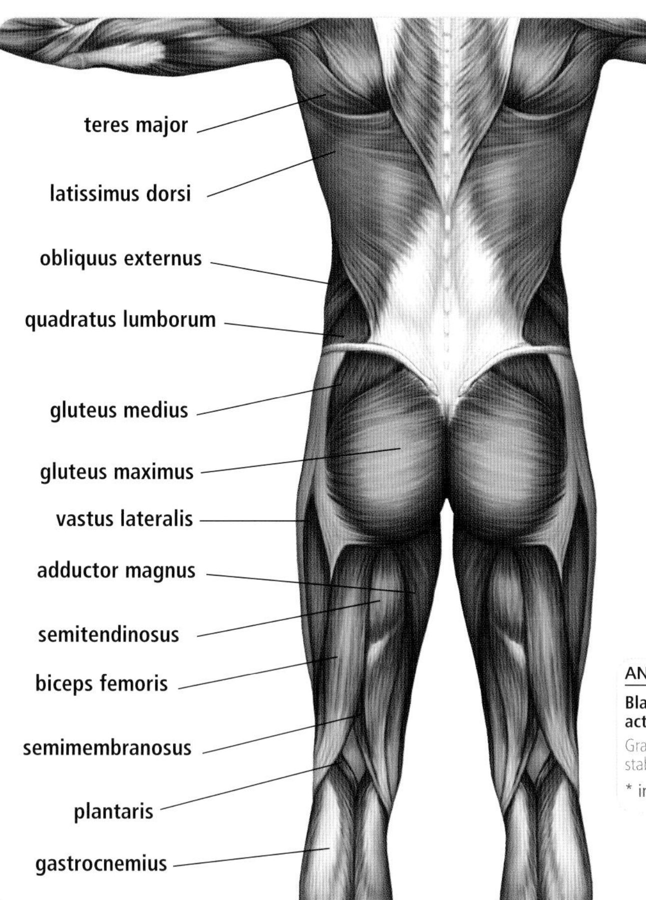

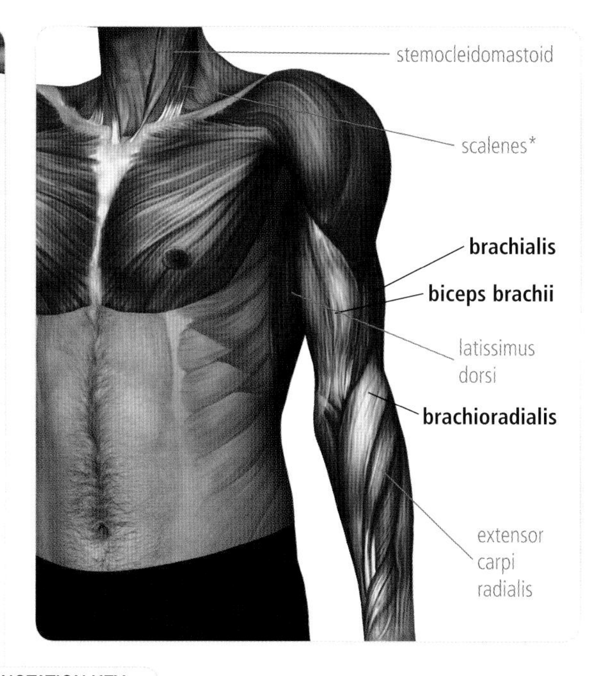

ANNOTATION KEY

Black text indicates active muscles

Gray text indicates stabilizing muscles

* indicates deep muscles

MUSCLES USED

- latissimus dorsi
- rhomboids
- trapezius
- erector spinae
- infraspinatus
- teres major
- teres minor
- posterior deltoid
- brachialis
- biceps brachii
- brachioradialis
- gluteus maximus
- biceps femoris
- semitendinosus
- semimembranosus
- gastrocnemius
- vastus lateralis
- vastus medialis
- vastus intermedius
- rectus femoris
- anterior tibialis
- soleus
- pectoralis major
- pectoralis minor
- coracobrachialis
- extensor carpi radialis
- flexor carpi radialis
- extensor digitorum
- flexor digitorum
- infraspinatus
- supscapularis
- levator scapulae
- medial deltoid
- triceps brachii
- serratus anterior
- transversus abdominis
- quadratus lumborum

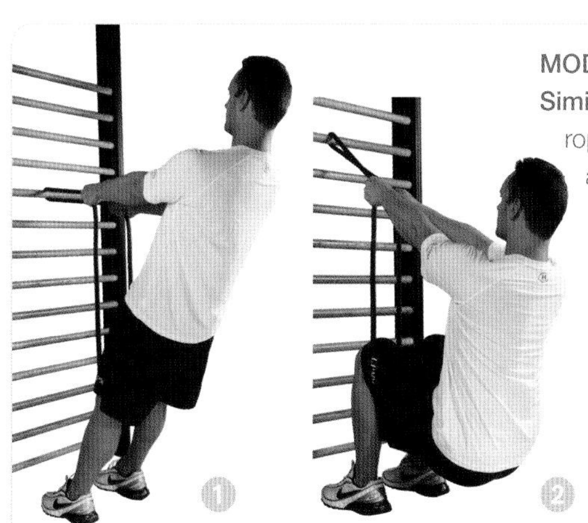

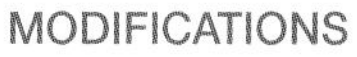

MODIFICATIONS

Similar Difficulty: Grasping a rope at chest height, stand with a slight lean backward. Sit down and backward with the hips, and keep tension on the rope as the arms extend forward and knees bend. Return by pulling upward and extending both knees and hips.

STEP CHIN

STABILIZE BY
- Keeping the chest high and shoulders down
- Keeping the hips and shoulders parallel

Starting Position: Begin with head higher than bar and your palms down, wider than shoulder-width grip. Place one foot on a step with only the ball of the foot bearing weight and the other leg straight and slightly behind the weight-bearing foot.

LOOK FOR
- Non–weight-bearing leg to remain in the same plane as the spine
- All joints to move at the same time

AVOID
- Allowing the shoulder to elevate
- Rotation in the hips
- Allowing the spine to deviate from vertical

Action: Begin by dropping and reaching downward with the free foot. Allow the arms to extend completely and the weight-bearing leg to bend at both hip and knee. During this movement, the non–weight-bearing foot should never touch the ground. Return by pulling the elbows down and pushing through the weight-bearing foot.

Movement Path: The spine travels downward and backward, arms extend upward and forward, hips retract and drop, and upper legs move upward toward the torso. Lower legs remain stationary.

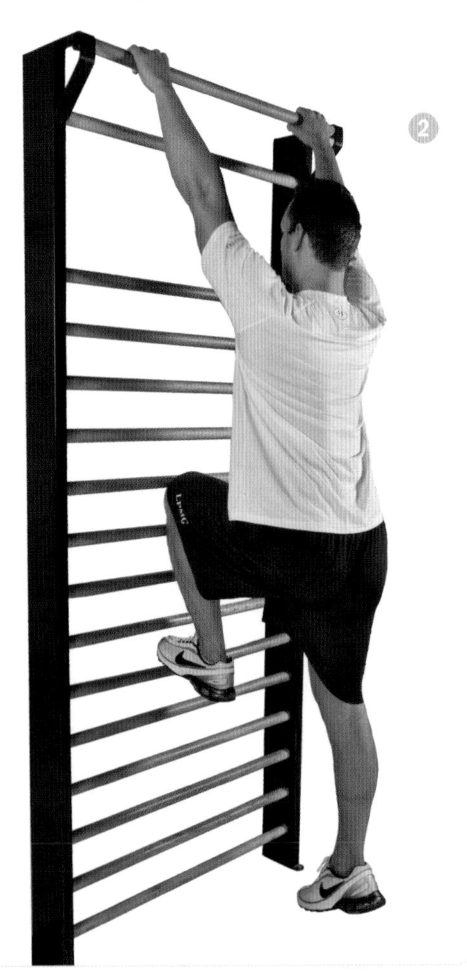

STEP CHIN • CHIN-UP

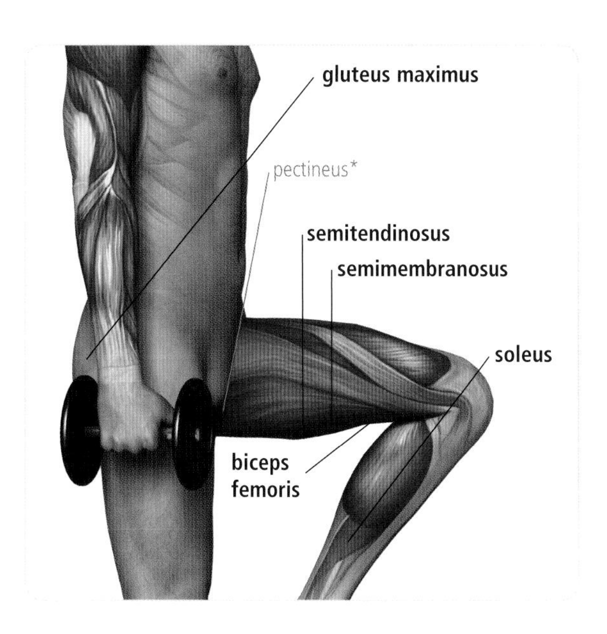

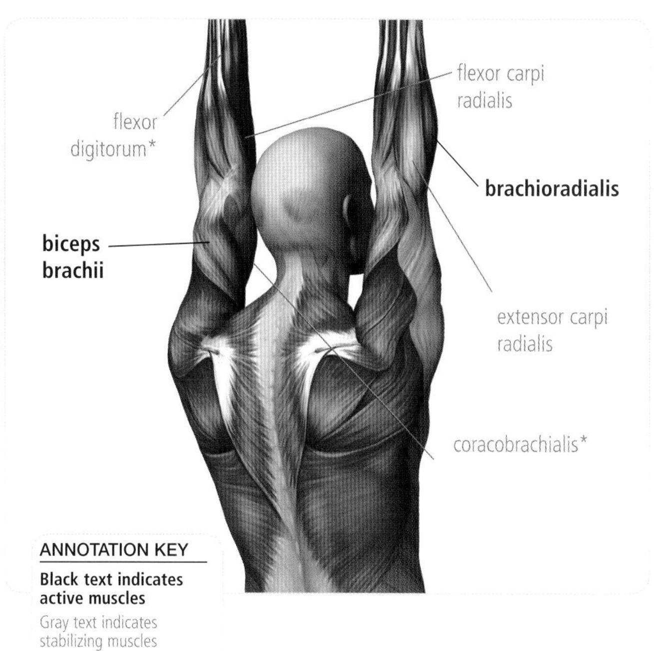

ANNOTATION KEY

Black text indicates active muscles

Gray text indicates stabilizing muscles

* indicates deep muscles

MUSCLES USED

- latissimus dorsi
- rhomboids
- erector spinae
- infraspinatus
- trapezius
- teres major
- teres minor
- posterior deltoid
- brachialis
- biceps brachii
- brachioradialis
- gluteus maximus
- biceps femoris
- semitendinosus
- semimembranosus
- gastrocnemius
- vastus lateralis
- vastus medialis
- vastus intermedius
- rectus femoris
- tibialis anterior
- biceps femoris
- semitendinosus
- semimembranosus
- soleus
- pectoralis major
- pectoralis minor
- coracobrachialis
- extensor carpi radialis
- flexor carpi radialis
- extensor digitorum
- flexor digitorum
- infraspinatus
- supscapularis
- levator scapulae
- medial deltoid
- triceps brachii
- serratus anterior
- transversus abdominis
- erector spinae
- quadratus lumborum

MODIFICATIONS

Similar Difficulty: Stand with feet directly under bar and slightly wider than hip-width. Grasp the bar at neck height with one hand slightly narrower than shoulder-width. Grasp a dumbbell with the other hand, the arm extended and relaxed adjacent to the hip.

Drop the hips downward and backward in a controlled manner, allowing the arm grasping the bar to extend fully while bending the knees and hips. Return by simultaneously pulling and standing, keeping the spine vertical and dumbbell arm straight and adjacent to the side.

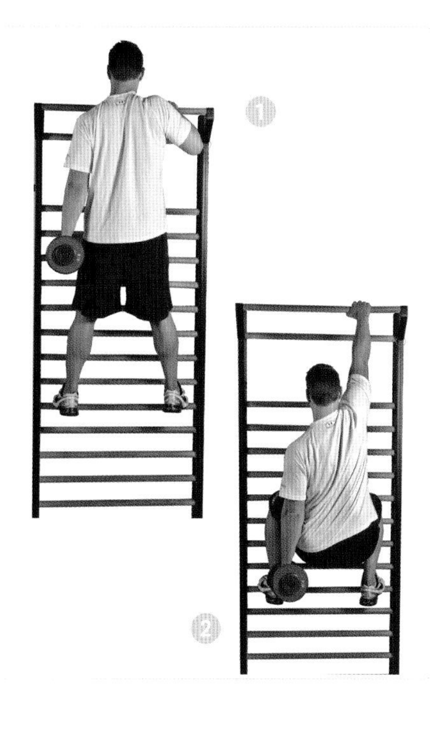

VERTICAL ROPE WITH ALTERNATE GRIP

1

Starting Position: Standing with a rope directly in front of you, grasp it with an alternating grip, one hand in front of your chin, and the other slightly above your head. Step forward so that the rope hangs to one hip, and place your heels on a bench. Knees and hips should be bent to 90-degree angles, and the chest should be slightly behind the rope, with arms extended.

Action: Pull down on the rope while simultaneously pushing down on your heels. Be sure to keep the knees bent and torso upright throughout the movement.

2

Movement Path: Arms move downward and inward toward the torso, spine ascends vertically, knees extend slightly as hips move upward.

LOOK FOR
- Hips to remain adjacent to rope
- Spinal position to remain consistent

AVOID
- Extending the knees excessively
- Allowing the torso to rotate

STABILIZE BY
- Pulling evenly with both arms
- Pushing evenly with both feet
- Keeping chest and head up

MODIFICATIONS
Similar Difficulty: Start seated on the ground with feet on floor, knees bent. Follow same action and movement path.

VERTICAL ROPE WITH ALTERNATE GRIP • CHIN-UP

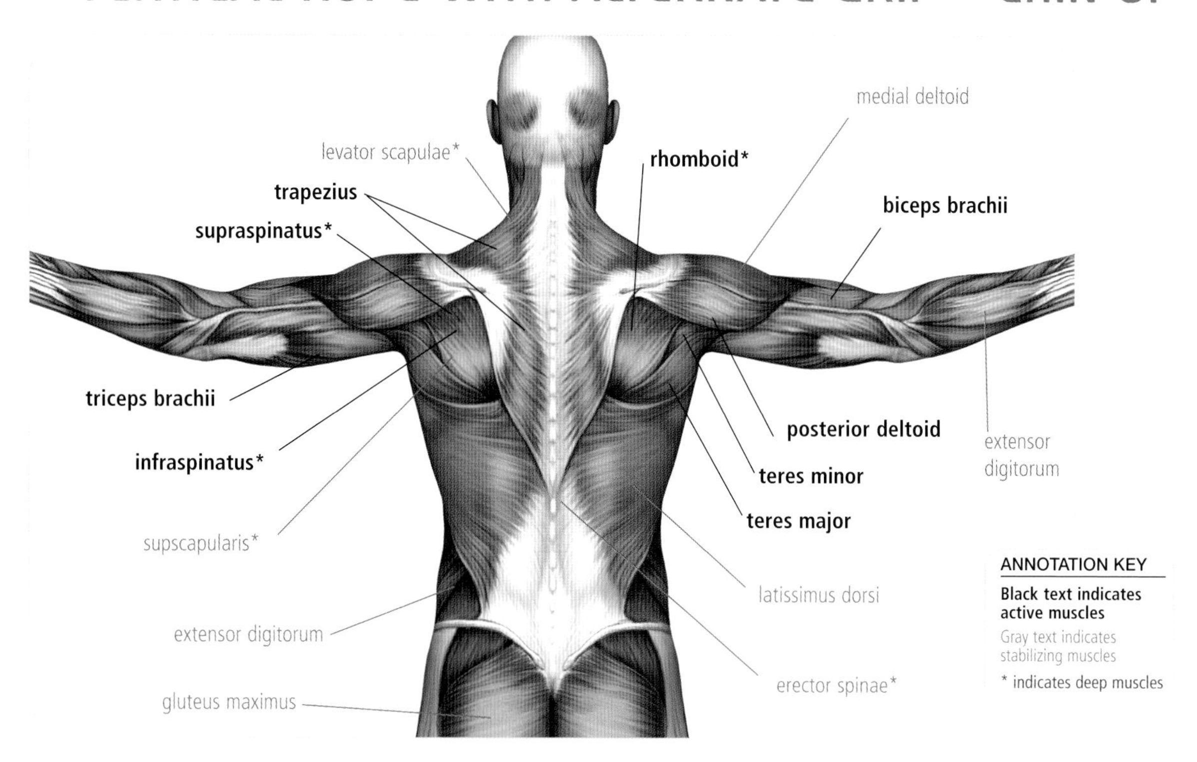

ANNOTATION KEY

Black text indicates active muscles

Gray text indicates stabilizing muscles

* indicates deep muscles

MUSCLES USED

- biceps brachii
- brachioradialis
- latissimus dorsi
- posterior deltoid
- rhomboid
- teres major
- trapezius
- biceps femoris
- gastrocnemius
- semimembranosus
- semitendinosus
- pronator teres
- flexor carpi radialis
- flexor digitorum
- pectoralis minor
- deltoideus
- triceps brachii
- brachialis
- flexor carpi ulnaris
- palmaris longus
- flexor carpi pollicis longus

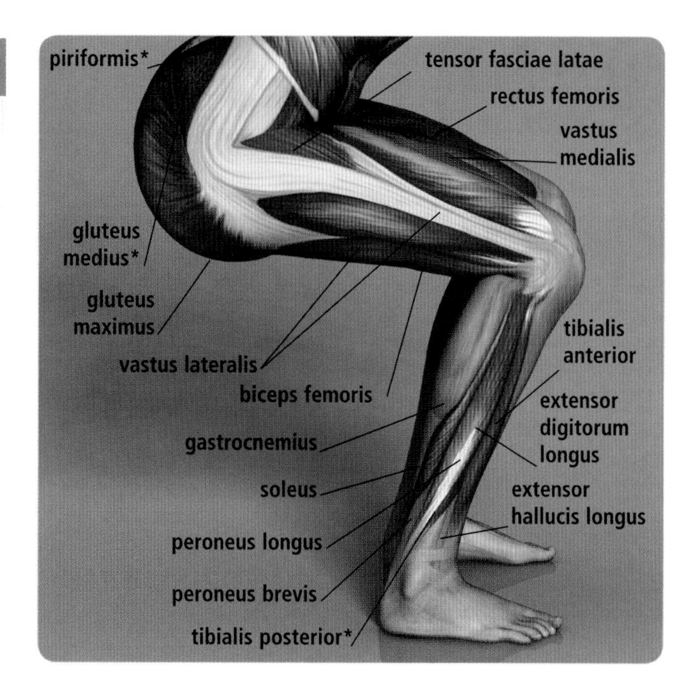

DROP & PULL

Starting Position: Grasp a rope with alternating grips, one hand in front of your face and the other your chest. Your body should be at an approximately 45-degree angle leaning on the rope in front of you.

STABILIZE BY
- Keeping legs, hips, and spine rigid
- Keeping weight on the edge of the shoe as the body rotates

LOOK FOR
- All body parts to move at once
- Feet to be involved in movement

AVOID
- Allowing hips to sag
- Segmental movement of knees, hips, and spine

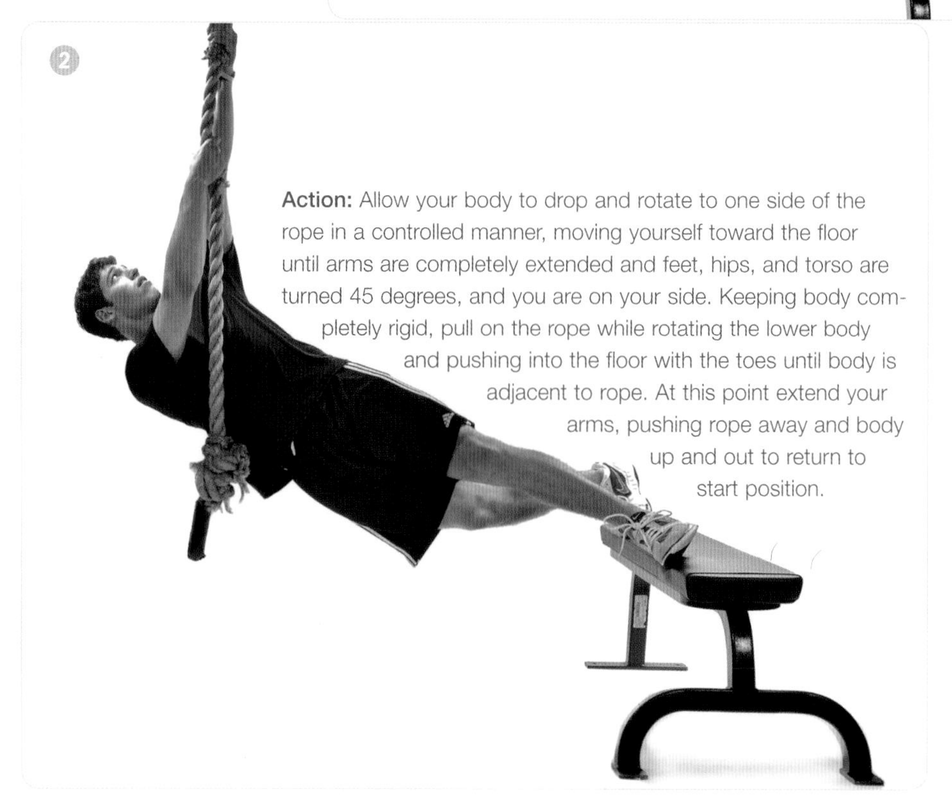

Action: Allow your body to drop and rotate to one side of the rope in a controlled manner, moving yourself toward the floor until arms are completely extended and feet, hips, and torso are turned 45 degrees, and you are on your side. Keeping body completely rigid, pull on the rope while rotating the lower body and pushing into the floor with the toes until body is adjacent to rope. At this point extend your arms, pushing rope away and body up and out to return to start position.

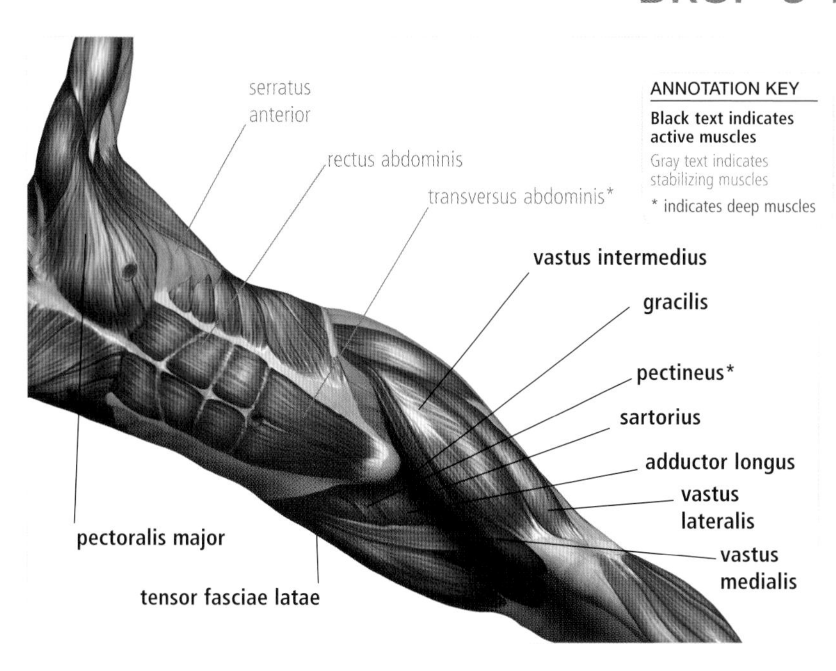

MUSCLES USED

- serratus anterior
- external oblique
- rectus abdominis
- posterior deltoid
- teres major
- teres minor
- supraspinatus
- infraspinatus
- subscapularis
- triceps brachii
- pectoralis major
- pectoralis minor
- latissimus dorsi
- transversus abdominis
- gluteus medius
- piriformis
- obturator externus
- obturator internus
- iliopsoas
- gluteus maximus
- pectineus
- vastus lateralis
- vastus medialis
- vastus intermedius
- rectus femoris
- biceps femoris
- semitendinosus
- semimembranosus
- tensor fasciae latae
- adductor longus
- adductor magnus
- gracilis
- quadratus lumborum
- erector spinae

Movement Path: Torso moves downward and rotates. Arms move toward and then away and across torso.

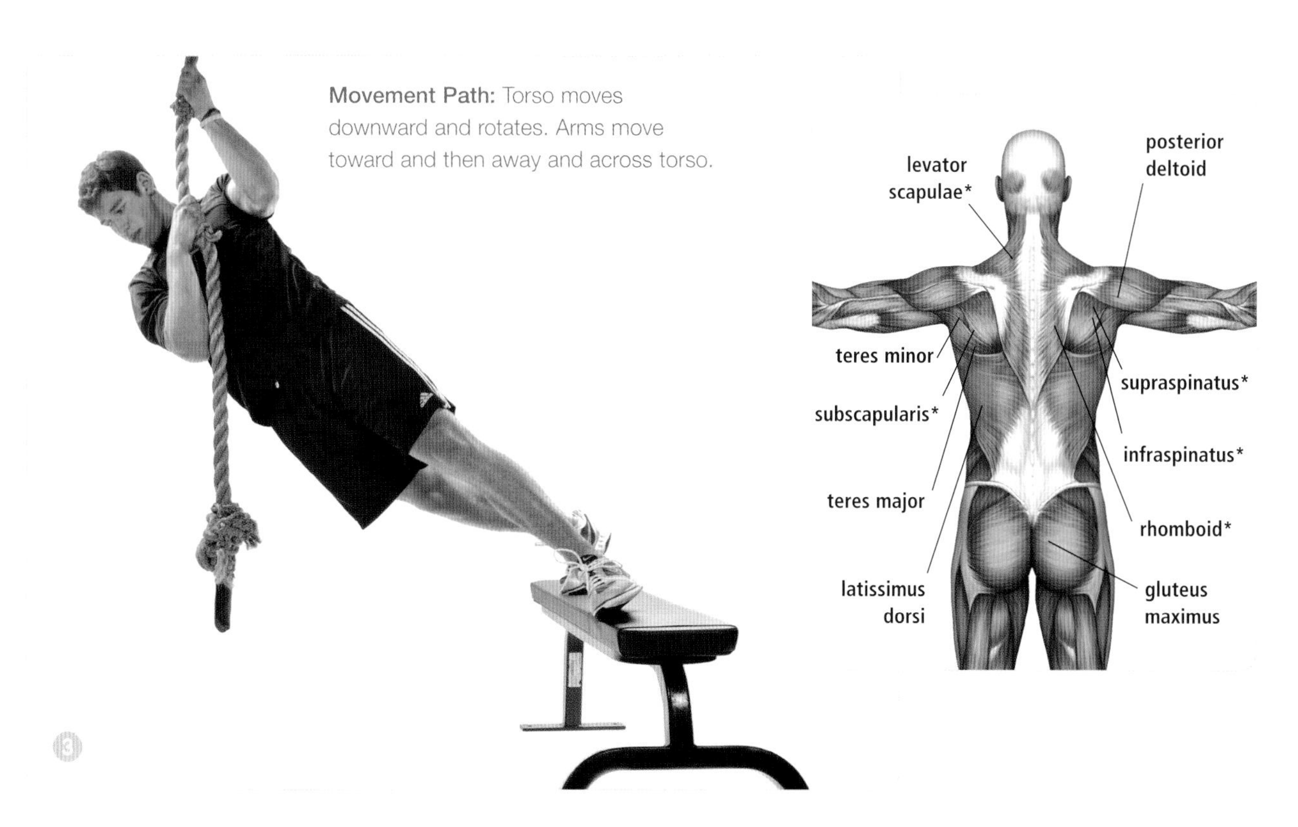

ROPE CHINS

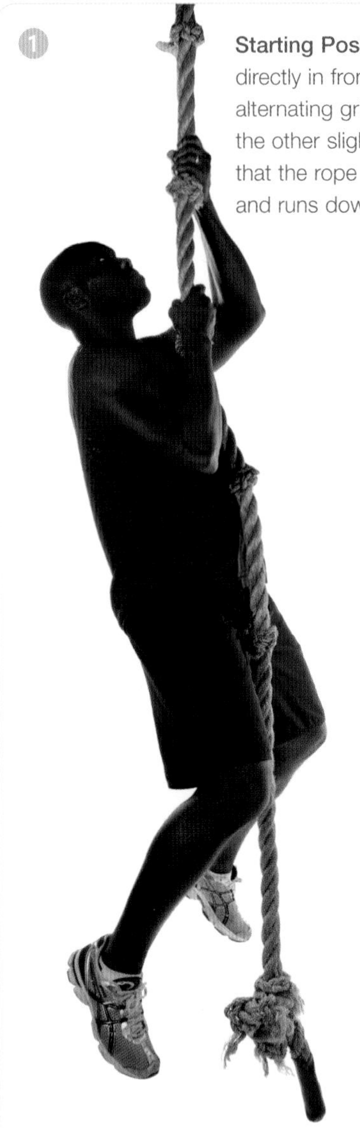

1

Starting Position: Standing on tiptoes with a rope directly in front of you, grasp the rope with an alternating grip, one arm completely extended, and the other slightly above your head. Step forward so that the rope hangs directly adjacent to your chest and runs down the middle of your body.

2

Action: Bend knees slightly and remove body weight from floor so that you are hanging onto the rope with only your hands. Pull down on the rope until your chin rises above your bottom hand. Be sure to keep the knees bent and torso upright throughout the movement. Let yourself down slowly and repeat.

Movement Path: Arms move downward and inward toward the torso, spine ascends vertically, knees remain slightly bent.

LOOK FOR
- Hips and chest to remain adjacent to rope
- Spinal position to remain consistent

AVOID
- Allowing the torso to rotate

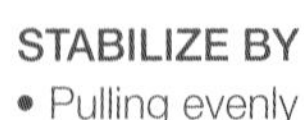
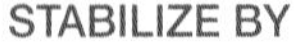

STABILIZE BY
- Pulling evenly with both arms
- Keeping chest and head up

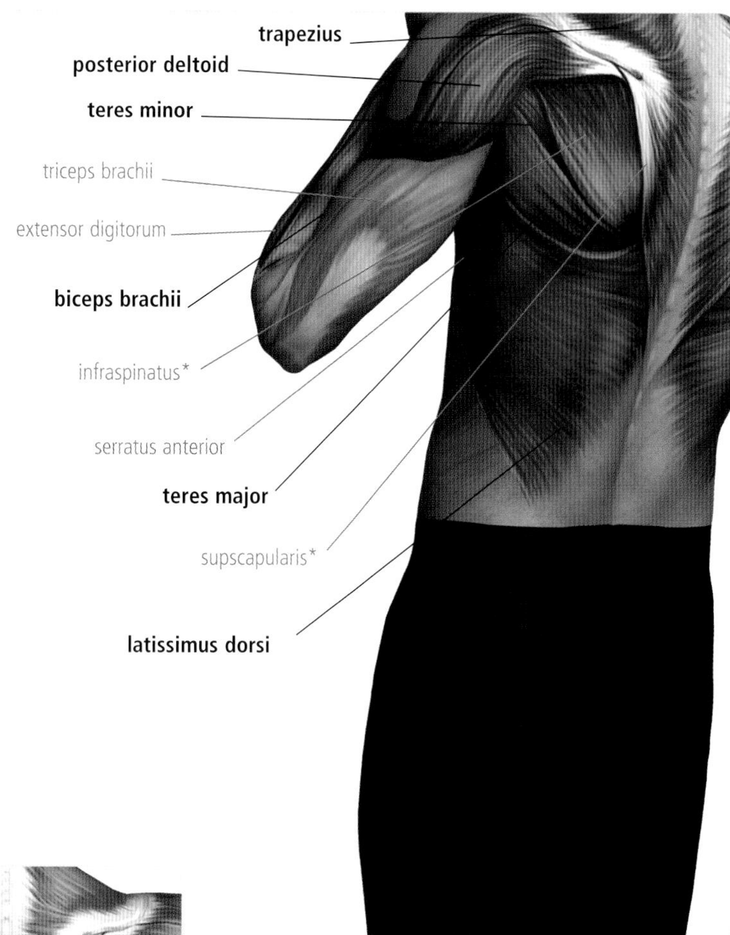

ANNOTATION KEY

Black text indicates active muscles

Gray text indicates stabilizing muscles

* indicates deep muscles

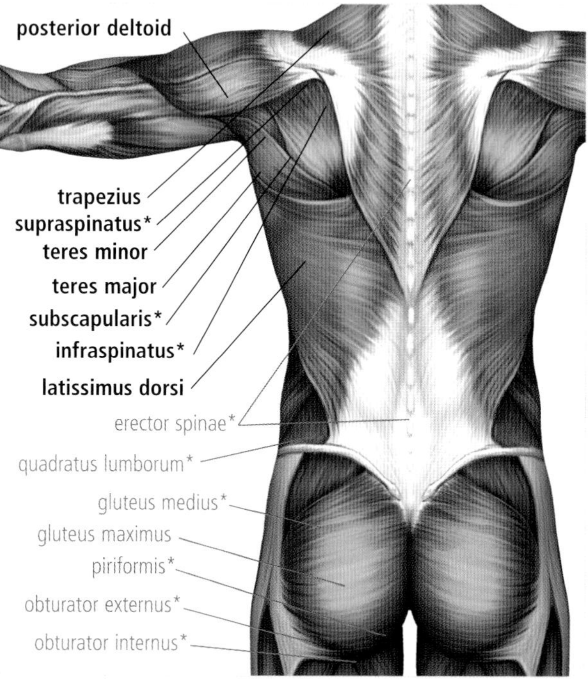

MUSCLES USED

- **biceps brachii**
- **brachioradialis**
- **latissimus dorsi**
- **posterior deltoid**
- **rhomboid**
- **teres major**
- **trapezius**
- biceps femoris
- gastrocnemius
- semimembranosus
- semitendinosus
- pronator teres
- flexor carpi radialis
- flexor digitorum
- pectoralis minor
- deltoideus
- triceps brachii
- brachialis
- flexor carpi ulnaris
- palmaris longus
- flexor carpi pollicis longus

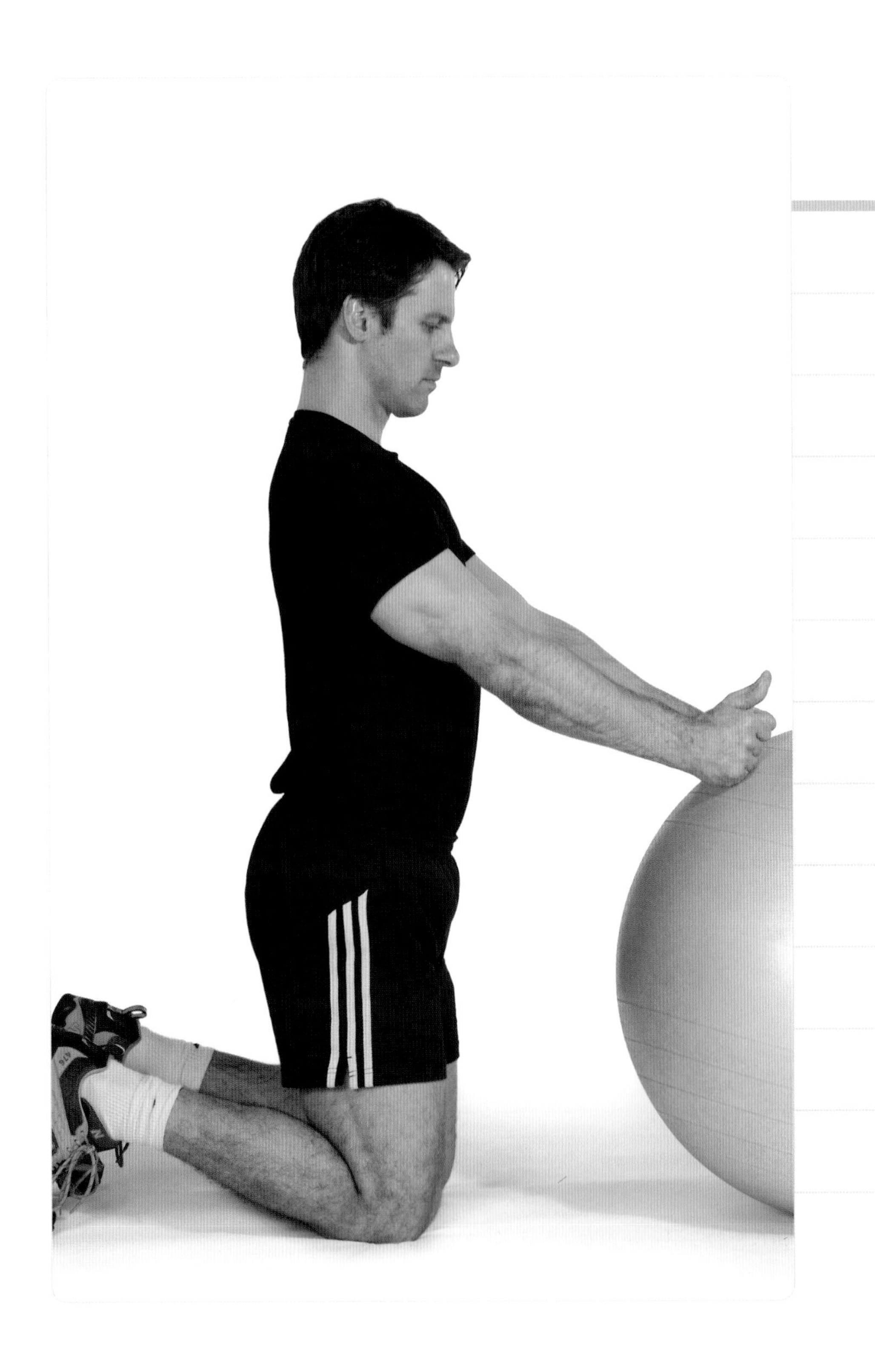

AB WHEEL

I chose this type of abdominal exercise for a very specific reason. Abdominals are the muscles that get the most amount of attention paid to them with the least amount of result. I have seen literally thousands of people perform hundreds of thousands of ab reps with very little to show for it, other than sore necks and sore backs.

The ab wheel, and variations I've chosen, generally involve a lot of muscle and, as far as bang for the buck, are without question the most effective movements I've seen. They produce results.

Joints involved are hip, shoulder, and knee. The primary muscles used are abdominals, obliques, and hip flexors. Muscles of the back and chest are all involved.

The primary benefit of this exercise is stomach and hip strength and flexibility, low-back flexibility, and spinal and shoulder stability.

AB WHEEL

Starting Position: On your knees, bend your torso forward at a 45 degree angle, with your spine in a neutral position. Extend your arms forward at a 45- to 90-degree angle to your torso, with your elbows straight and your hands grasping the wheel.

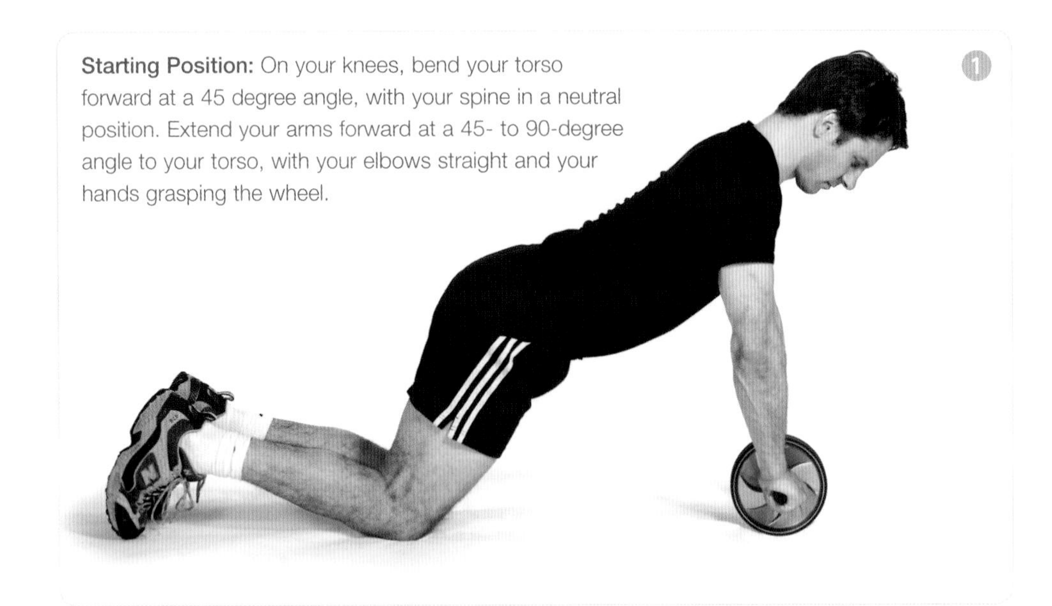

LOOK FOR
- All joints to move at the same time
- Your head and spine to remain aligned

AVOID
- Rounding or arching your spine
- Allowing your joints to move sequentially
- Moving quickly in either direction

Action: Inhale and extend your arms forward, allowing your torso to drop until your chest is almost parallel to the floor, rolling the wheel in a straight line away from you. Your hips move forward, following your torso, but your knees remain stationary. Exhale, and draw your arms and hips back simultaneously; your torso elevates and returns to the starting position.

Movement Path: Your center of mass is translated forward and downward as your arms and hips extend into a linear position, with your knees as the fulcrum.

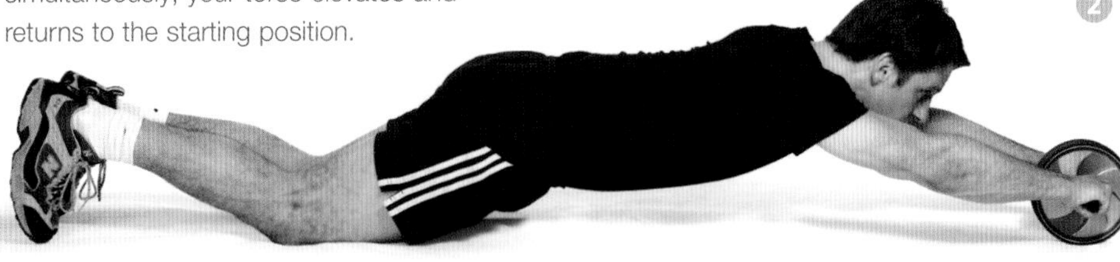

STABILIZE BY
- Pulling your abdomen up and in
- Keeping your shoulders down and back throughout the movement
- Keeping your arms extended and your wrists solid
- Maintaining a neutral spinal position throughout the movement

AB WHEEL • AB WHEEL

MUSCLES USED

- iliacus
- iliopsoas
- latissimus dorsi
- obliquus externus
- obliquus internus
- pectoralis major
- rectus abdominis
- rectus femoris
- serratus anterior
- teres major
- triceps brachii

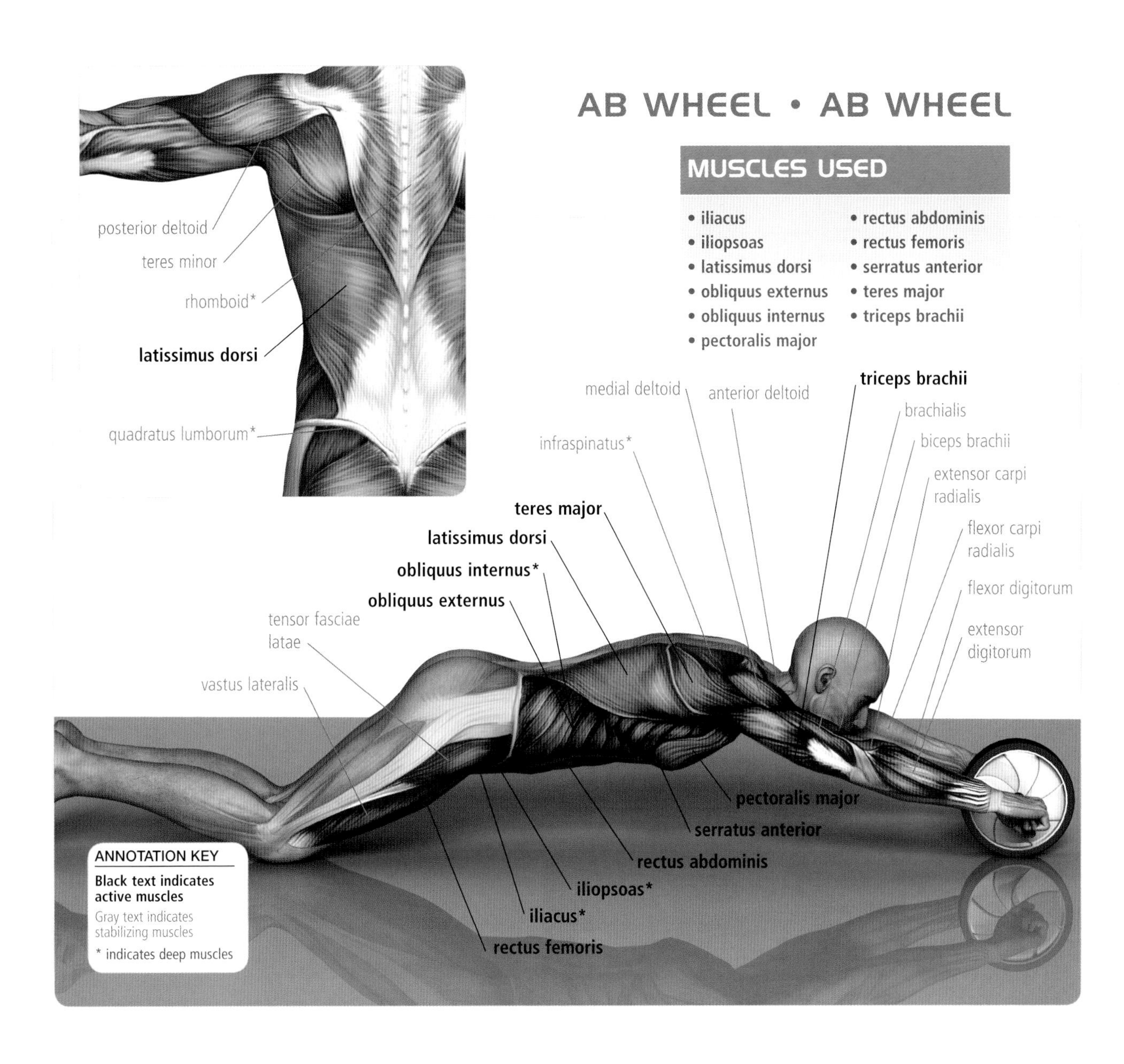

MODIFICATIONS
Similar Difficulty: Replace the wheel with a Swiss ball; your hands begin higher up.

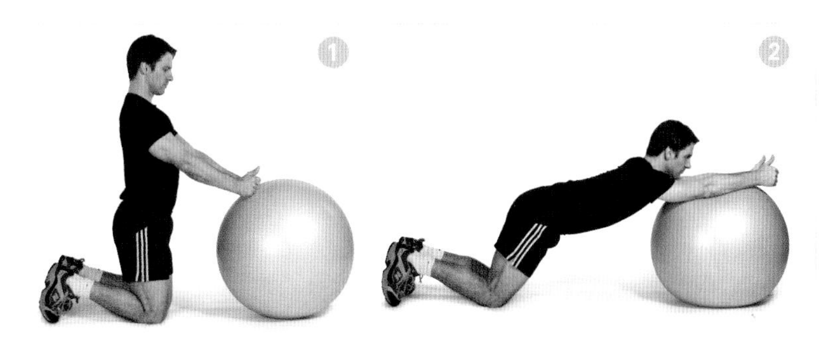

PLOUGH ON PHYSIO BALL

Starting Position: Place your hands on the ground, with your legs extended so that the tops of your shoes are on top of a physio ball in a push-up position. Keep your spine neutral.

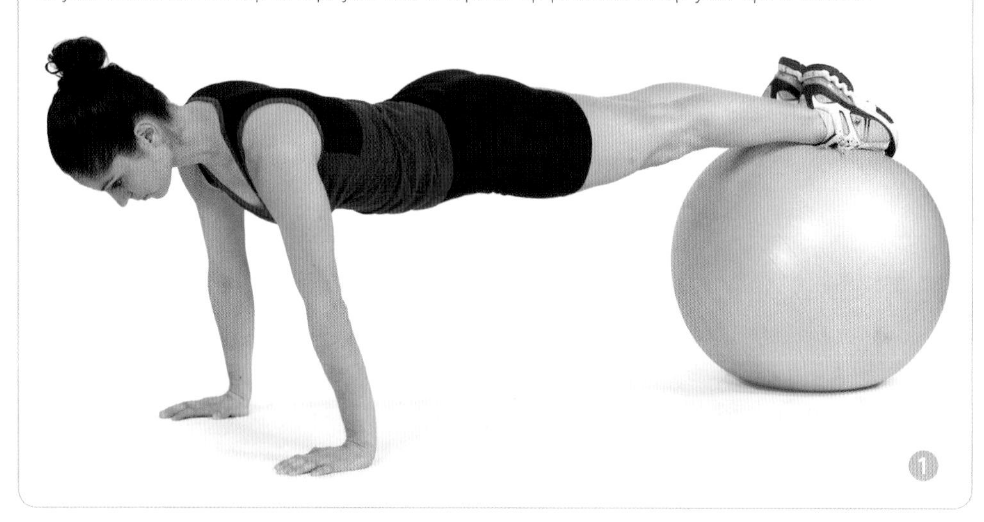

1

LOOK FOR
- A simultaneous movement while your hips raise, so that your spine is at a 45-degree angle from your hip to your shoulder from the ground

AVOID
- Dropping your knees toward the floor
- Bending your elbows
- Allowing your shoulders to either elevate toward your ears or round forward

Action: Pull your knees up toward your chest while flexing your feet, balancing your toes on the ball, driving your hips toward the ceiling, and retracting your abdomen.

Movement Path: Your torso flexes in a straight line and a single plane. Your feet move up toward your midline in a horizontal plane.

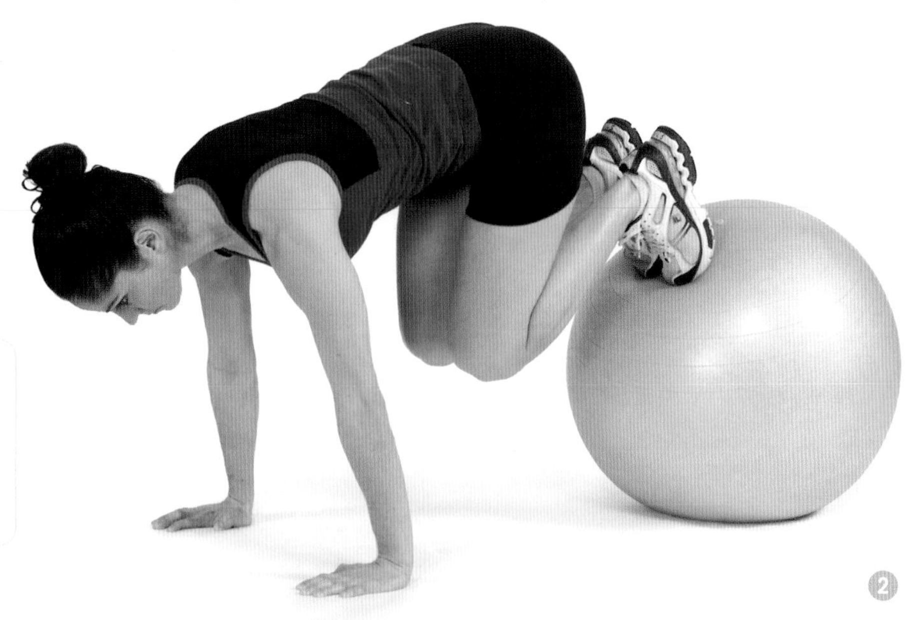

2

STABILIZE BY
- Keeping your chest high and contracted
- Elongating your neck and extending your elbows throughout the movement

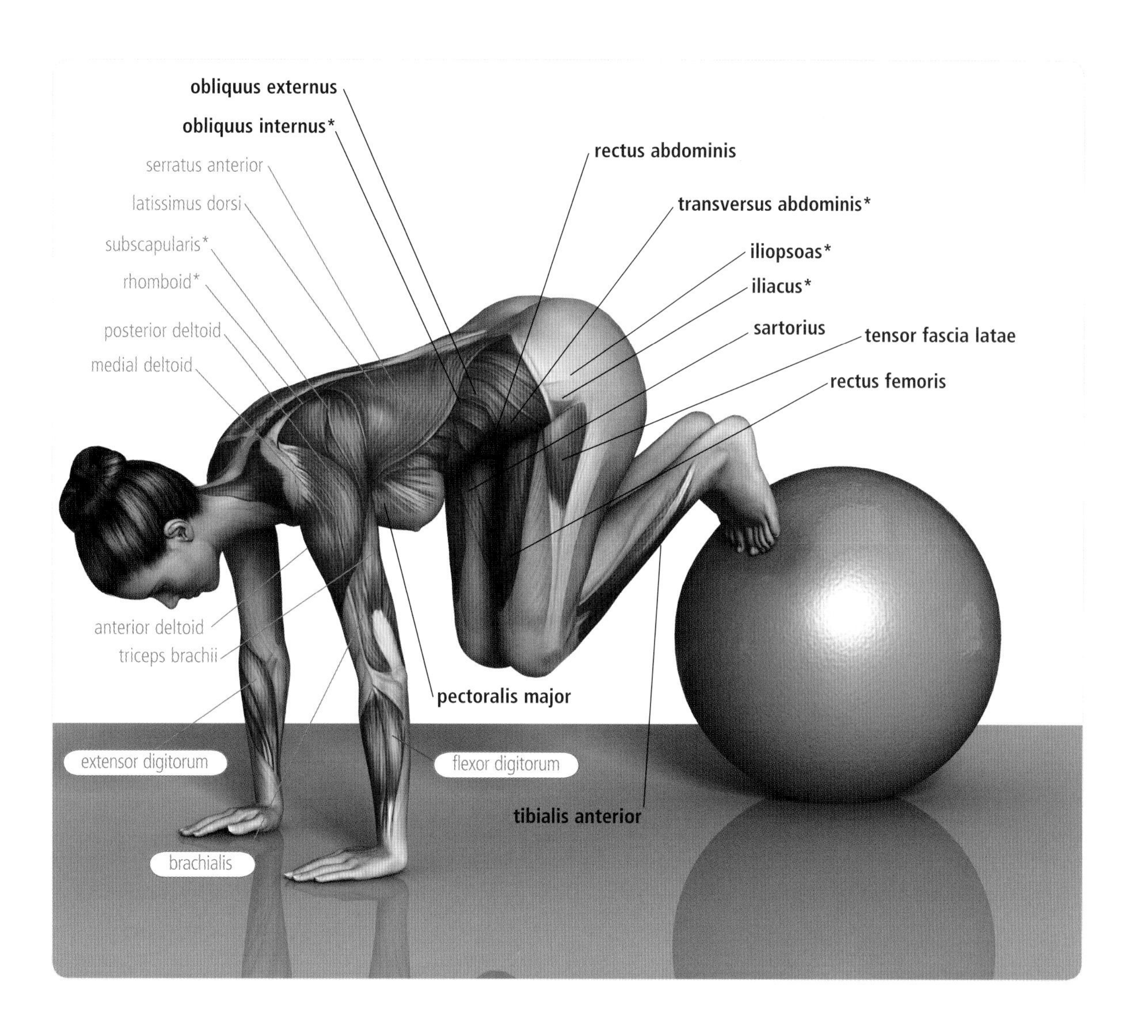

ANNOTATION KEY

Black text indicates active muscles

Gray text indicates stabilizing muscles

* indicates deep muscles

MUSCLES USED

- iliacus
- iliopsoas
- obliquus externus
- obliquus internus
- rectus abdominis
- sartorius
- tibialis anterior
- transversus abdominis

PLOUGH WITH ROTATION

1 **Starting Position:** Assume the top of a push-up position with hands slightly wider than shoulder-width with feet on one towel (or a small physio ball).

Action: Keeping shoulder girdle solid, draw both knees upward while simultaneously rotating the hips and lower body until ankle is rotated 90 degrees and both feet are on edge and pointing to one side. Extend knees and hips, and rotate back to starting position. Repeat on other side.

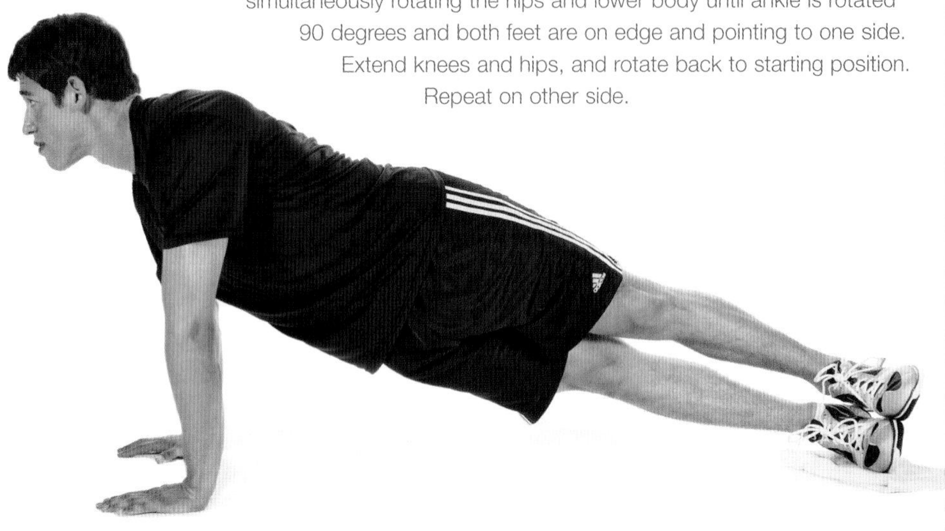

Movement Path: Torso remains stationary, while hips and knees flex and rotate.

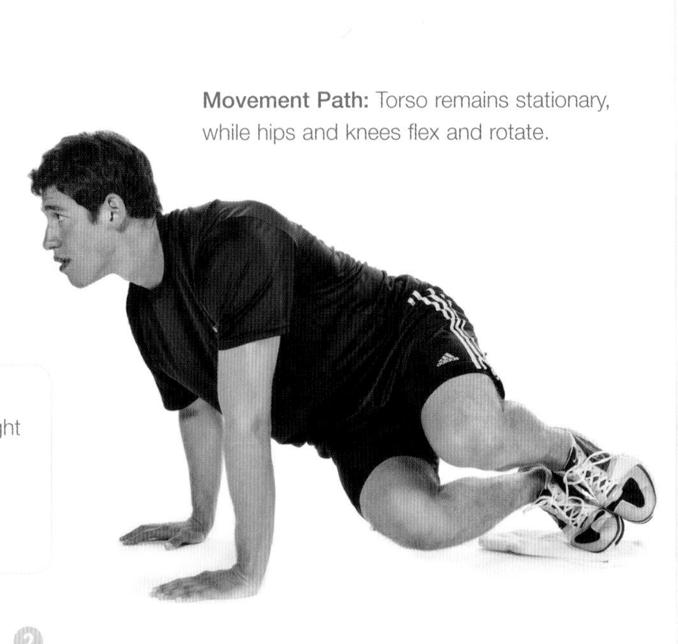

2

LOOK FOR
- A smooth and even movement
- Hips to remain at same height throughout the movement
- Feet to be solid and weight bearing on edge of shoe
- Knees to remain parallel

AVOID
- Allowing back to either arch or sag
- Shoulders to remain motionless
- Separating either knees or feet

STABILIZE BY
- Keeping elbows straight
- Keeping spine high
- Allowing weight to be evenly distributed on support

PLOUGH WITH ROTATION • AB WHEEL

MUSCLES USED

- rectus abdominis
- internal oblique
- external oblique
- transversus abdominis
- rectus femoris
- tibialis anterior
- sartorius
- iliopsoas
- iliacus
- triceps brachii
- anterior deltoid
- medial deltoid
- posterior deltoid
- rhomboids
- subscapularis
- latissimus dorsi
- pectoralis major

ANNOTATION KEY

Black text indicates active muscles

Gray text indicates stabilizing muscles

* indicates deep muscles

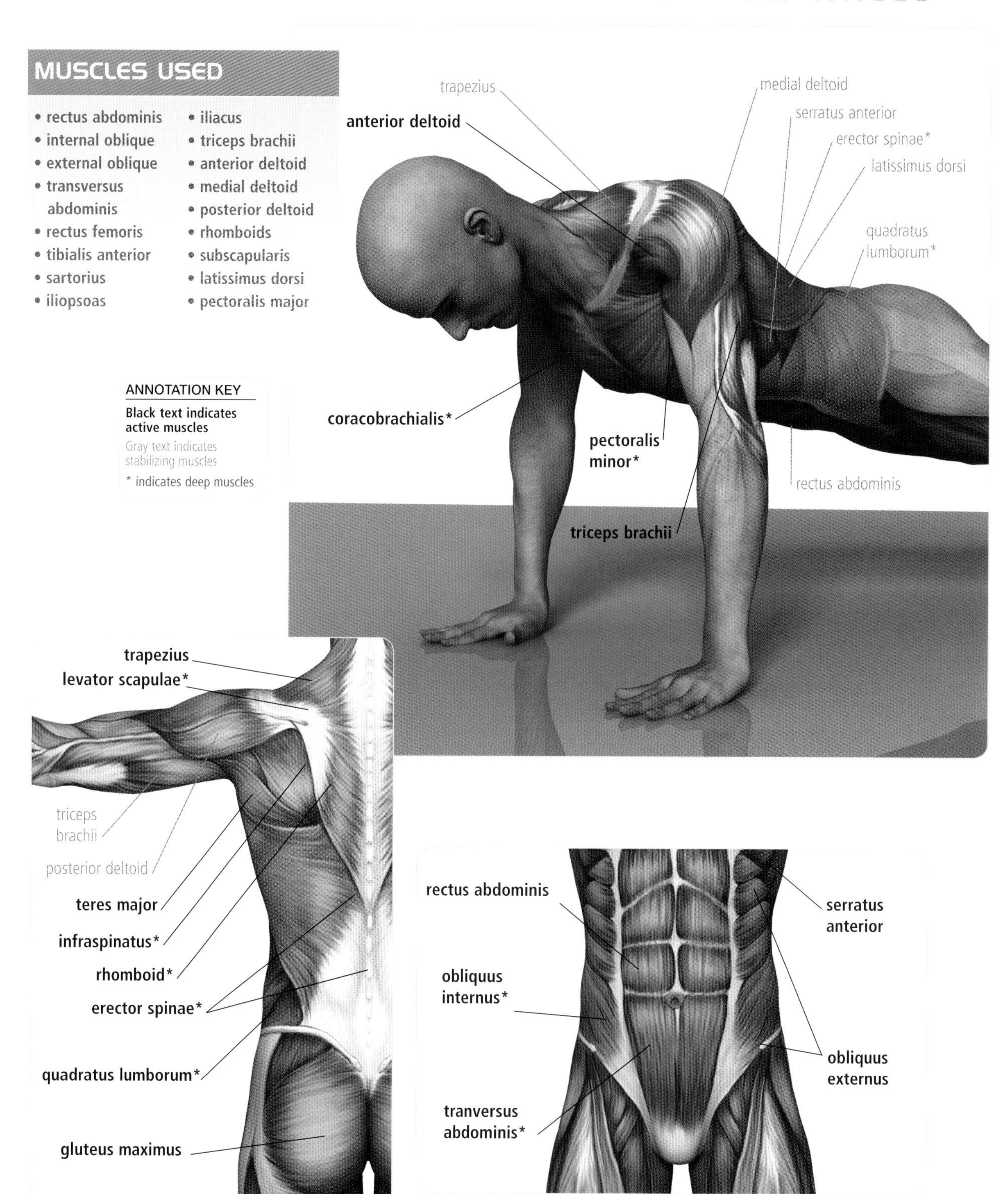

STRAIGHT-LEG HKR

Starting Position: Grab a bar with palms facing forward and preferably with back against a wall. Feet should not be contacting the ground.

Action: Pulling on the bar so that the shoulders are down and away from ears, keep legs straight (knees and ankles taut). Kick forward, bringing both legs up to horizontal, keeping low back flat, and exhaling. Slowly allow legs to drop in a controlled manner until they are directly beneath you.

Movement Path: Torso remains motionless and lower body flexes and moves upward and forward in a curvilinear fashion to 90 degrees at hip joint.

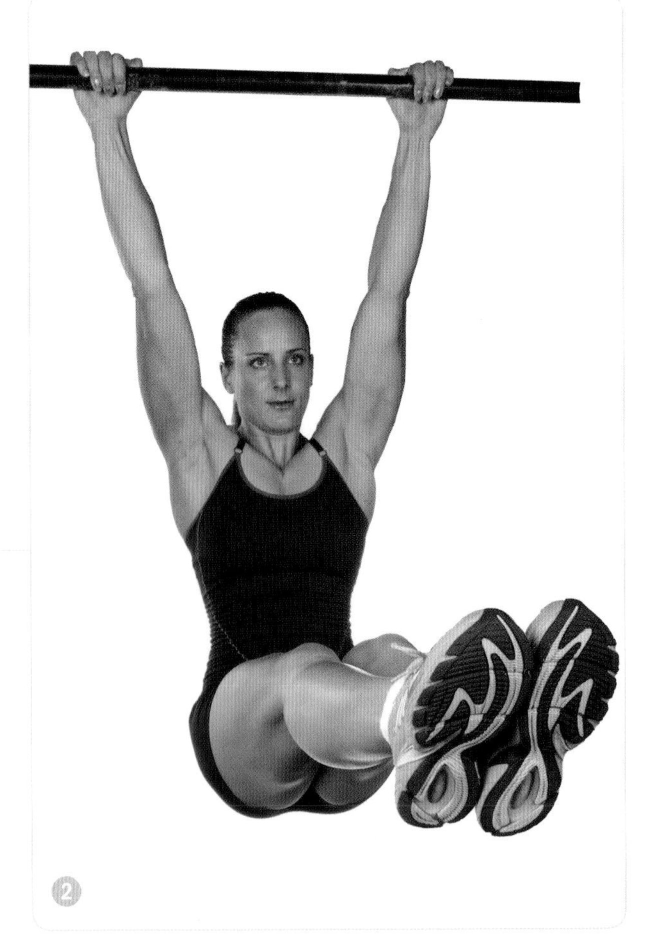

LOOK FOR
- Legs to move in a controlled manner
- A 90-degree angle in torso/hip
- Shoulders to remain down

AVOID
- Swinging and creating momentum
- Allowing hips to roll upward and forward
- Arching the back

STABILIZE BY
- Keeping stomach tight
- Chest up
- Legs completely rigid

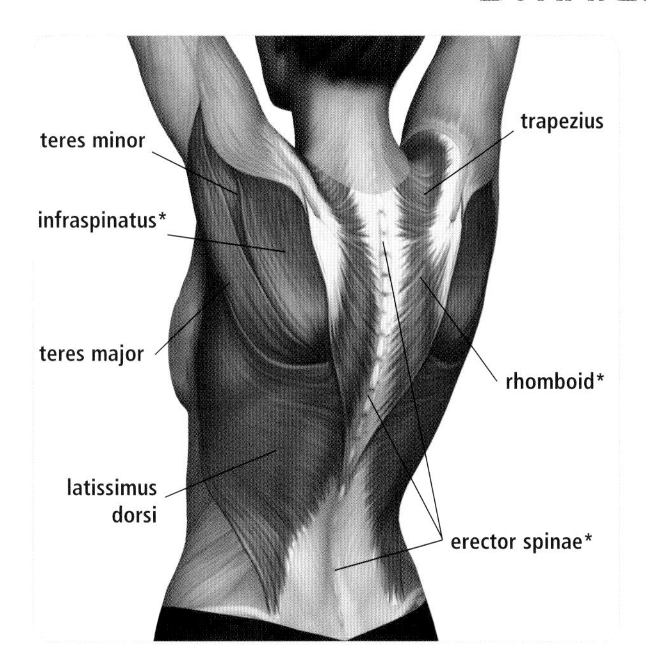

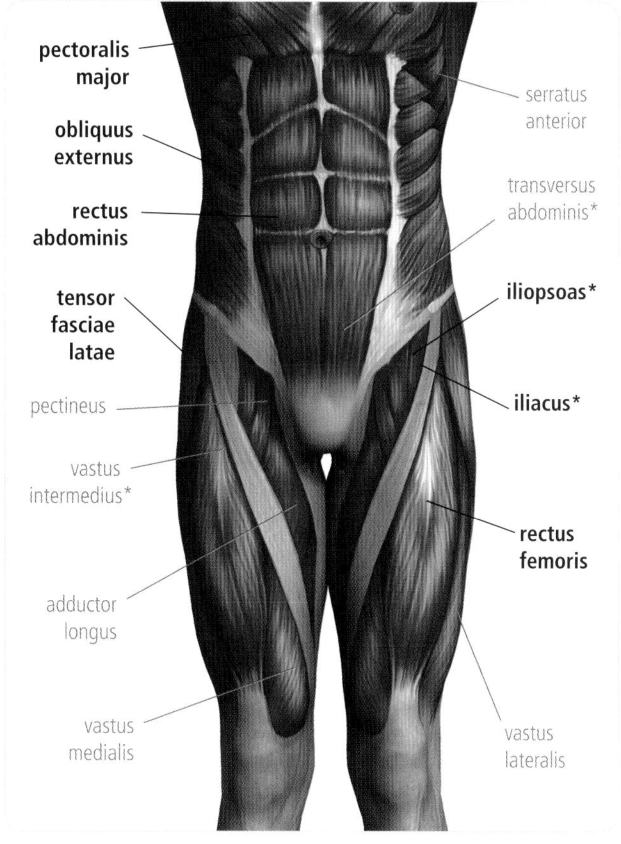

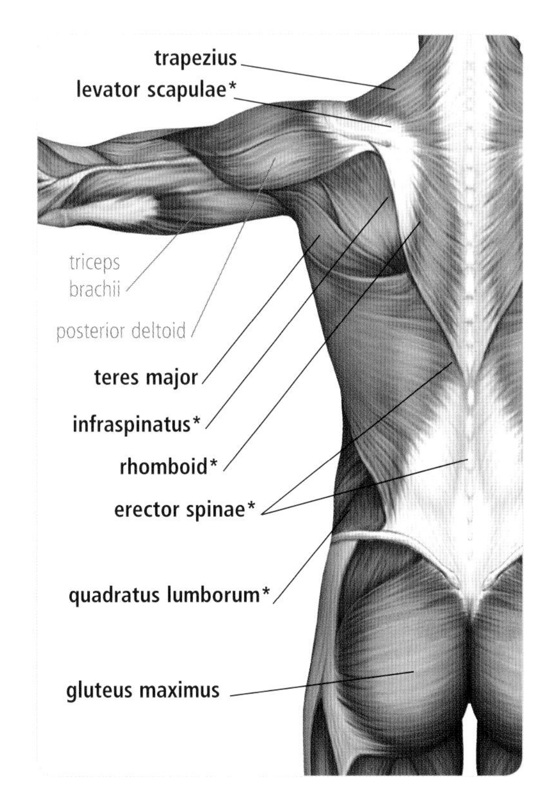

MUSCLES USED

- rectus abdominis
- external oblique
- iliopsoas
- iliacus
- rectus femoris
- tensor fasciae latae
- pectoralis major
- latissimus dorsi
- teres major
- triceps brachii
- trapezius
- rhomboids
- subscapularis
- teres minor
- infraspinatus
- transversus abdominis
- vastus lateralis
- vastus medialis
- vastus intermedius
- rectus femoris

ANNOTATION KEY

Black text indicates active muscles

Gray text indicates stabilizing muscles

* indicates deep muscles

BENT-KNEE HKR WITH MEDICINE BALL

STABILIZE BY
- Keeping your upper arms parallel and your shoulders down
- Gripping the stirrups firmly
- Keeping your legs parallel

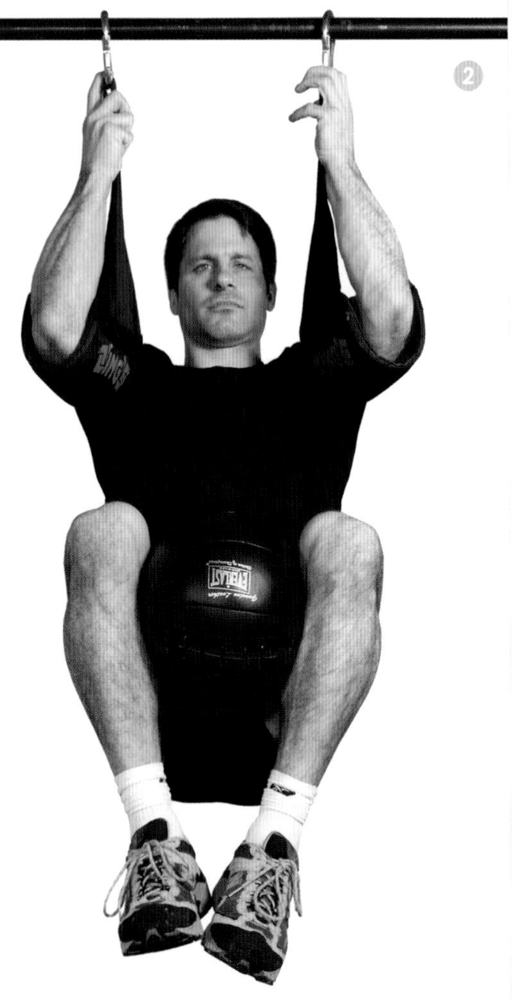

LOOK FOR
- Your knees to bend as your upper legs are raised (your lower legs remain vertical)
- Your legs to move upward together

AVOID
- Swinging
- Extending your arms upward to more than 5 degrees above horizontal
- Moving your hips backward

Starting Position: Clasping a medicine ball between your knees, hang with your upper arms in stirrups, with your elbows bent at 90-degree angles, pointing forward just above shoulder height. Grasp the stirrups with your hands and make sure your torso, legs, and hips are straight.

Action: Pull your upper arms and elbows downward and your upper legs and knees upward toward your elbows, flexing at the hips. Tuck your hips forward and bring your chest forward slightly. Return to the starting position in a slow and controlled manner. Exhale as you rise and inhale as you return to the starting position.

Movement Path: You torso rounds slightly as your hips flex upward and your upper arms are pulled downward. Your center of mass makes no appreciable movement.

BENT-KNEE HKR WITH MEDICINE BALL • AB WHEEL

MUSCLES USED

- iliacus
- iliopsoas
- rectus abdominis
- rectus femoris
- tensor fasciae latae

ANNOTATION KEY

Black text indicates active muscles

Gray text indicates stabilizing muscles

* indicates deep muscles

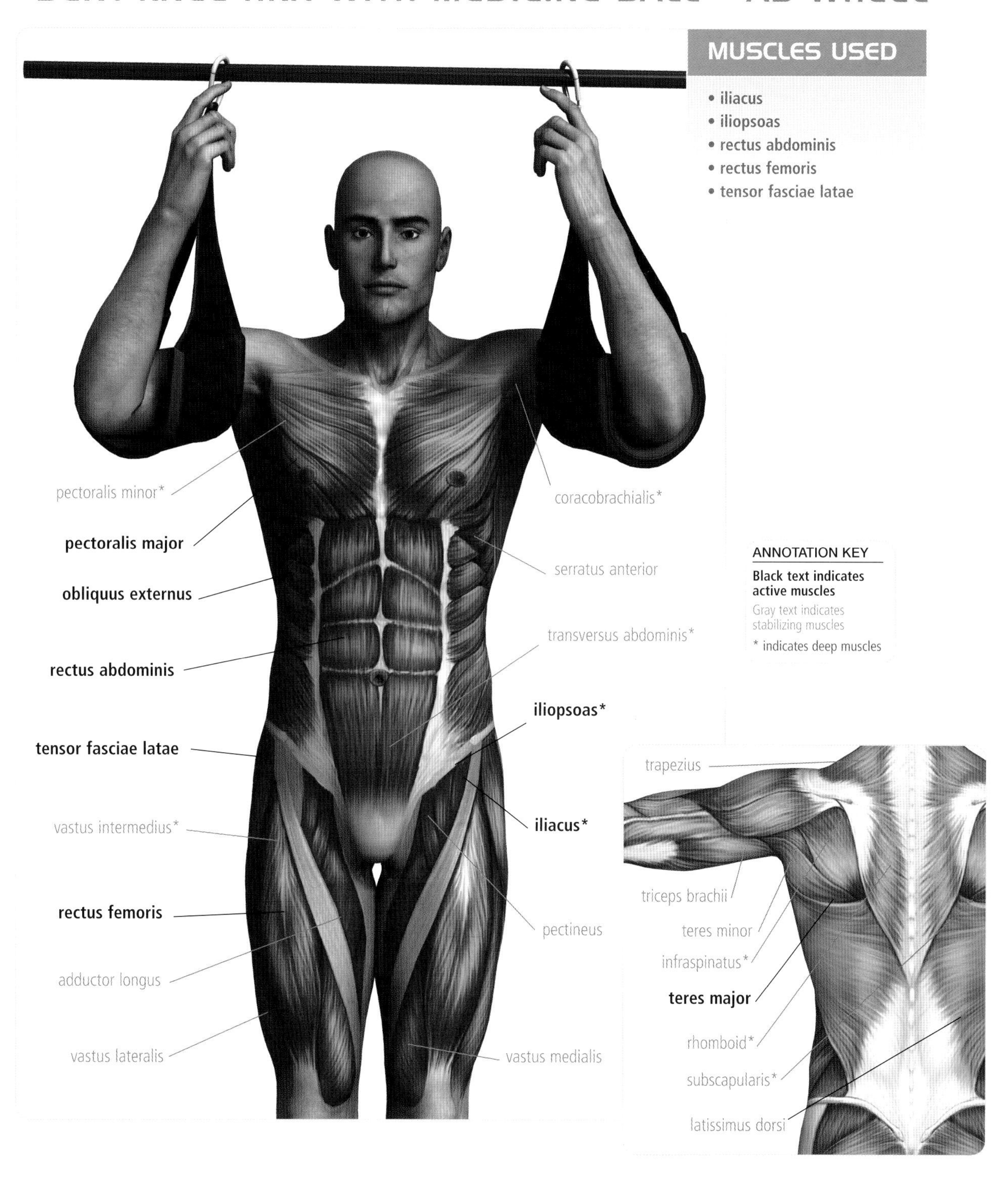

HKR WITH ROTATION

1

Starting Position: Hang with your upper arms in stirrups, with your elbows bent at 90-degree angles, pointing forward just above shoulder height. Grasp the stirrups with your hands and make sure that your torso, legs, and hips are straight.

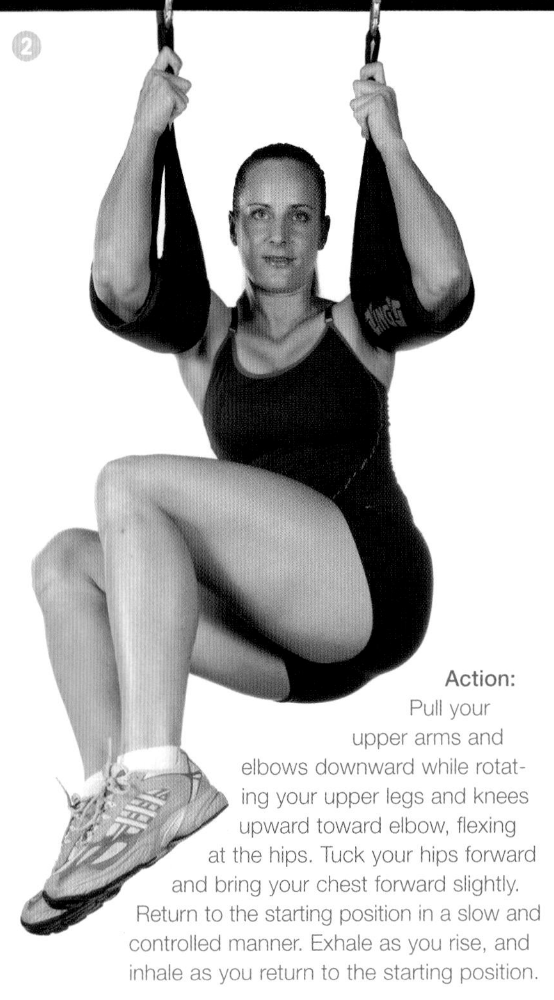

2

Action: Pull your upper arms and elbows downward while rotating your upper legs and knees upward toward elbow, flexing at the hips. Tuck your hips forward and bring your chest forward slightly. Return to the starting position in a slow and controlled manner. Exhale as you rise, and inhale as you return to the starting position.

LOOK FOR
- Your knees to bend as your upper legs are raised (your lower legs remain vertical)
- Your legs to move upward together
- Legs to remain parallel

AVOID
- Swinging
- Extending your arms upward to more than 5 degrees above horizontal
- Moving your hips backward

STABILIZE BY
- Keeping your upper arms parallel and your shoulders down
- Gripping the stirrups firmly
- Keeping your legs parallel

MUSCLES USED

- iliacus
- iliopsoas
- rectus abdominis
- rectus femoris
- tensor fasciae latae
- pectoralis minor
- pectineus
- vastus intermedius
- adductor longus
- vastus lateralis
- vastus medialis
- coracobrachialis
- serratus anterior
- trapezius
- triceps brachii
- teres minor
- infraspinatus
- rhomboid
- subscapularis
- transverses abdominis

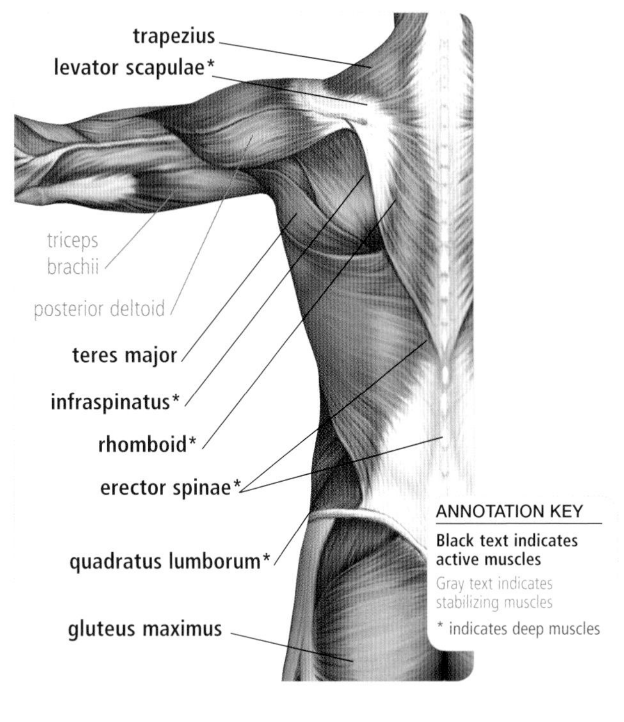

ANNOTATION KEY
Black text indicates active muscles
Gray text indicates stabilizing muscles
* indicates deep muscles

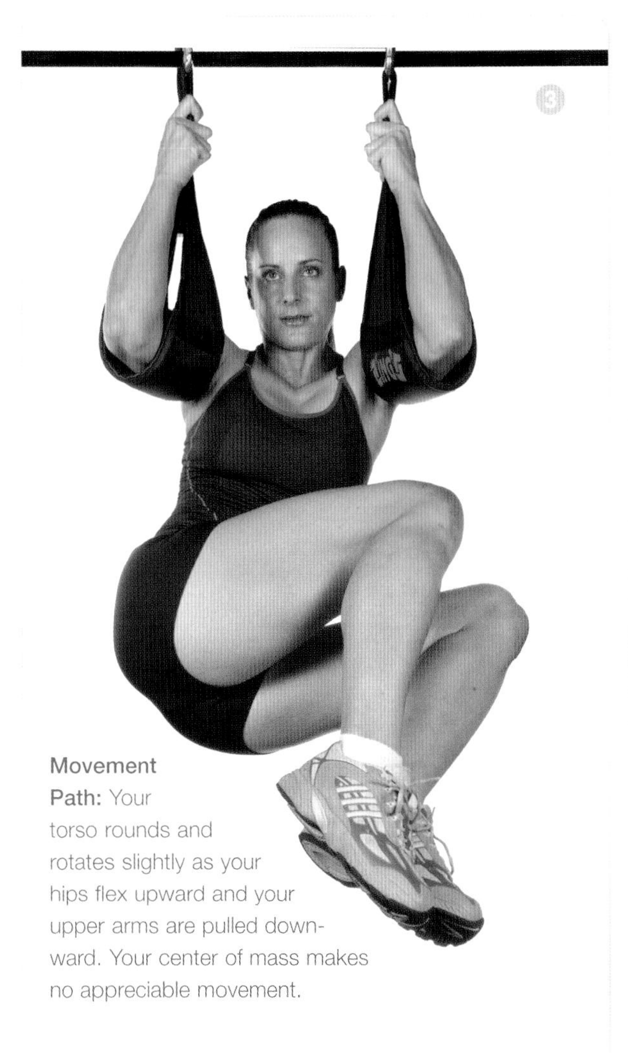

Movement Path: Your torso rounds and rotates slightly as your hips flex upward and your upper arms are pulled downward. Your center of mass makes no appreciable movement.

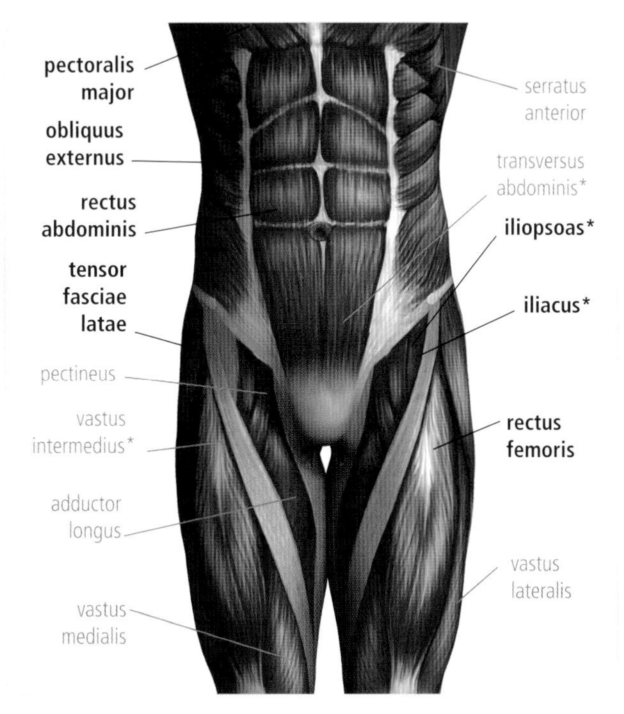

V-UPS WITH PHYSIO BALL

Starting Position: Extend your arms above your head while lying flat on the ground. Bend your knees slightly so that your feet are slightly off the floor, keeping your spine long. Grasp a physio ball with your lower legs.

Action: Push your lower back into the ground, keeping your spine long. Contract your abdominal muscles, and lift your upper back off the ground and forward, exhaling as you come up. Simultaneously reach upward with both arms and legs by folding the torso. Transfer the ball from feet to hands, and slowly return to start position. Repeat, and return ball to feet.

Movement Path: Your torso curves from your mid-low back to the top of your head, in a straight line up toward the knees.

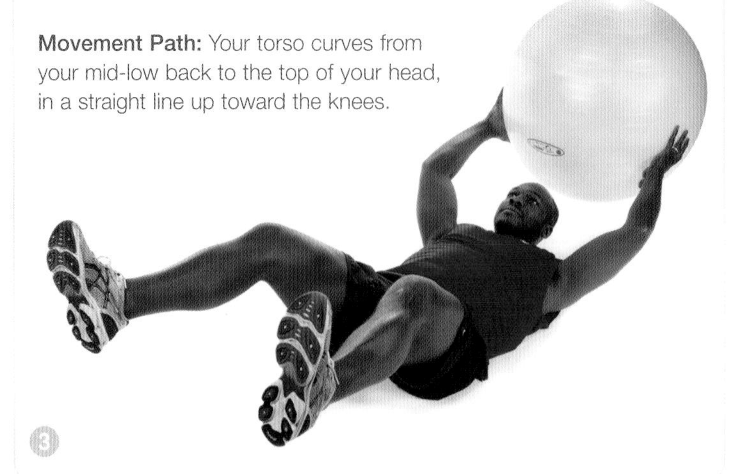

LOOK FOR
- A slight pause at the top of the movement
- A smooth movement throughout the entire length of your spine
- Your abdominal muscles to contract and pull in
- Your hips to remain stable
- Knees to remain in same position

AVOID
- Bending the knees excessively
- Using momentum for any part of the movement
- Arching your back, or elevating your feet

STABILIZE BY
- Keeping your shoulders down with your elbows widely spread
- Keeping your hips even and your feet flat

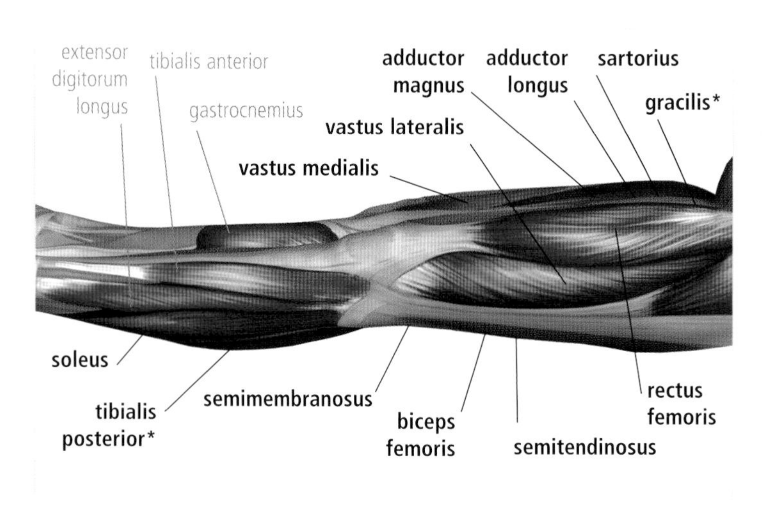

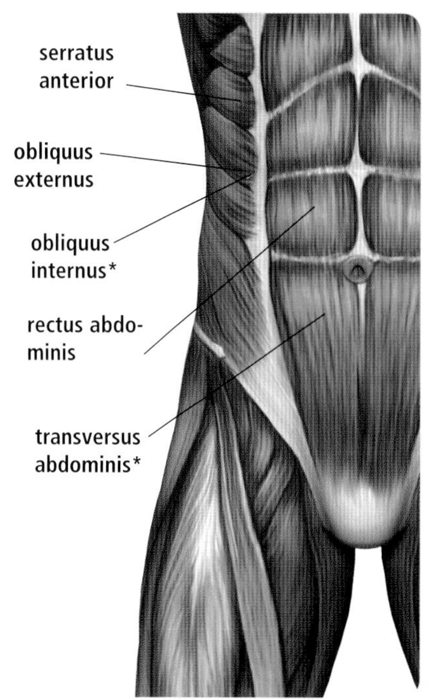

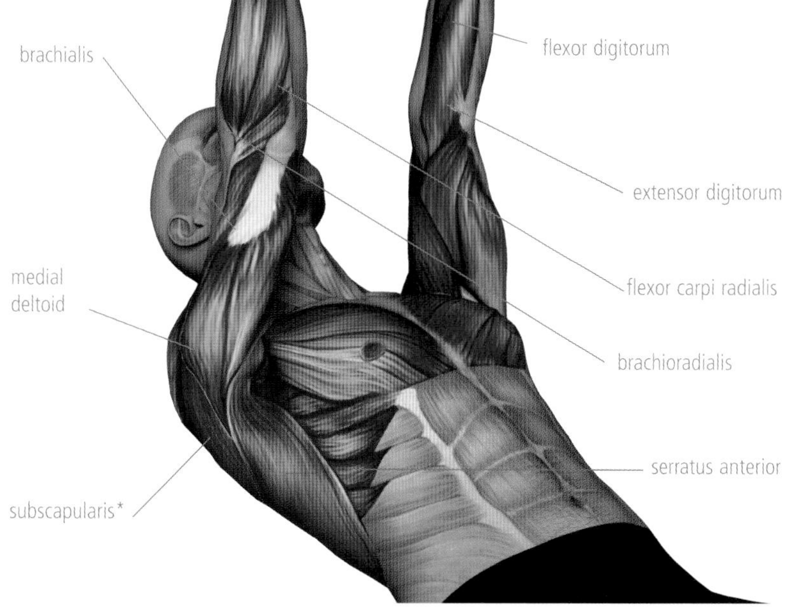

ANNOTATION KEY

Black text indicates active muscles

Gray text indicates stabilizing muscles

* indicates deep muscles

MUSCLES USED

- obliques externus
- rectus abdominis
- rectus femoris
- scalenes
- splenius
- sternocleidomastoideus
- trapezius
- biceps brachii
- pectoralis major
- medial deltoid
- serratus anterior
- latissimus dorsi
- iliopsoas

HAND WALK-OUT

Starting Position: From a standing position, bend forward from the waist, and place your hands on the ground in front of you and slightly wider than your feet. Keep knees as straight as possible.

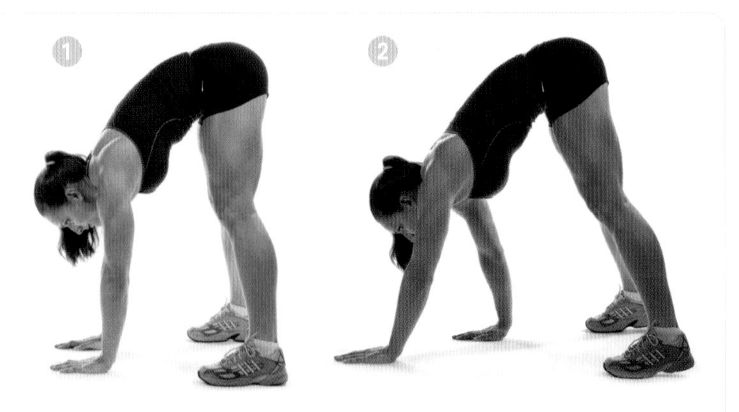

Action: Shift weight to hands and slowly "walk" them forward while keeping knees straight and hips up and spine straight. Continue dropping out until you've reached horizontal or "push-up" position. Return by walking hand back toward the start position and pushing hips upward folding the torso at the hips.

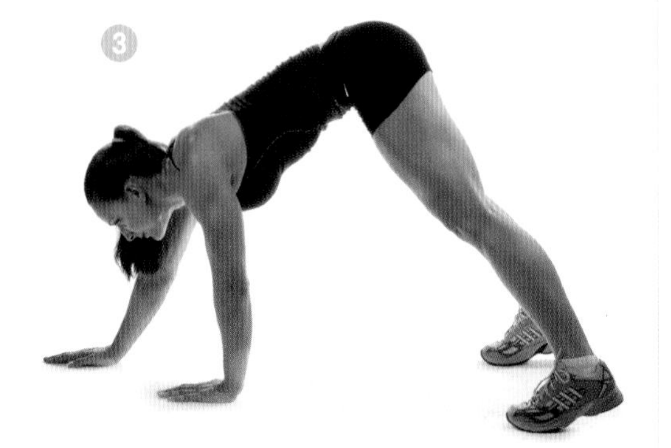

LOOK FOR
- Spine and legs to remain straight
- Slow, steady movement

AVOID
- Bending the knees or spine
- Allowing the elbows to bend

Movement Path: Shoulders move forward as hips and legs move downward.

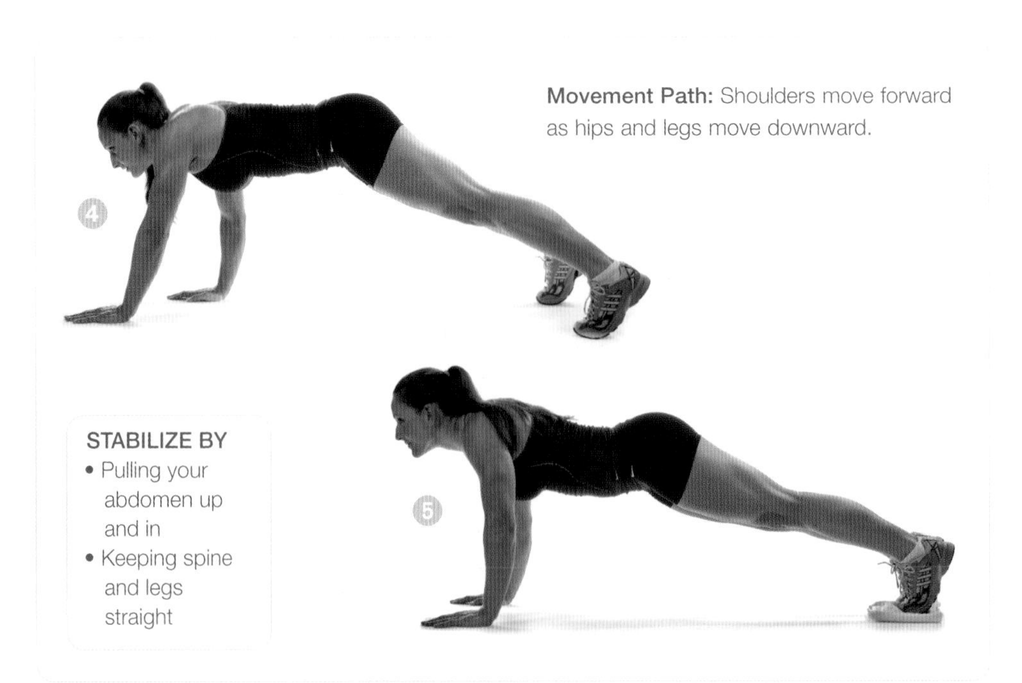

STABILIZE BY
- Pulling your abdomen up and in
- Keeping spine and legs straight

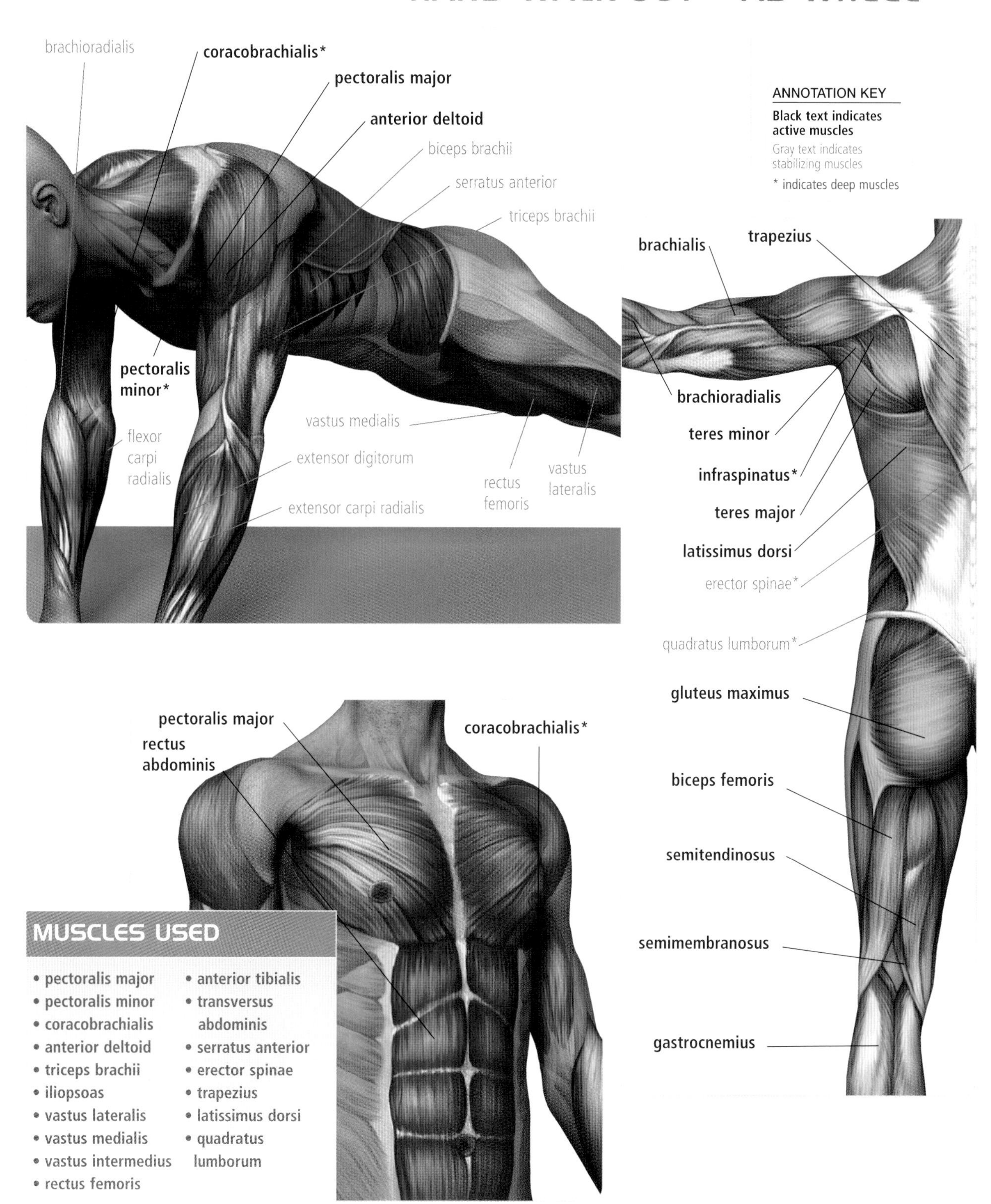

MUSCLES USED

- pectoralis major
- pectoralis minor
- coracobrachialis
- anterior deltoid
- triceps brachii
- iliopsoas
- vastus lateralis
- vastus medialis
- vastus intermedius
- rectus femoris
- anterior tibialis
- transversus abdominis
- serratus anterior
- erector spinae
- trapezius
- latissimus dorsi
- quadratus lumborum

FRONT PLANK

Starting Position: Lie face down on the ground and fold your hands directly beneath your chin with your elbows by your sides and your feet on your toes.

Action: Raise the length of your torso to a horizontal position with a slight arch in your lower back. Your shoulder blades should be flat and your spine long.

Movement Path: None.

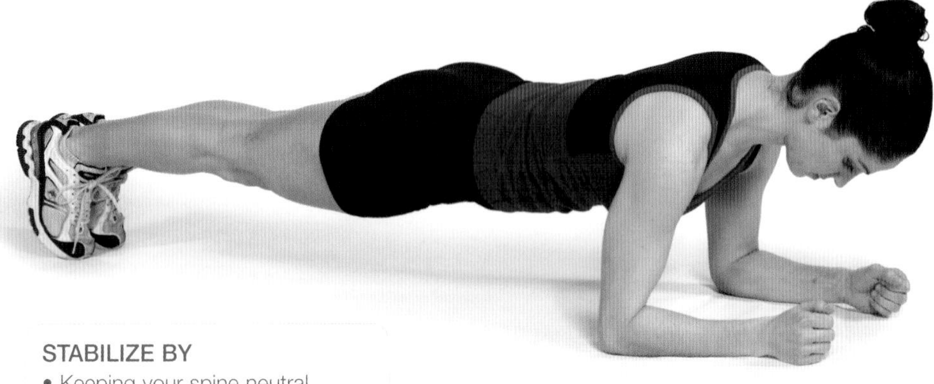

LOOK FOR
- A neutral spinal position
- Locked knees, with your ankles at 90-degree angles and your elbows directly under your shoulder joints

AVOID
- Rounding your spine, dropping your hips, and elevating your shoulders toward your ears

STABILIZE BY
- Keeping your spine neutral
- Keeping your shoulders down and your head up
- Maintaining the contraction of your gluteals and legs
- Keeping your legs straight and your ankles bent at 90 degree angles, with your toes pointing directly into the ground

MODIFICATIONS
Easier: Raise your forelegs and rest your weight on your knees to shorten the lever.

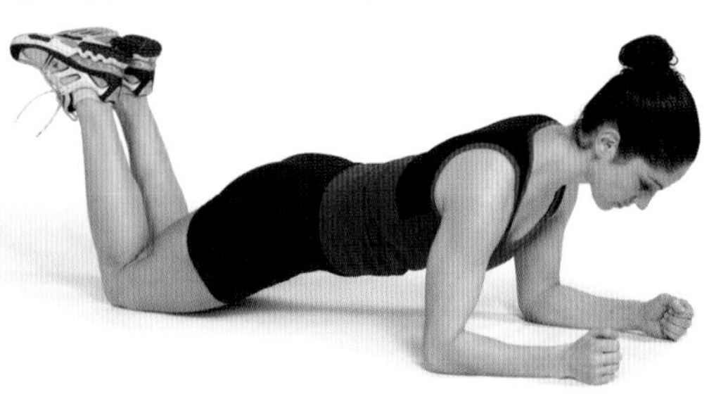

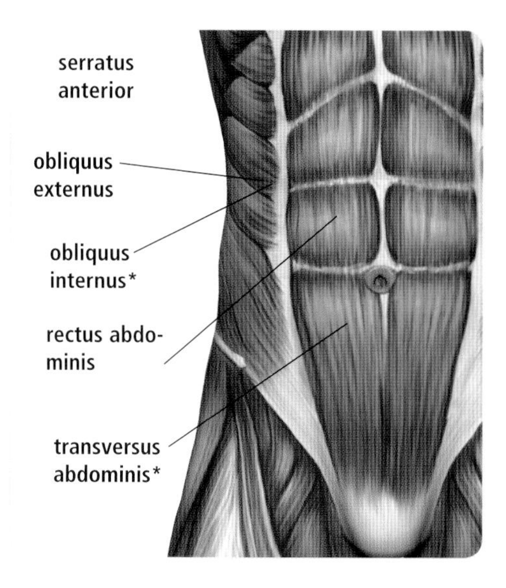

MUSCLES USED

- erector spinae
- iliacus
- iliopsoas
- obliquus internus
- rectus abdominis
- rectus femoris
- serratus anterior
- splenius
- tibialis anterior
- transversus abdominis
- vastus intermedius

ANNOTATION KEY
Black text indicates active muscles
Gray text indicates stabilizing muscles
* indicates deep muscles

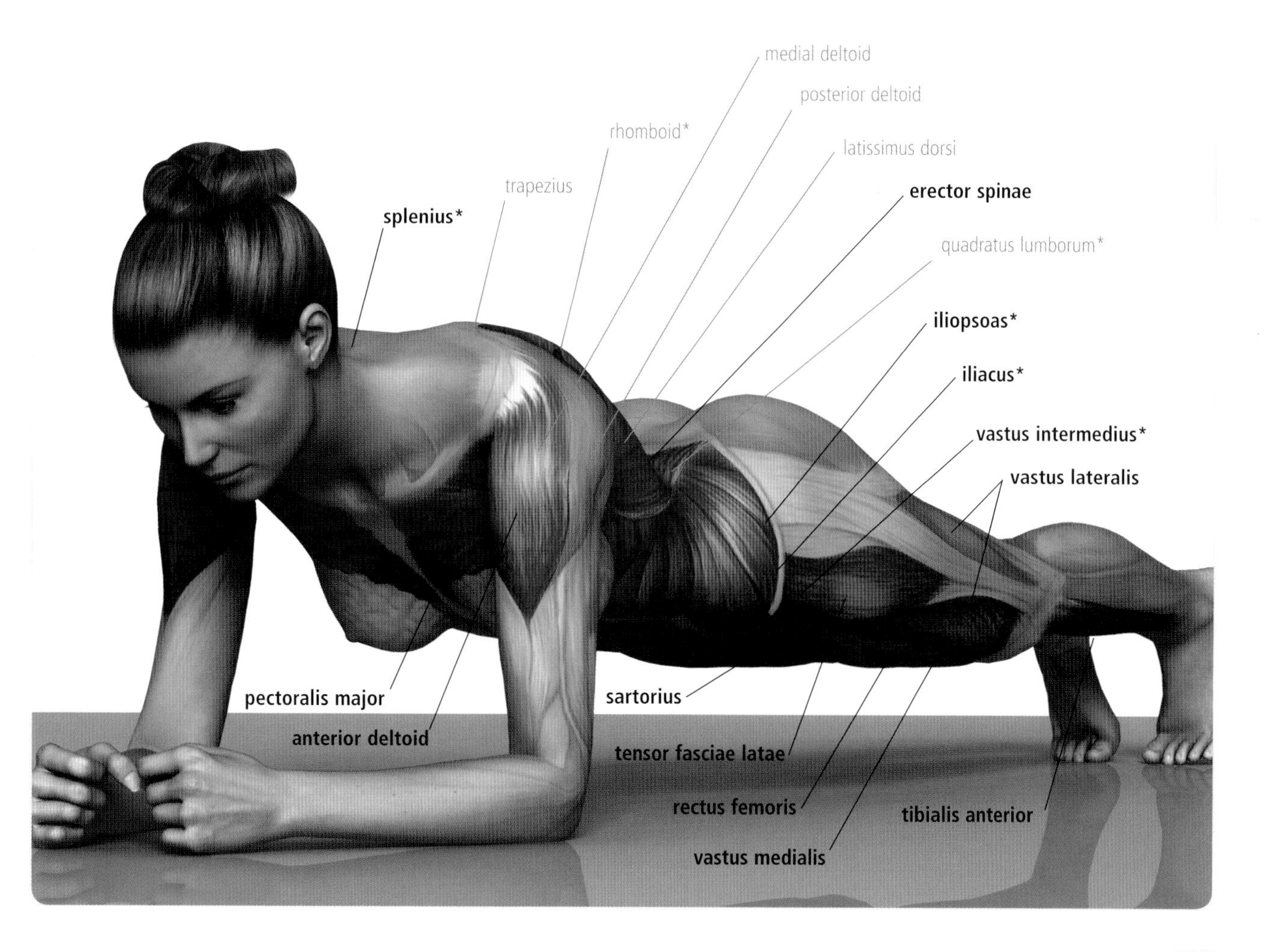

PLANK TO PIKE

Starting Position: Place hands on ground, and place feet with ankles fixed at 90-degree angles, toes down on physio ball so that body is horizontal. Hands are wider than shoulder-width, and fingertips are parallel to collarbone. Feet are placed on ball with top of foot (shoelaces) contacting the ball, and toes are pointed.

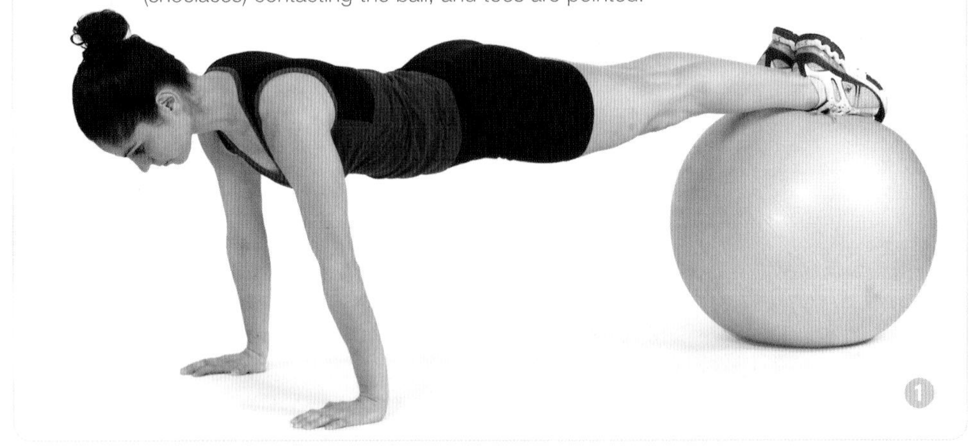

LOOK FOR

- A single plane of movement, i.e., a straight line from head to ankle

AVOID

- A segmental elevation, i.e., your shoulders rising before your hips or vice versa
- Elevating your shoulders toward your ears
- Moving your head forward
- Allowing the ankles to change position
- Allowing the ball or body to migrate laterally

Action: Lower your entire body by allowing the elbows to bend until your torso has dropped into a position where the chest is at the level of your hands. Return by extending the elbows and pushing into the ground, elevating entire body simultaneously. From top position, pull ball forward by flexing foot and drawing the toes and hips upward so that the torso is bent at the hips. Toes are on top of the ball and both feet are at 90-degree angles. Upper body and head are facing downward. Return by dropping hips and extending toes until body returns to horizontal.

Movement Path: The plane of your body rotates upward in an arc. Use your feet as a lever.

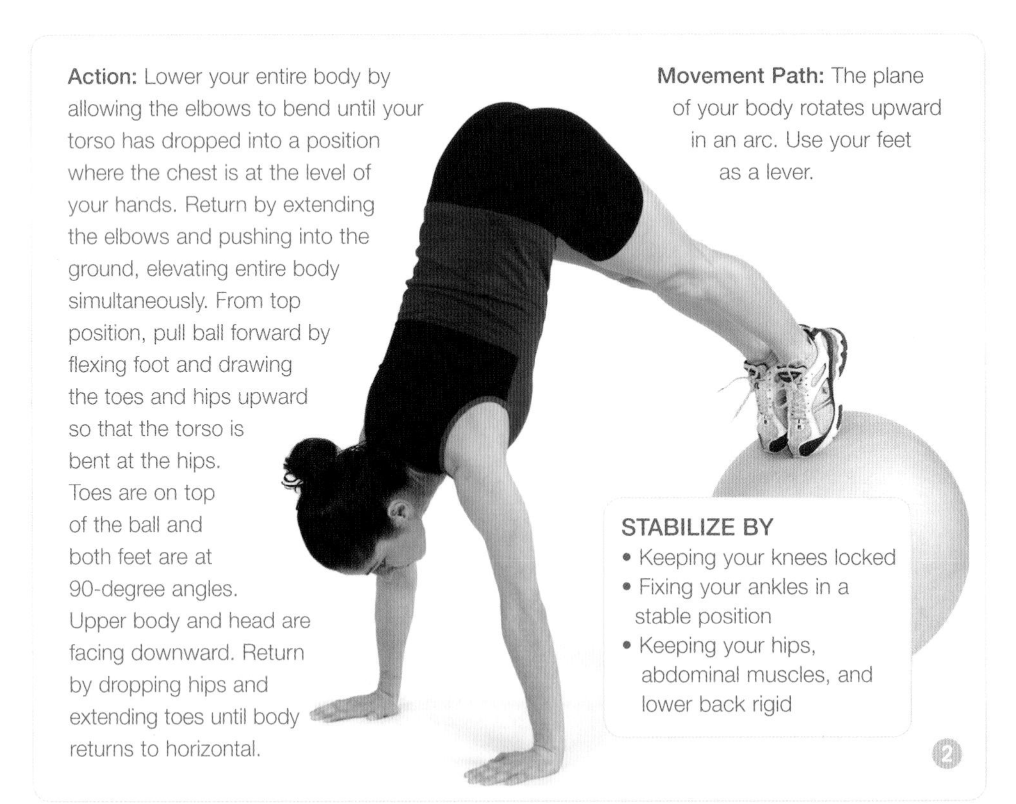

STABILIZE BY

- Keeping your knees locked
- Fixing your ankles in a stable position
- Keeping your hips, abdominal muscles, and lower back rigid

PLANK TO PIKE • AB WHEEL

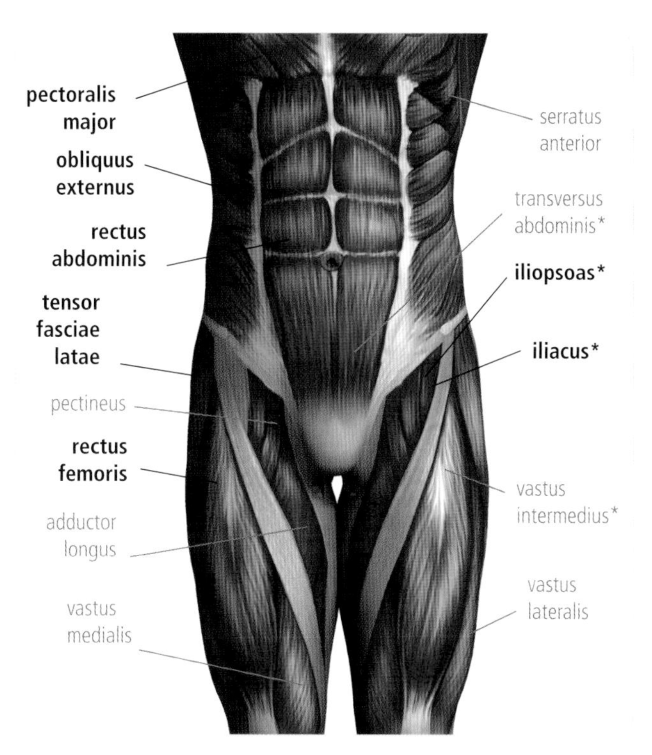

MUSCLES USED

- pectoralis major
- pectoralis minor
- coracobrachialis
- anterior deltoid
- triceps brachii
- iliopsoas
- vastus lateralis
- vastus medialis
- vastus intermedius
- rectus femoris
- anterior tibialis
- transversus abdominis
- serratus anterior
- erector spinae
- trapezius
- latissimus dorsi
- quadratus lumborum

ANNOTATION KEY

Black text indicates active muscles

Gray text indicates stabilizing muscles

* indicates deep muscles

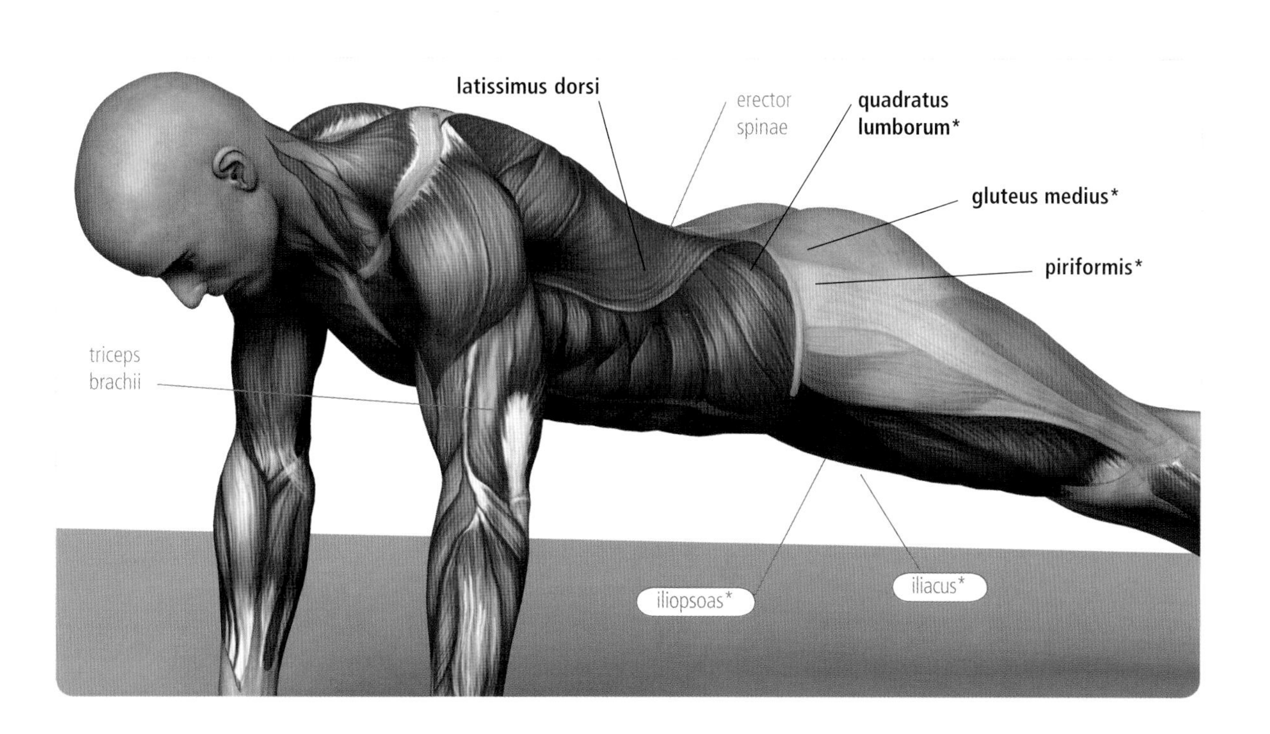

LAYOUT ON RINGS

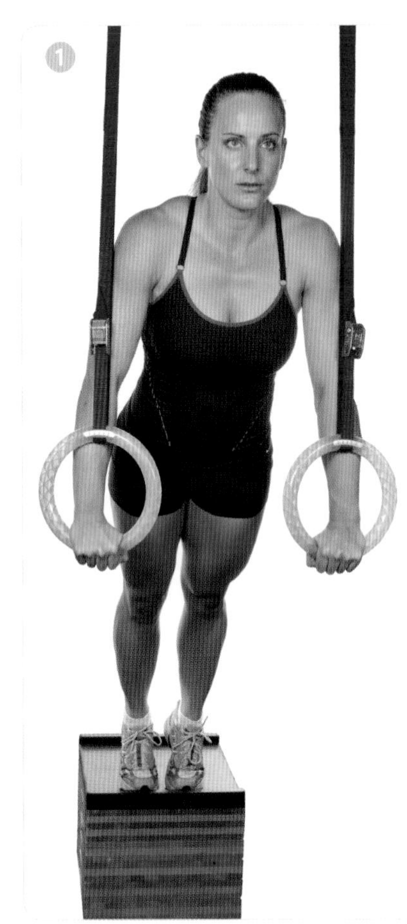

Starting Position: With body rigid and at a 45-degree angle to the floor, grasp rings directly under the shoulder with a palms-down grip, so that rings are parallel and directly beneath the chest. Legs, hips, and spine form a straight line.

Action: Allowing the entire body to descend in a controlled manner with arms straight, push the hands forward and outward, using toes as a fulcrum. While descending, keep hands parallel, allowing the body to descend until arms are in a horizontal position. Return by pulling arms back toward the floor until body returns to start position.

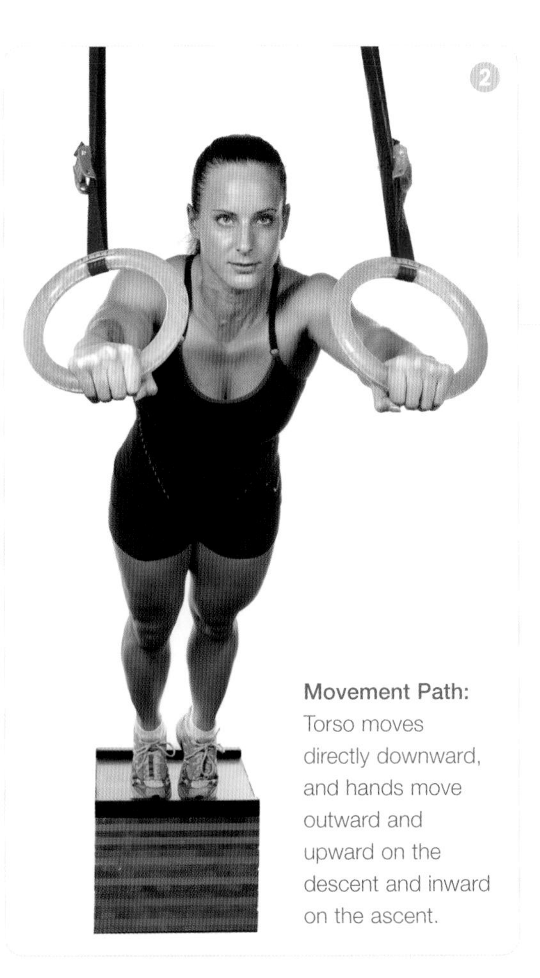

Movement Path: Torso moves directly downward, and hands move outward and upward on the descent and inward on the ascent.

LOOK FOR

- Arms to remain straight and parallel
- A single plane of movement, i.e., a straight line from head to ankle

AVOID

- Segmental elevation, i.e., your shoulders rising before your hips or vice versa
- Elevating your shoulders toward your ears
- Moving your head forward

STABILIZE BY

- Keeping shoulders down
- Keeping your knees locked
- Fixing your ankles in a stable position
- Keeping your hips, abdominal muscles, and lower back rigid

LAYOUT ON RINGS • AB WHEEL

MUSCLES USED

- latissimus dorsi
- pectoralis major
- pectoralis minor
- coracobrachialis
- anterior deltoid
- rectus abdominis
- serratus anterior
- triceps brachii
- iliopsoas
- vastus lateralis
- vastus medialis
- vastus intermedius
- rectus femoris
- anterior tibialis
- transversus abdominis
- serratus anterior
- erector spinae
- trapezius
- quadratus lumborum

ANNOTATION KEY

Black text indicates active muscles

Gray text indicates stabilizing muscles

* indicates deep muscles

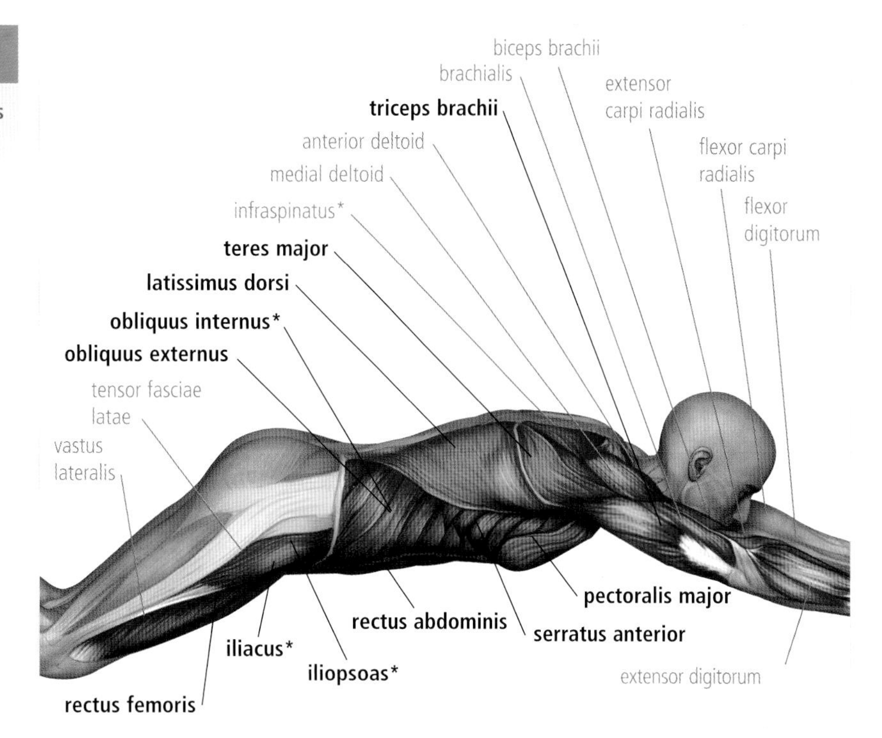

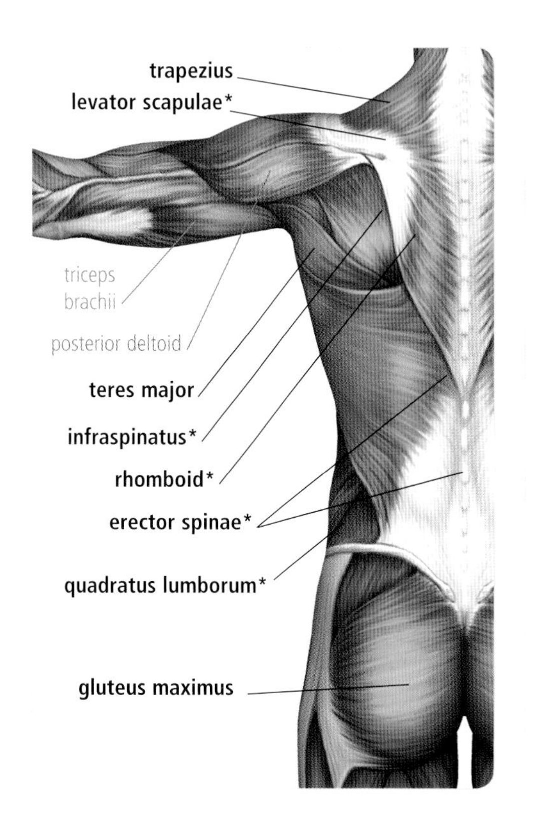

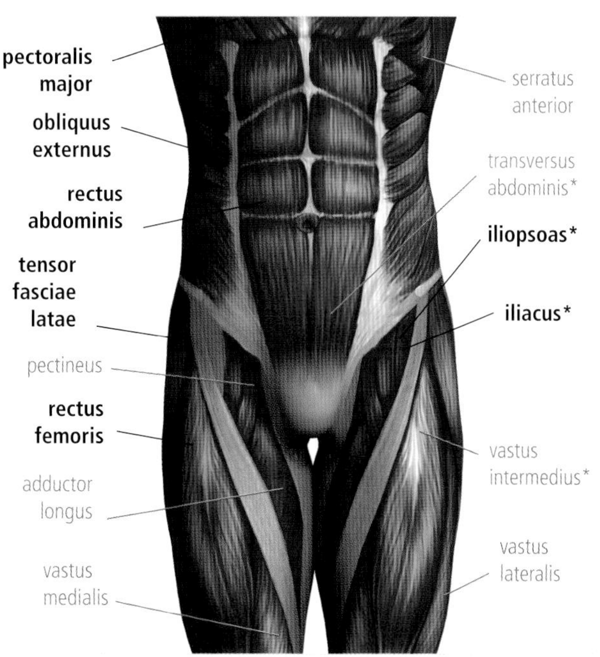

PROGRAMS

The following pages contain 12 sample exercise programs: 4 beginner, 4 intermediate, and 4 advanced. Each program consists of two pages. Included are:

- Specific exercise groupings, or "workouts"
- A visual representation of each exercise to be performed, with its page reference
- The weeks the workouts are to be performed in
- A program overview, detailing both times per week and workouts to be performed
- A Prescription box, giving weekly volume and rest periods for a given workout
- An Exercise Sequence box, showing the order of exercises for a given workout
- A Notes section, which gives basic information on how the program should be used
- Space for user notes

Below are Legend and Programs Glossary boxes defining the elements and nomenclature used in the programs section. Opposite is a master list that includes all 12 programs. On page 135 there is a sample of how a workout may be logged.

Please remember that these workouts only address musculoskeletal conditioning. Warm-up, cardiovascular components, and flexibility are not addressed here. Before beginning any exercise program, you should always consult with your physician.

LEGEND

Numbers = days per week

Letters = specific workouts

Roman Numerals = programs or prescription

Level: Subjective categorization of both exercises and workouts based on technical difficulty and complexity

PROGRAMS GLOSSARY

5 Ingredients: category or type of exercise

Exercise: specific movement from a given category

Workout: group of exercises

Programs: group of workouts

Sequence: order in which 5 Ingredients are reinforced in a given workout

	BEGINNER					INTERMEDIATE					ADVANCED				
	Program I (6 weeks)					Program II (8 weeks)					Program III (8 weeks)				
Weeks	Days					Days					Days				
	1	2				1	2				1	2			
1	A	B				A	B				A	E			
2	A	B				C	D				B	D			
3	A	B				A	B				F	A			
4	B	A				C	D				C	D			
5	B	A				B	A				B	E			
6	B	A				D	C				F	C			
7						B	A				D	F			
8						D	C				E	A			

	Program IV (6 weeks)					Program V (6 weeks)					Program VI (4 weeks)				
Weeks	Days					Days					Days				
	1	2	3			1	2	3			1	2	3		
1	C	A	D		A	A	B	C			D	E	F		
2	C	A	D		D	D	E	F			D	E	F		
3	C	A	D		A	A	B	C			D	E	F		
4	D	C	A		D	D	E	F			D	E	F		
5	D	C	A		A	A	B	C							
6	D	C	A		D	D	E	F							

	Program VII (4 weeks)					Program VIII (4 weeks)					Program IX (4 weeks)				
Weeks	Days					Days					Days				
	1	2	3	4		1	2	3	4		1	2	3	4	
1	G	H	G	H		I	J	K	L		M	N	O	D	
2	G	H	G	H		I	J	K	L		M	N	O	D	
3	H	G	H	G		I	J	K	L		M	N	O	D	
4	H	G	H	G		I	J	K	L		M	N	O	D	

	Program X (4 weeks)					Program XI (4 weeks)					Program XII (4 weeks)				
Weeks	Days					Days					Days				
	1	2	3	4	5	1	2	3	4	5	1	2	3	4	5
1	Q	S	R	U	T	I	J	K	P	Z	V	W	X	Y	Z
2	Q	S	R	U	T	I	J	Z	K	P	V	W	X	Y	Z
3	Q	S	R	U	T	I	J	K	P	Z	V	W	X	Y	Z
4	Q	S	R	U	T	I	J	Z	P	K	V	W	X	Y	Z

PROGRAM I

BEGINNER

WORKOUTS

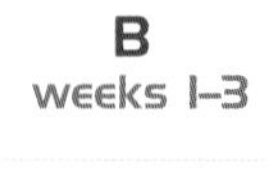

A weeks 1–3	B weeks 1–3	B weeks 4–6	A weeks 4–6
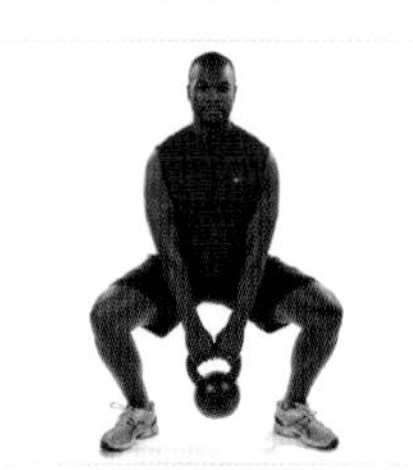 Sumo with Kettlebell page 18	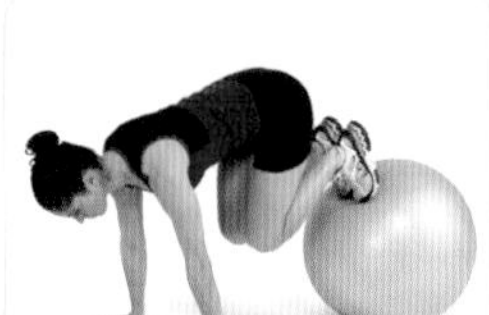 Plough on Physio Ball page 112	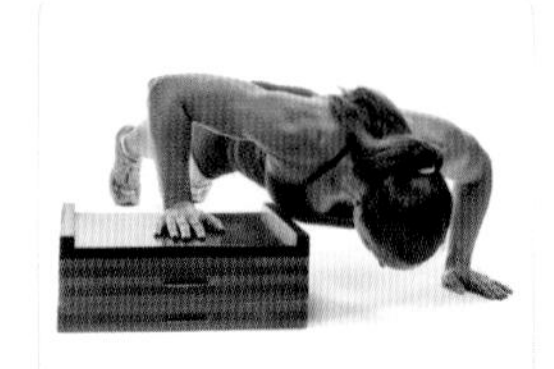 Hand Walkover page 78	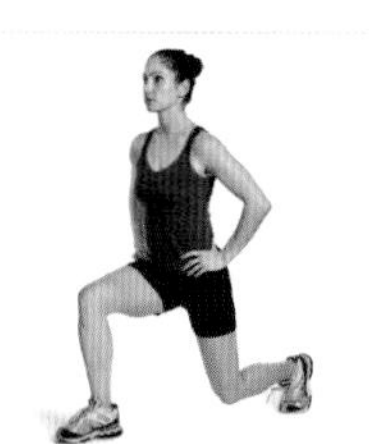 Stationary Lunge page 38
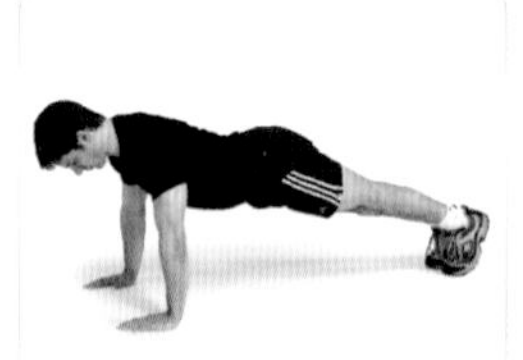 Basic Push-up page 60	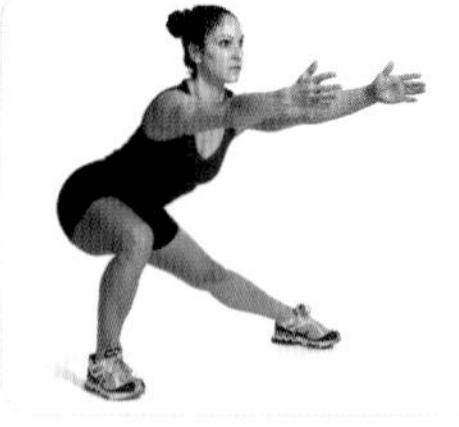 Lateral Lunge page 42	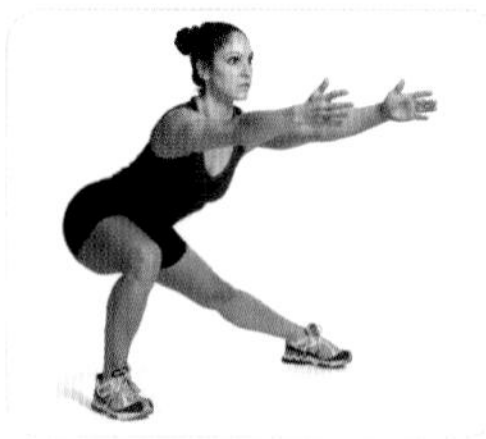 Lateral Lunge page 42	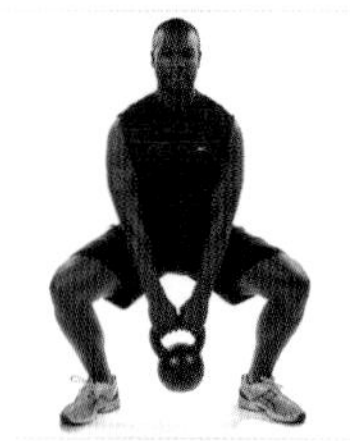 Sumo with Kettlebell page 18
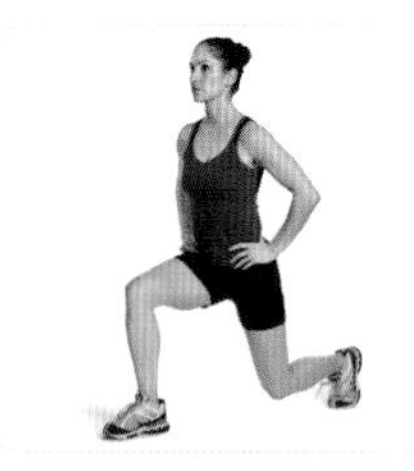 Stationary Lunge page 38	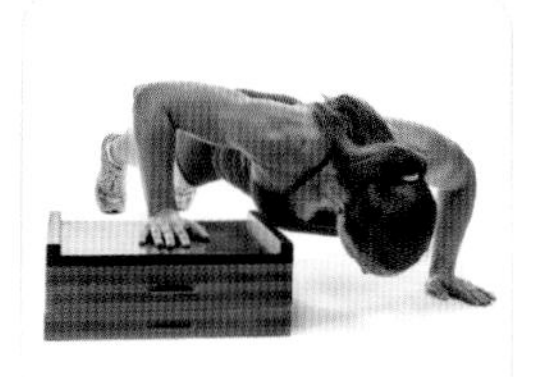 Hand Walkover page 78	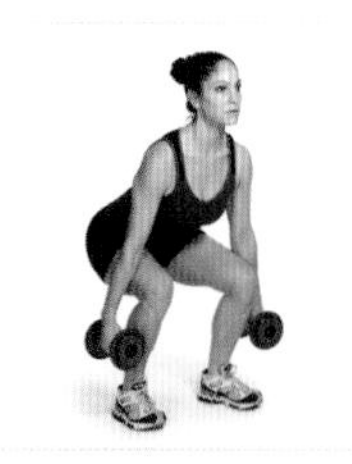 Full with Dumbbells page 15	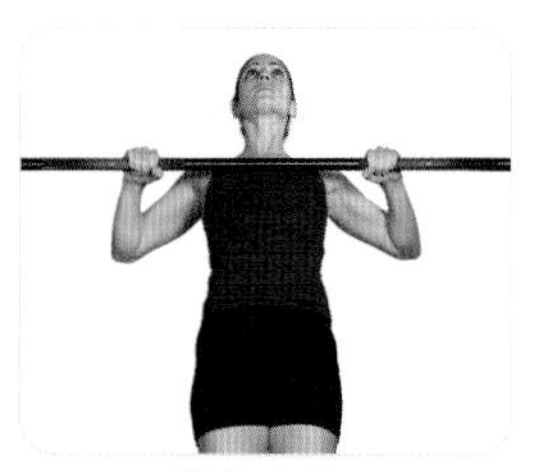 45° Body Row page 90
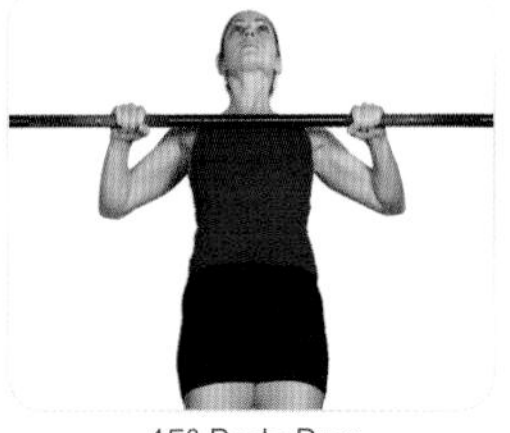 45° Body Row page 90	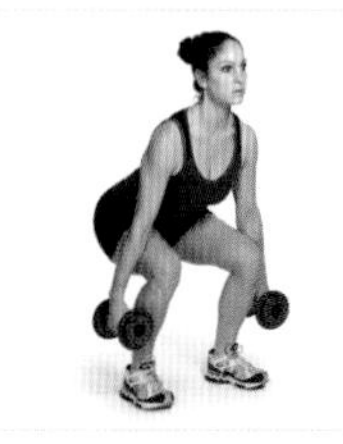 Full with Dumbbells page 15	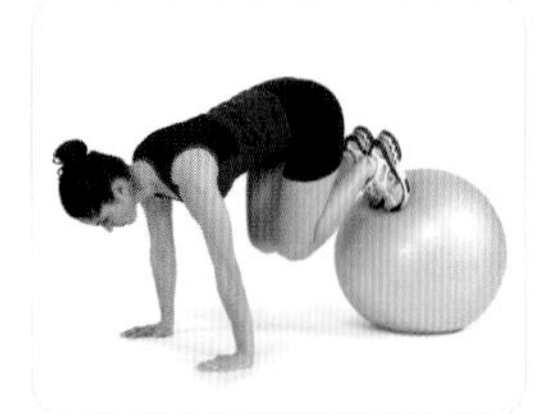 Plough on Physio Ball page 112	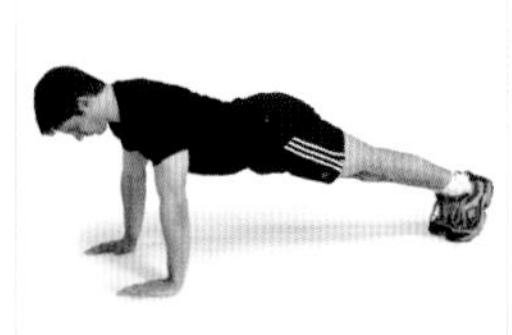 Basic Push-up page 60
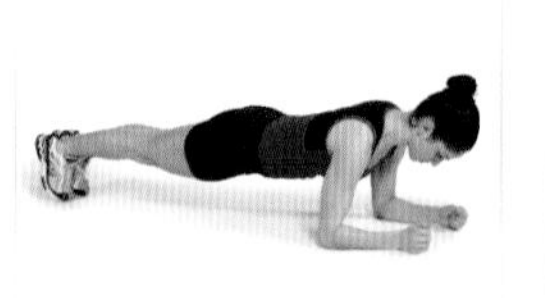 Front Plank page 126	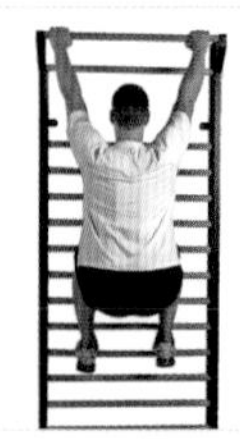 Stand-Pull page 98	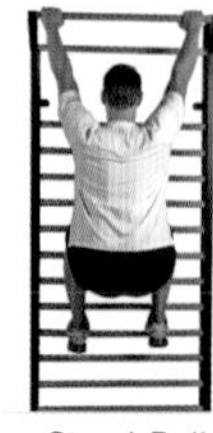 Stand-Pull page 98	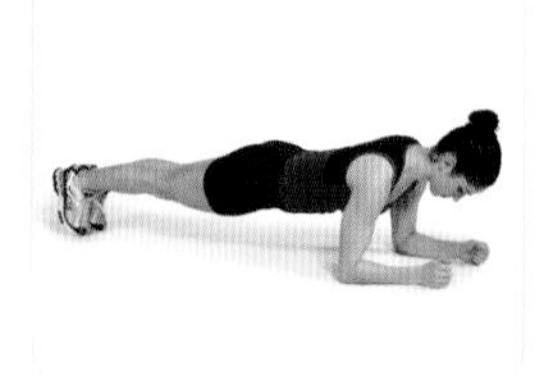 Front Plank page 126

PROGRAM I • BEGINNER

SAMPLE PROGRAM LOG

		Week 1				Week 2				Week 3				Week 4			
		Sets	Reps	Weight	Rest	Sets	Reps	Weight	Rest	Sets	Reps	Weight	Rest	Sets	Reps	Weight	Rest
A	Sumo																
	Stationary																
	Basic																
	45° Body Row																
	Front Plank																

PROGRAM: I DURATION: 6 WEEKS

Days per week: 3
Total weeks: 6
Type: Intermediate
Endurance

Weeks	Day 1	Day 2
1	A	B
2	A	B
3	A	B
4	B	A
5	B	A
6	B	A

PRESCRIPTION

Week	Sets	Repetitions	Weight/Progression	Rest Set/Exercise
1	3	8	T.B.D.	:75 / :90
2	3	10	Same as week 1	:60 / :75
3	3	12	Same as week 1	:45 / :60
4	3	10	Increase 10% BW (2–5 reps)	:60 / :90
5	3	8	Increase 10% BW (2–5 reps)	:75 / :90
6	3	6	Increase 10% BW (2–5 reps)	:75 / :90

EXERCISE SEQUENCE

Order	Workout A	Workout B	Workout B	Workout A
1	Dead Lift	Ab Wheel	Push-up	Lunge
2	Push-up	Lunge	Lunge	Dead Lift
3	Lunge	Push-up	Dead Lift	Chin-up
4	Chin-up	Dead Lift	Ab Wheel	Push-up
5	Ab Wheel	Chin-up	Chin-up	Ab Wheel

Notes: In weeks 1–3 the exercise order remains consistent. In weeks 4–6 both the exercise sequence and workout schedule (workout B is done first) change.

PROGRAM II

INTERMEDIATE

WORKOUTS

A weeks 1, 3, 5, 7	B weeks 1, 3, 5, 7	C weeks 2, 4, 6, 8	D weeks 2, 4, 6, 8
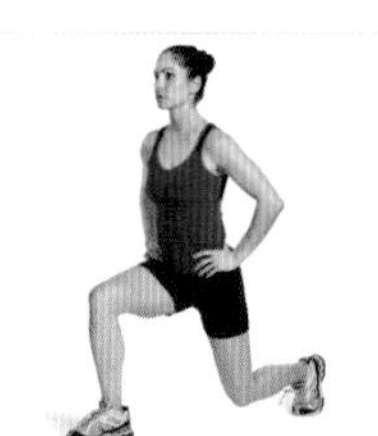 Stationary Lunge page 38	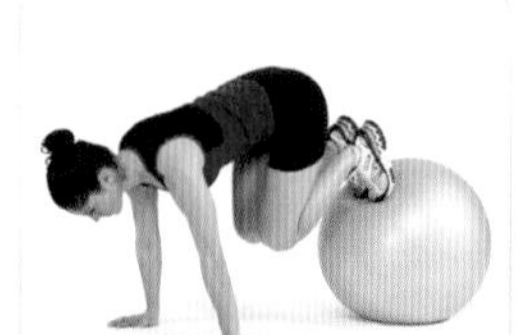 Plough on Physio Ball page 112	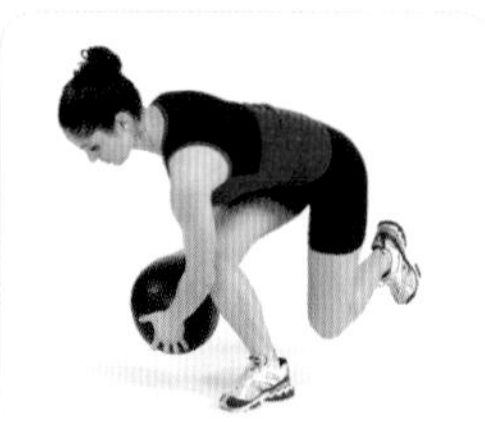 PNF Raise with Medicine Ball page 26	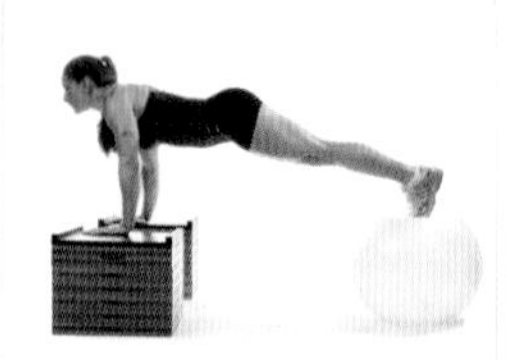 On Physio Ball & Blocks page 64
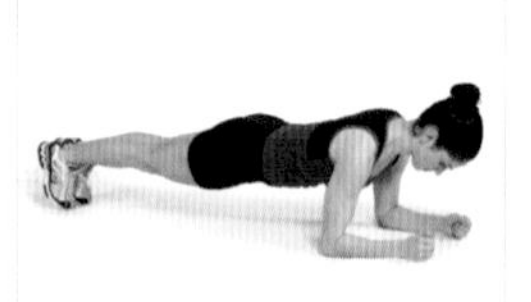 Front Plank page 126	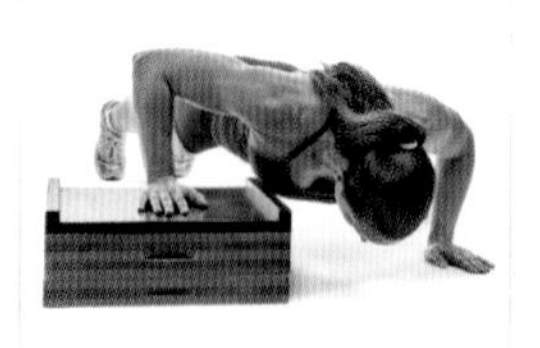 Hand Walkover page 78	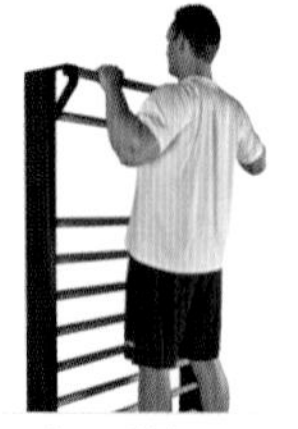 Step Chin page 100	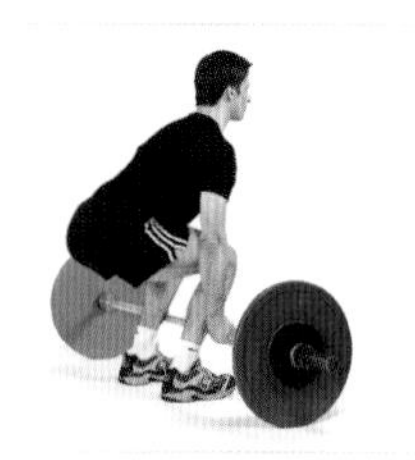 Full with Barbells page 14
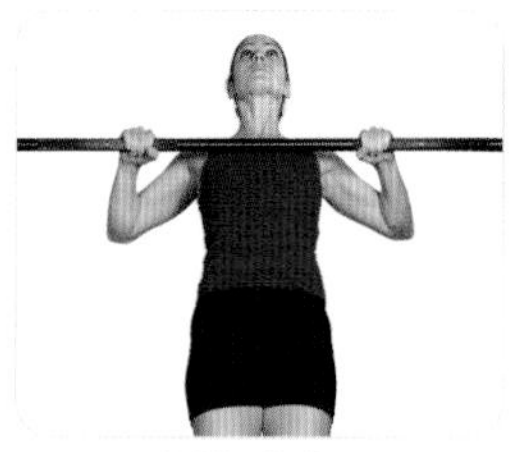 45º Body Row page 90	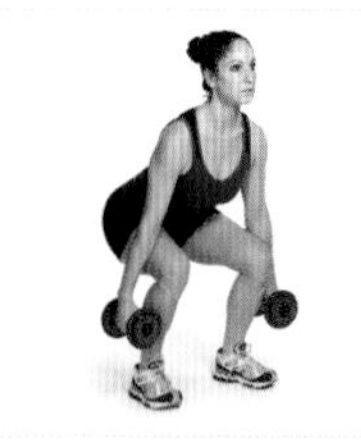 Full with Dumbbells page 15	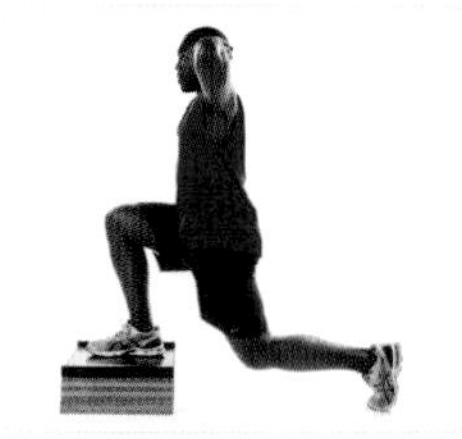 Up to Box page 54	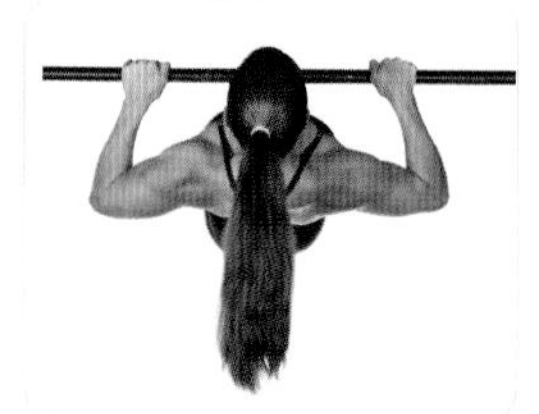 Horizontal Body Row page 92
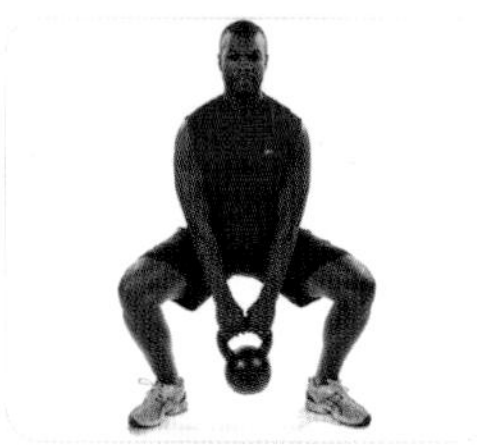 Sumo with Kettlebell page 18	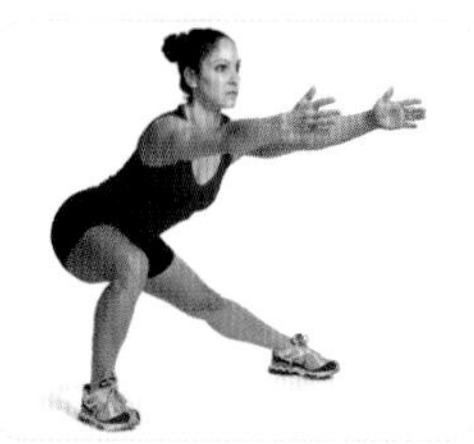 Lateral Lunge page 42	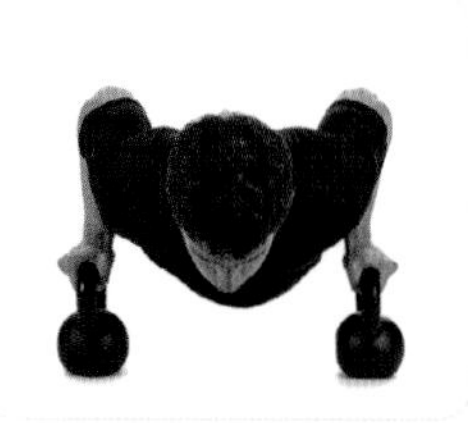 Push-up on Kettlebells page 76	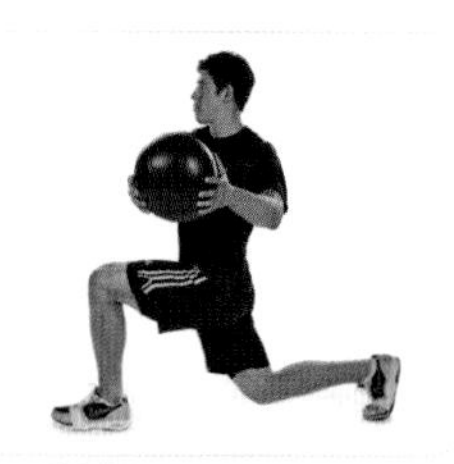 Walking with Rotation page 40
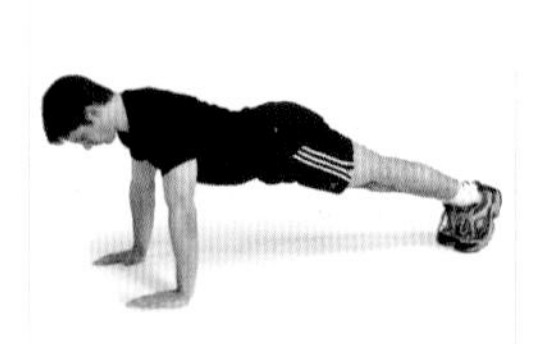 Basic Push-up page 60	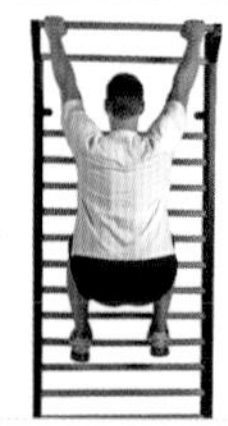 Stand-Pull page 98	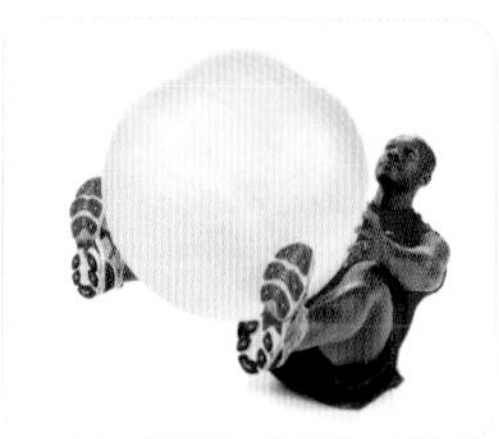 V-ups with Physio Ball page 122	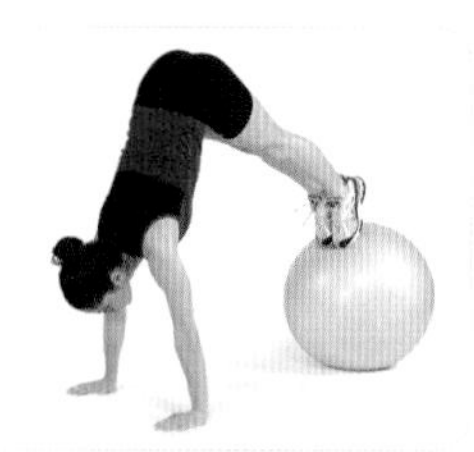 Plank to Pike page 128

USER NOTES

PROGRAM II • INTERMEDIATE

PROGRAM: II DURATION: 8 WEEKS

Days per week: 2
Total weeks: 8
Type: Endurance

Weeks	1	2
1	A	B
2	C	D
3	A	B
4	C	D

Weeks	1	2
5	B	A
6	D	C
7	B	A
8	D	C

PRESCRIPTION

Week	Sets	Repetitions	Weight/Progression	Rest Set/Exercise
1	3	8	T.B.D.	:75 / :90
2	3	10	Same	:75 / :75
3	3	12	Same	:75 / :75
4	3	15	Same	:90 / :75
5	4	6	Up weight 10%	:75 / :90
6	4	8	Same	:75 / :90
7	4	10	Same	:75 / :90
8	4	12	Same	:90 / :90

EXERCISE SEQUENCE

Order	Workout A	Workout B	Workout C	Workout D
1	Lunge	Ab Wheel	Dead Lift	Push-up
2	Ab Wheel	Push-up	Chin-up	Dead Lift
3	Chin-up	Dead Lift	Lunge	Chin-up
4	Dead Lift	Lunge	Push-up	Lunge
5	Push-up	Chin-up	Ab Wheel	Ab Wheel

Notes: There must be at least 1 day between workouts; 2–3 is optimal (e.g., Mon-Thurs or Tues-Fri).

PROGRAM III

ADVANCED

WORKOUTS

A weeks 1, 3, 8	B weeks 2, 5	C weeks 4, 6	D weeks 2, 4, 7
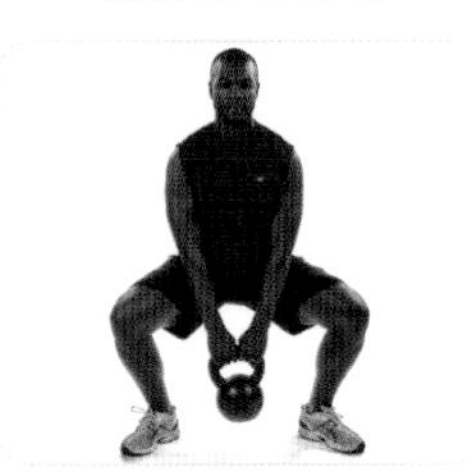 Sumo with Kettlebell page 18	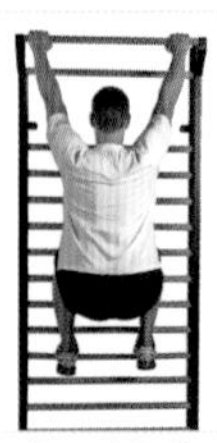 Stand-Pull page 98	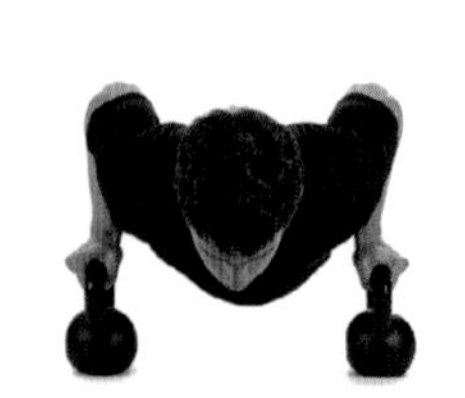 Push-up on Kettlebells page 76	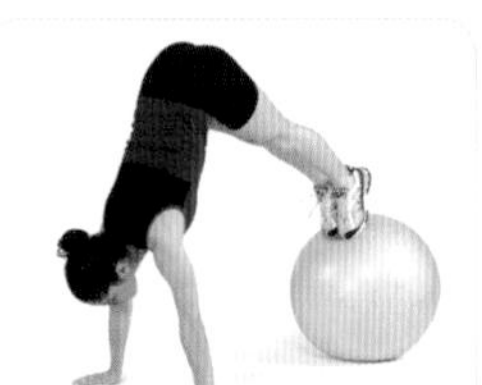 Plank to Pike page 128
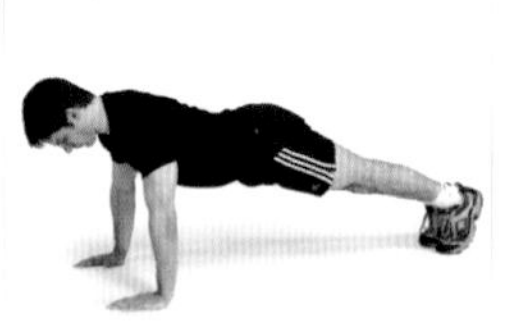 Basic Push-up page 60	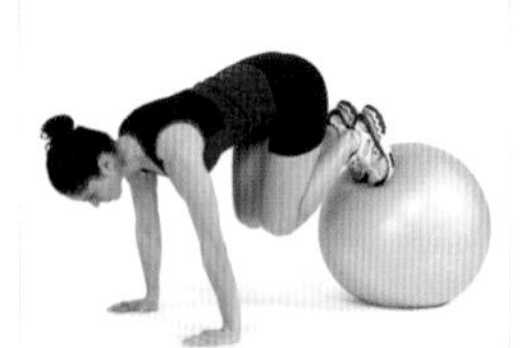 Plough on Physio Ball page 112	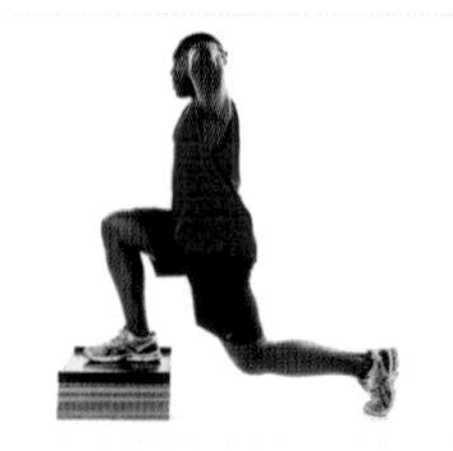 Up to Box page 54	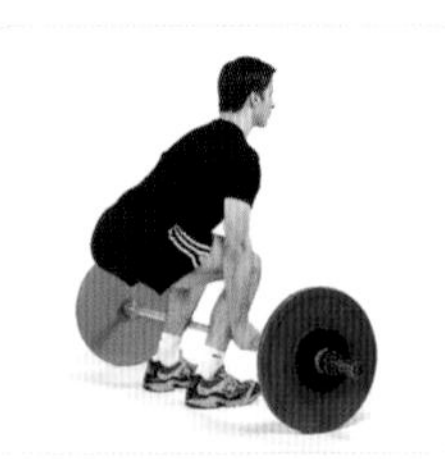 Full with Barbells page 14
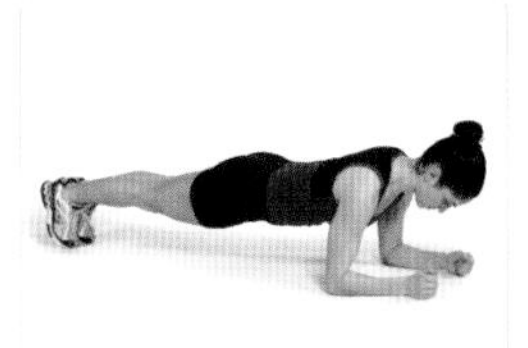 Front Plank page 126	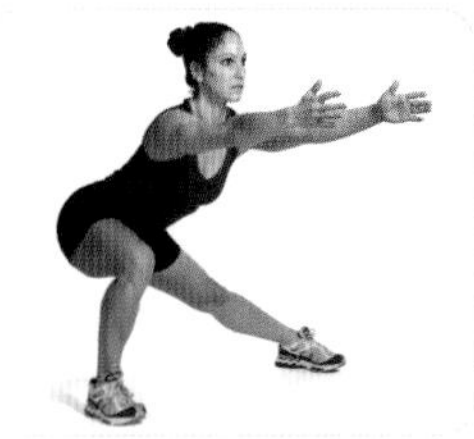 Lateral Lunge page 42	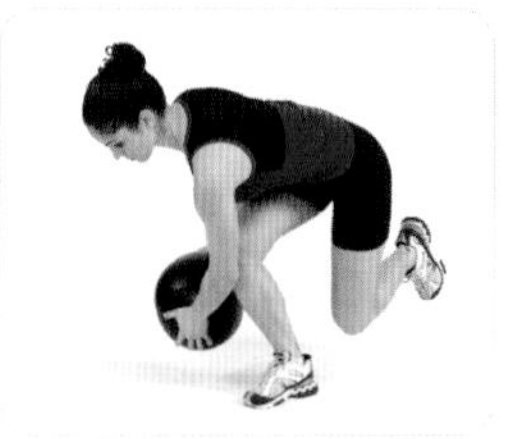 PNF Raise with Medicine Ball page 26	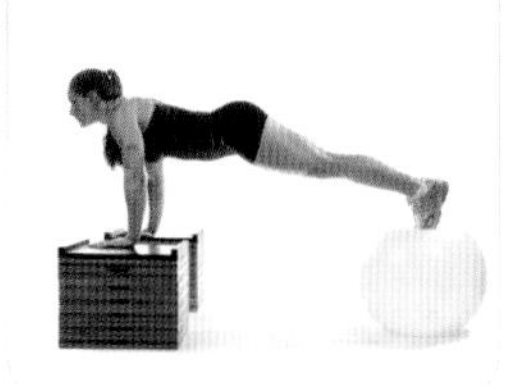 On Physio Ball & Blocks page 64
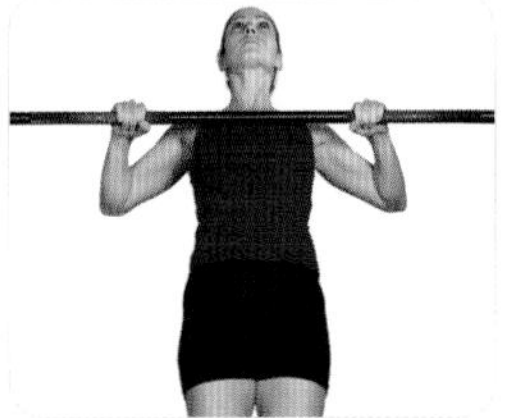 45° Body Row page 90	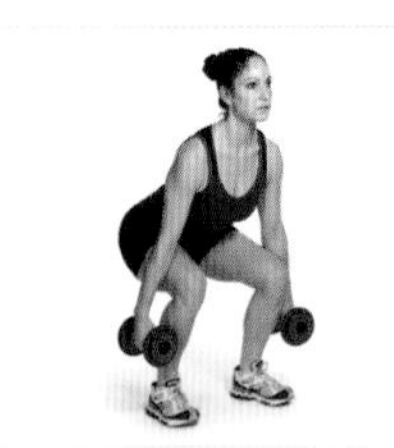 Full with Dumbbells page 15	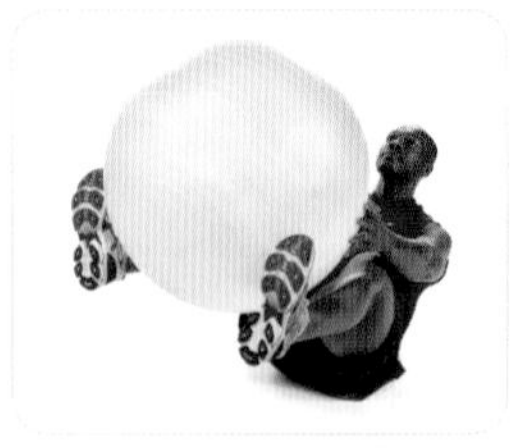 V-ups with Physio Ball page 122	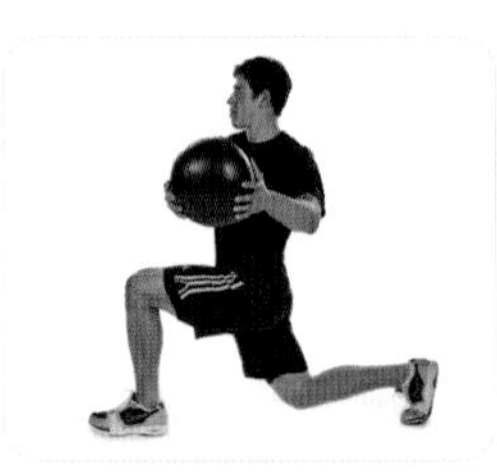 Walking with Rotation page 40
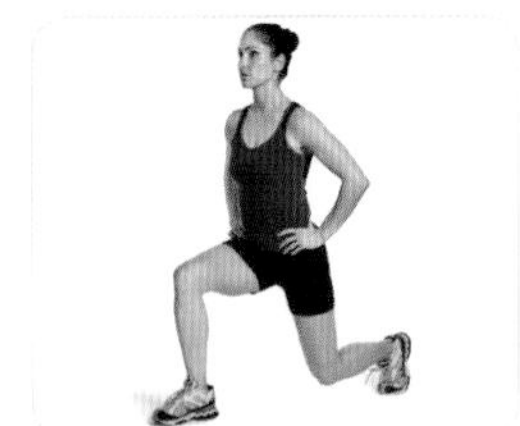 Stationary Lunge page 38	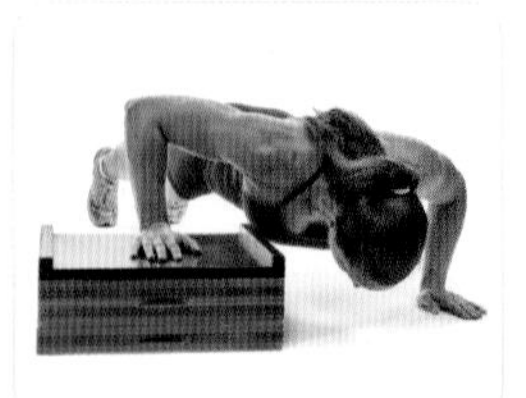 Hand Walkover page 78	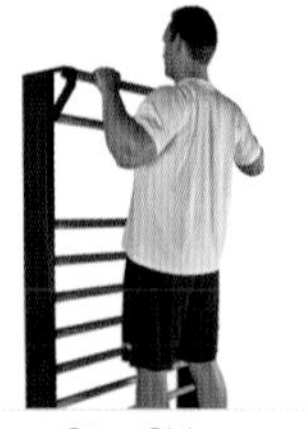 Step Chin page 100	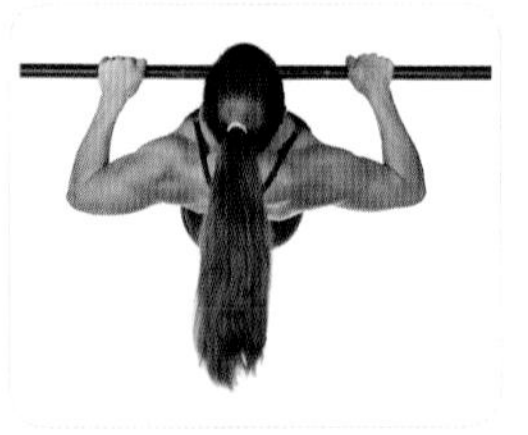 Horizontal Body Row page 92

E
weeks 1, 5, 8

F
weeks 3, 6, 7

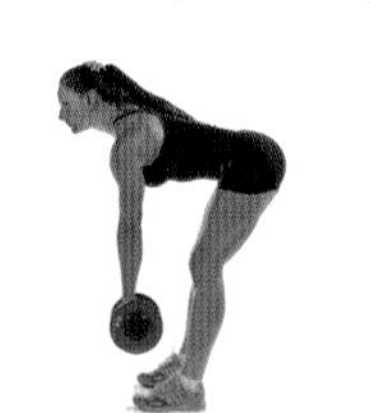

Straight-leg with Dumbbell
page 22

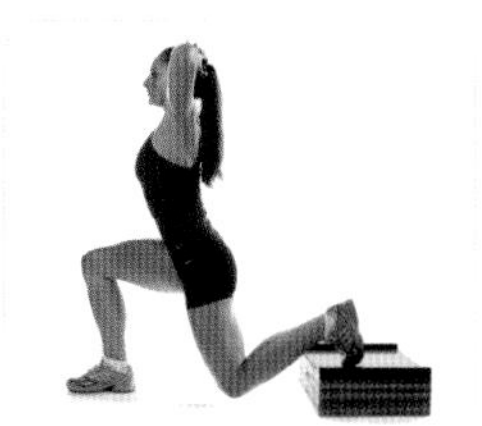

Off Box
page 56

Plough with Rotation
page 114

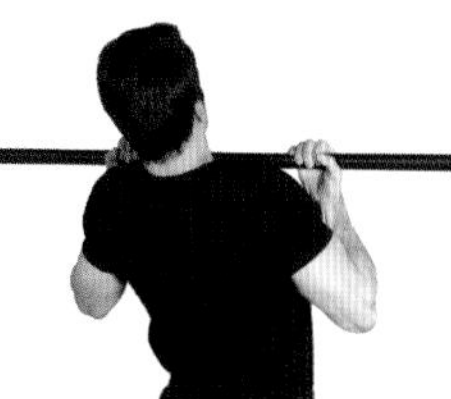

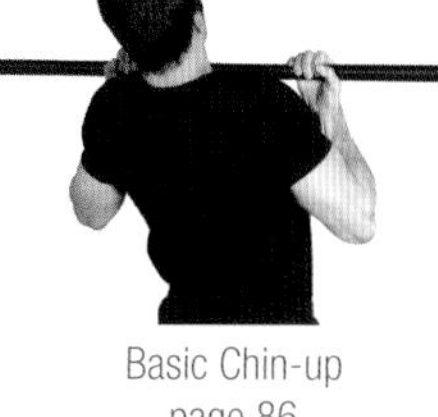

Basic Chin-up
page 86

45° Towel Slide
page 44

Hands on Rings
page 80

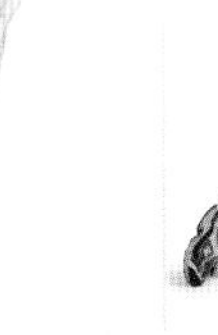

Pull-up Grip
page 88

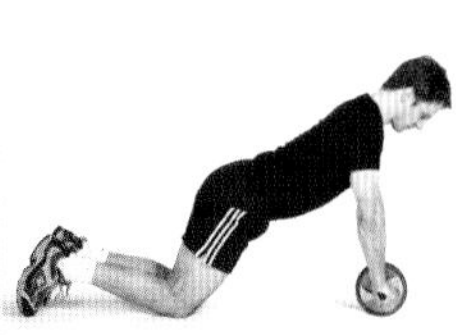

Ab Wheel
page 110

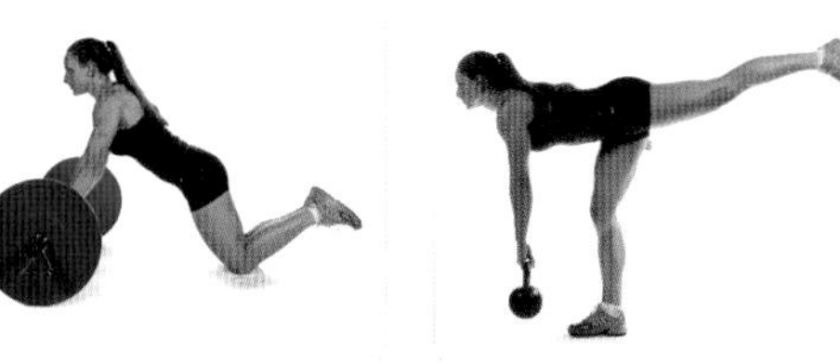

Push-up & Roll-out
page 62

Single-leg / Straight Leg with Kettlebell page 24

PROGRAM III • ADVANCED

PROGRAM: III DURATION: 8 WEEKS

Days per week: 2
Total weeks: 8
Type: Advanced Cardiovascular Endurance

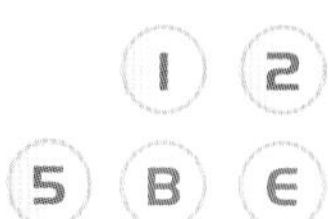

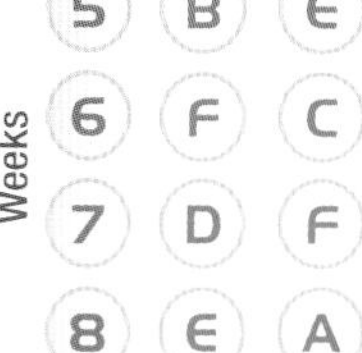

Weeks	1	2
1	A	E
2	B	D
3	F	A
4	C	D

Weeks	1	2
5	B	E
6	F	C
7	D	F
8	E	A

PRESCRIPTION

Week	Sets	Repetitions	Weight/Progression	Rest Set/Exercise
1	5	6	T.B.D.	:60 / 0
2	5	6	Same	:45 / 0
3	5	8	Same	:60 / 0
4	5	8	Same	:45 / 0
5	5	10	Same	:60 / 0
6	5	10	Same	:45 / 0
7	5	12	Same	:60 / 0
8	5	12	same	:45 / 0

EXERCISE SEQUENCE

Workout

Order	A	B	C	D	E	F
1	Dead Lift	Chin-up	Push-up	Ab Wheel	Dead Lift	Lunge
2	Push-up	Ab Wheel	Lunge	Dead Lift	Ab Wheel	Chin-up
3	Ab Wheel	Lunge	Dead Lift	Push-up	Lunge	Push-up
4	Chin-up	Dead Lift	Ab Wheel	Lunge	Chin-up	Ab Wheel
5	Lunge	Push-up	Chin-up	Chin-up	Push-up	Dead Lift

Notes: Exercises in this program are to be done in "circuit" fashion. There is no rest between exercises. All 5 movements are to be done consecutively with rest to be taken between rounds or groups.

PROGRAM IV

BEGINNER

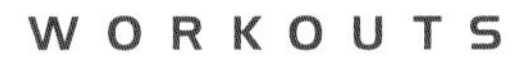

WORKOUTS

A
weeks 1–6

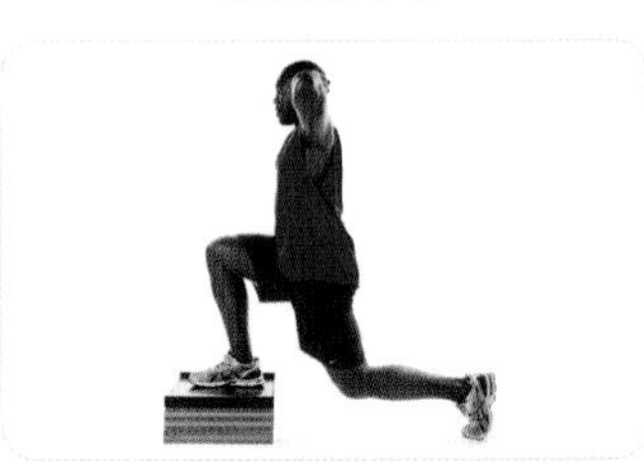

Up to Box
page 54

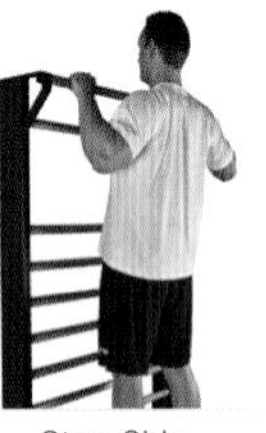

Step Chin
page 100

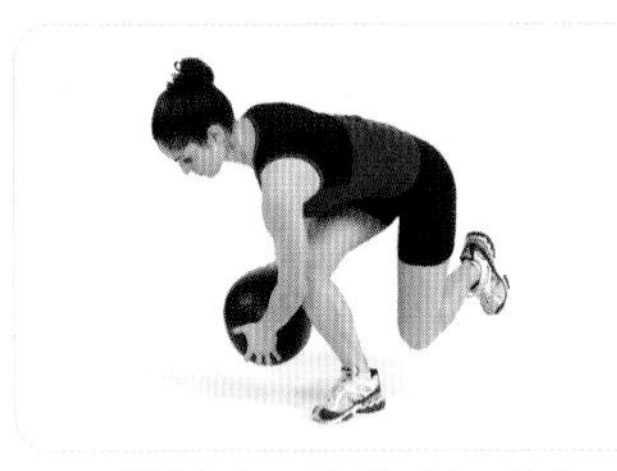

PNF Raise with Medicine Ball
page 26

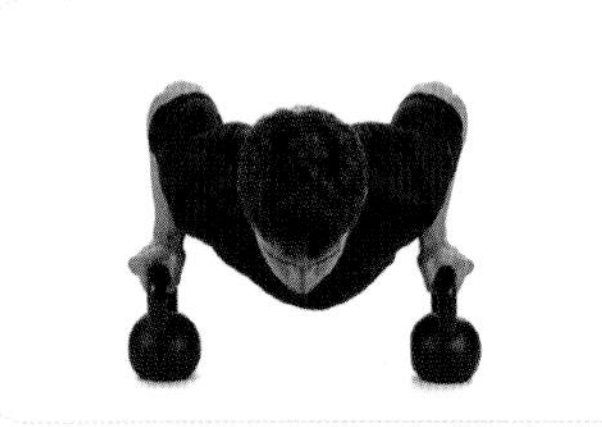

Push-up on Kettlebells
page 76

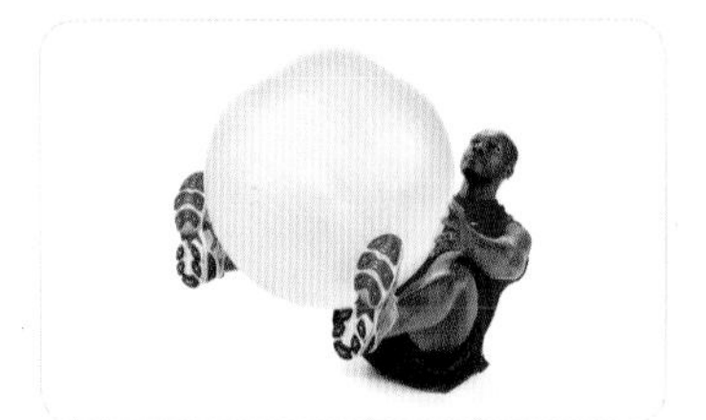

V-ups with Physio Ball
page 122

B
weeks 1–6

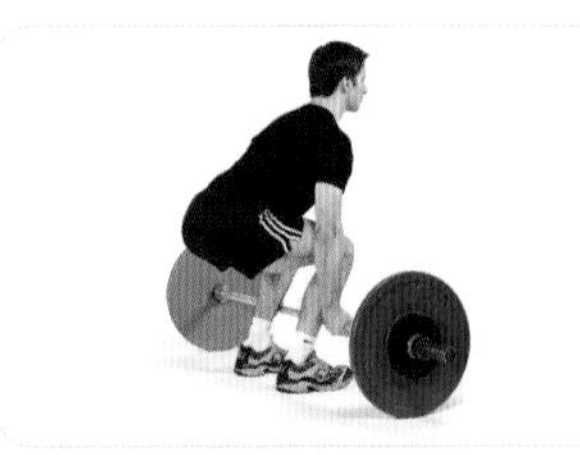

Full with Barbells
page 14

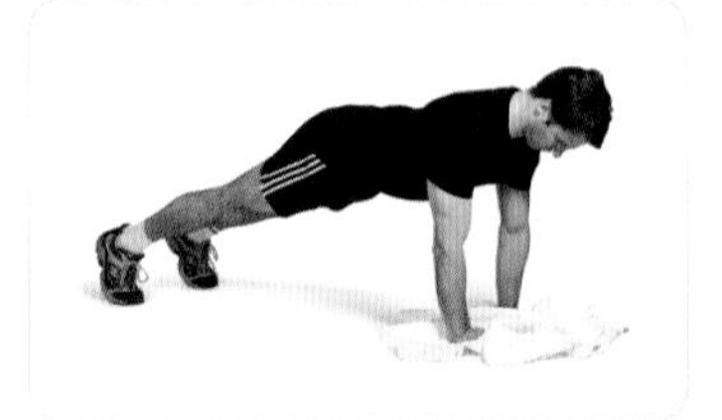

Towel Fly
page 68

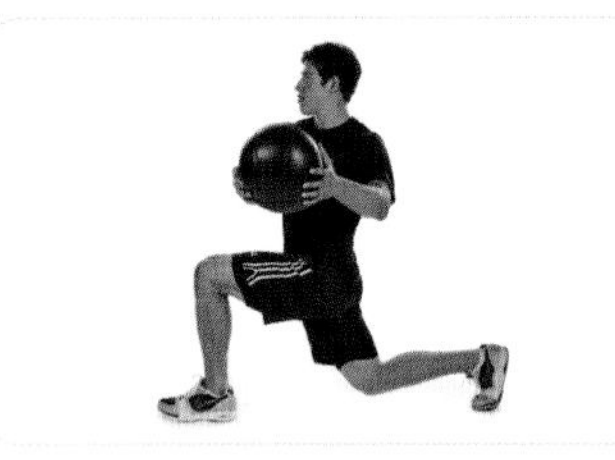

Walking Lunge with Rotation
page 40

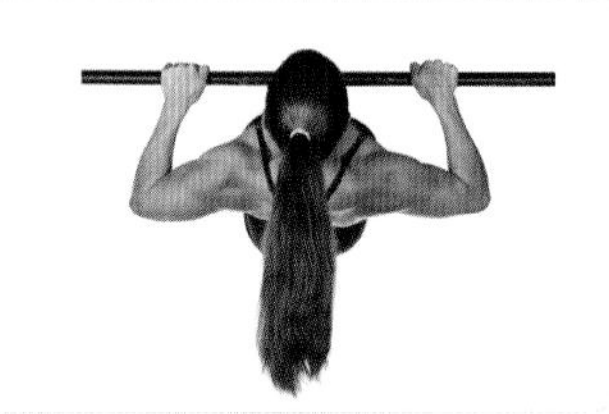

Horizontal Body Row
page 92

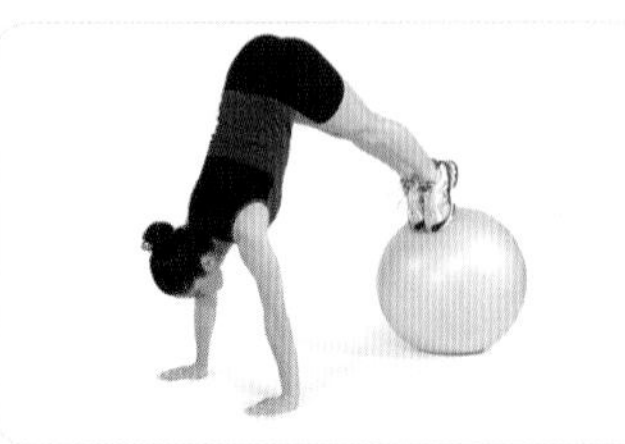

Plank to Pike
page 128

C
weeks 1–6

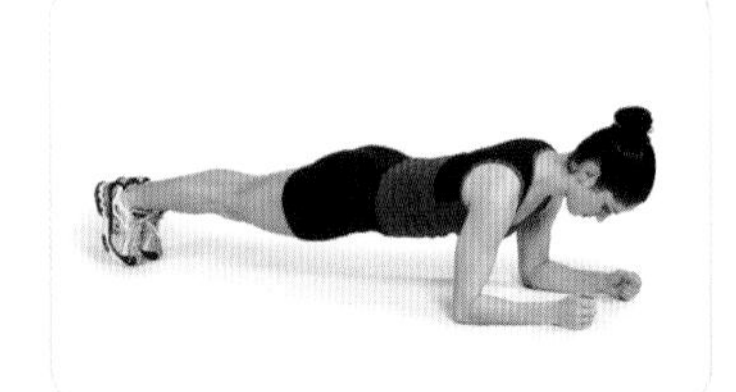

Front Plank
page 126

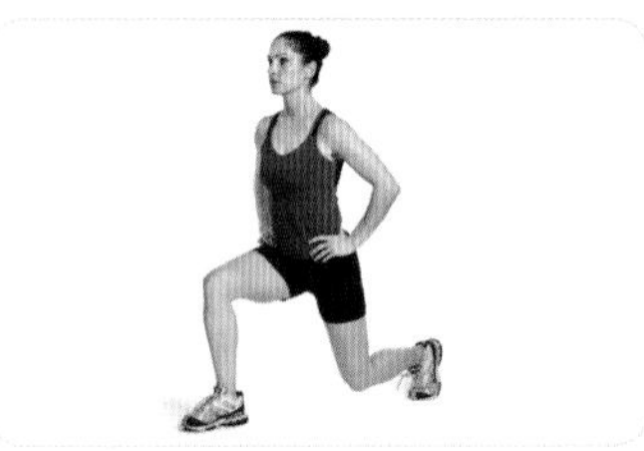

Stationary Lunge
page 38

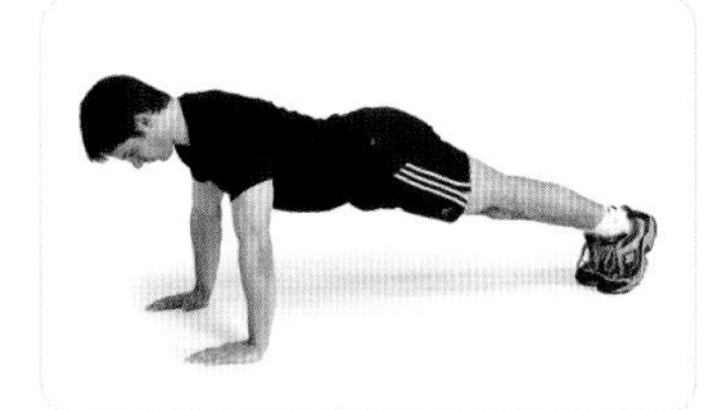

Basic Push-up
page 60

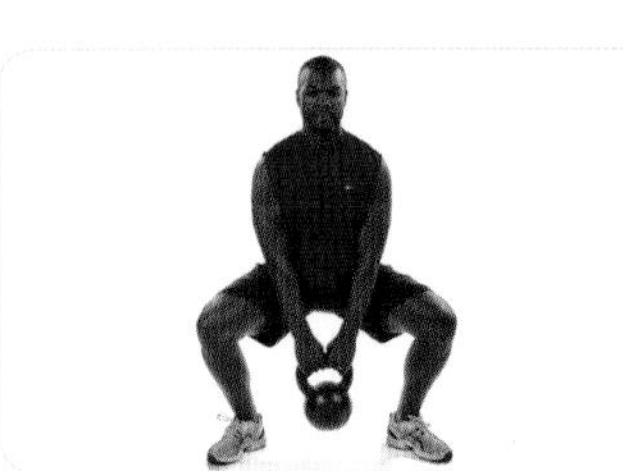

Sumo with Kettlebell
page 18

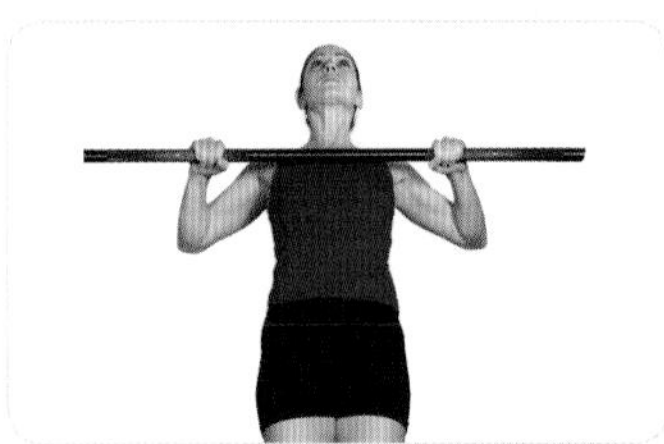

45° Body Row
page 90

PROGRAM IV • BEGINNER

USER NOTES

PROGRAM: IV DURATION: 6 WEEKS

Days per week: 3
Total weeks: 6
Type: Strength/Endurance

Weeks	Day 1	Day 2	Day 3
1	C	A	D
2	C	A	D
3	C	A	D
4	D	C	A
5	D	C	A
6	D	C	A

PRESCRIPTION

Week	Sets	Repetitions	Weight/Progression	Rest Set/Exercise
1	3	10	T.B.D.	:120 / :120
2	3	8	Increase 10% BW 2–5 reps	:90 / :120
3	3	6	Increase 10% BW 2–5 reps	:120 / :120
4	3	8	Same as week 3	:90 / :120
5	3	10	Same as week 3	:90 / :90
6	3	12	Same as week 3	:75 / :90

EXERCISE SEQUENCE

Order	Workout A	Workout B	Workout C
1	Lunge	Dead Lift	Ab Wheel
2	Chin-up	Push-up	Lunge
3	Dead Lift	Lunge	Push-up
4	Push-up	Chin-up	Dead Lift
5	Ab Wheel	Ab Wheel	Chin-up

Notes: There must be at least 1 day between workouts. This program is optimally suited for Mon-Wed-Fri training.

INTERMEDIATE

PROGRAM V

WORKOUTS

A
weeks 1, 3, 5

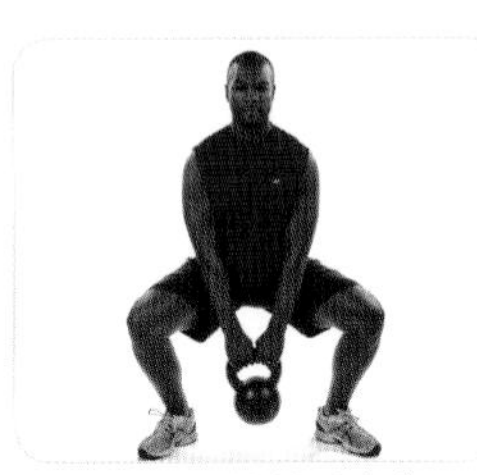
Sumo with Kettlebell
page 18

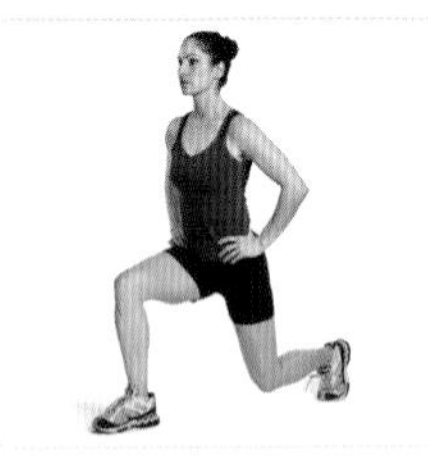
Stationary Lunge
page 38

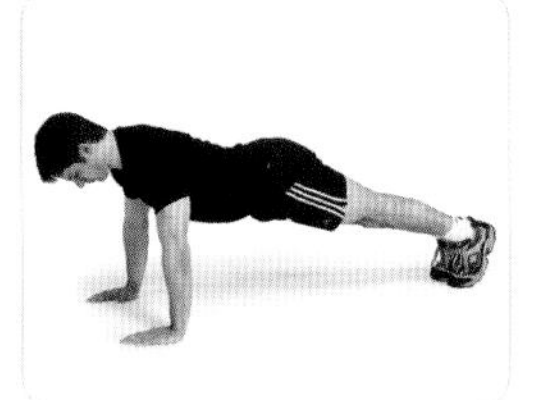
Basic Push-up
page 60

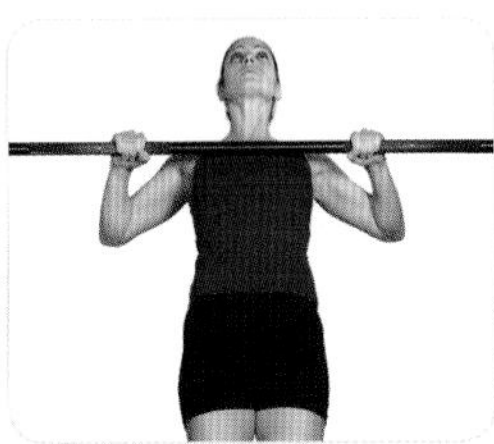
45° Body Row
page 90

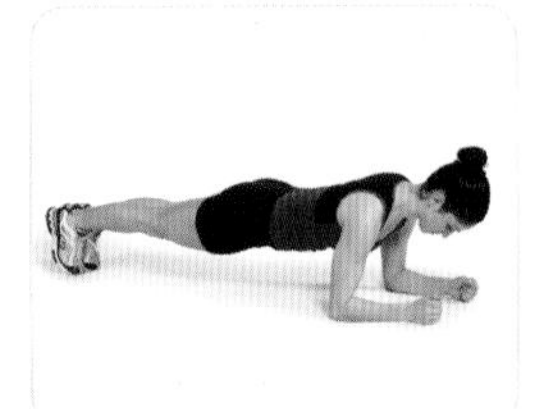
Front Plank
page 126

B
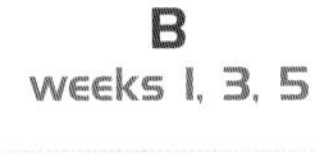
weeks 1, 3, 5

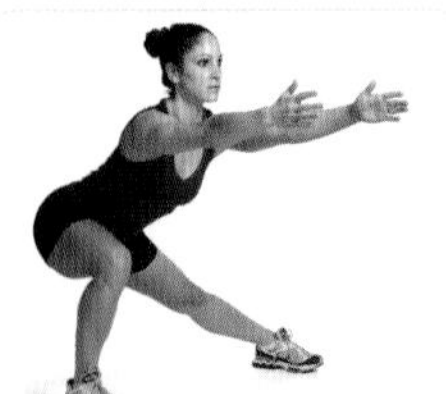
Lateral Lunge
page 42

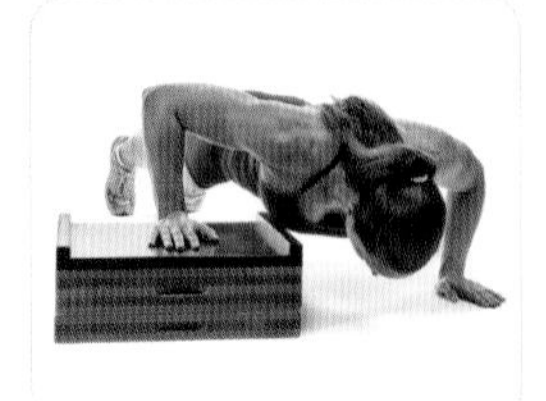
Hand Walkover
page 78

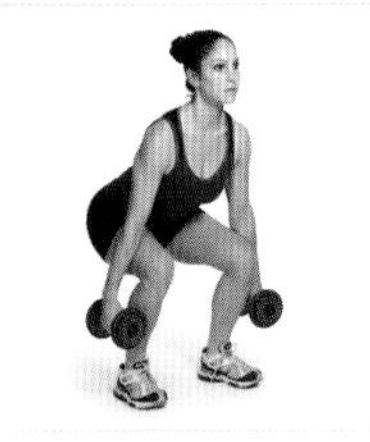
Full ith Dumbbells
page 15

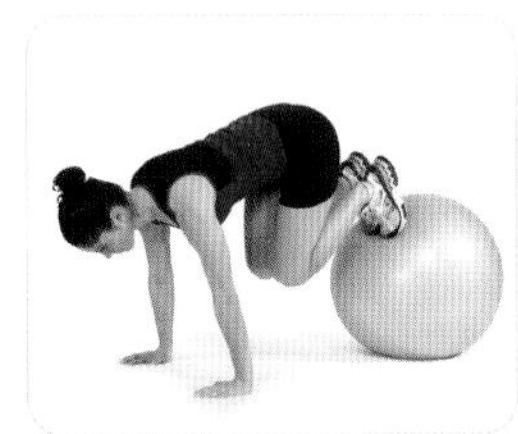
Plough on Physio Ball
page 112

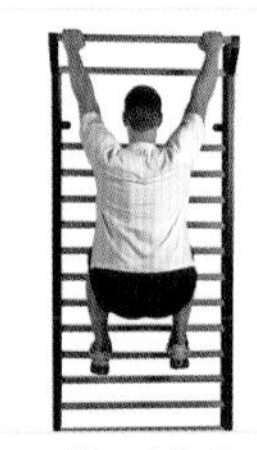
Stand-Pull
page 98

C
weeks 1, 3, 5

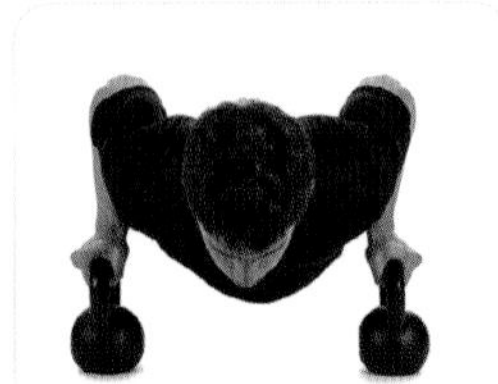
Push-up on Kettlebells
page 76

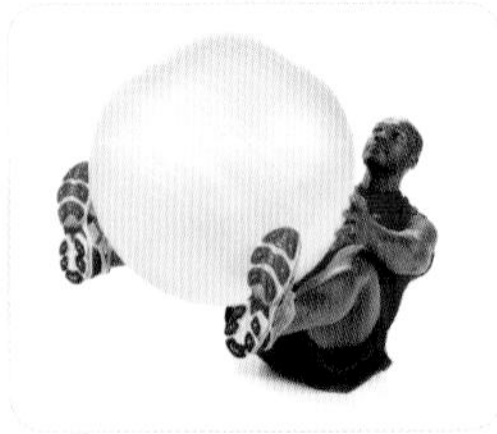
V-ups with Physio Ball
page 122

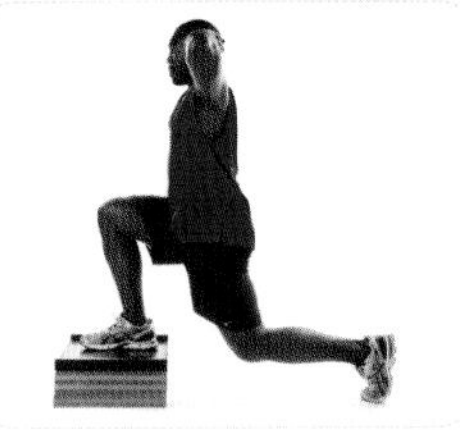
Up to Box
page 54

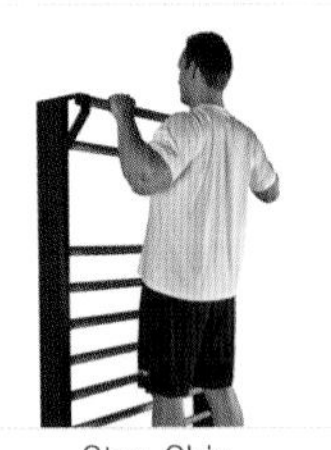
Step Chin
page 100

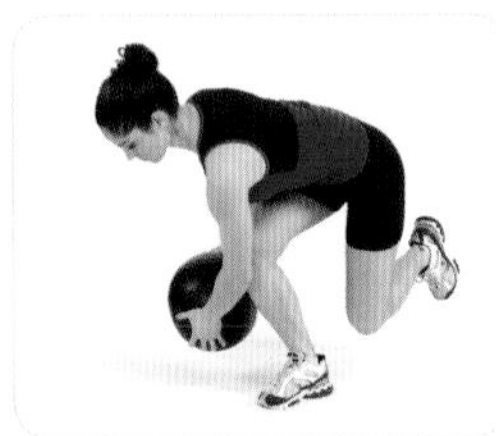
PNF Raise with Medicine Ball
page 26

D
weeks 2, 4, 6

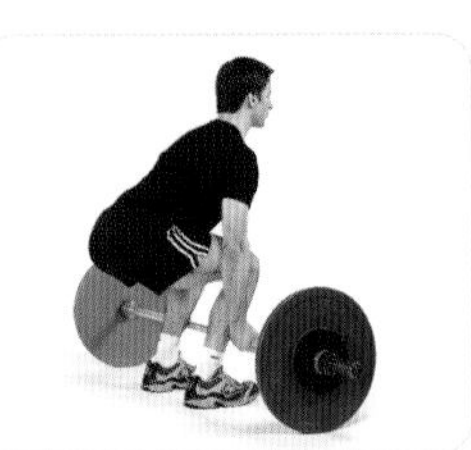
Full with Barbells
page 14

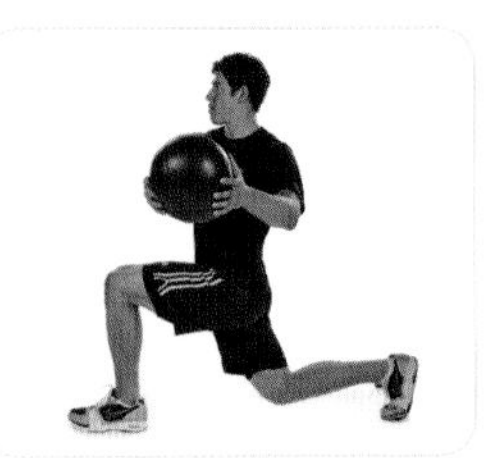
Walking with Rotation
page 40

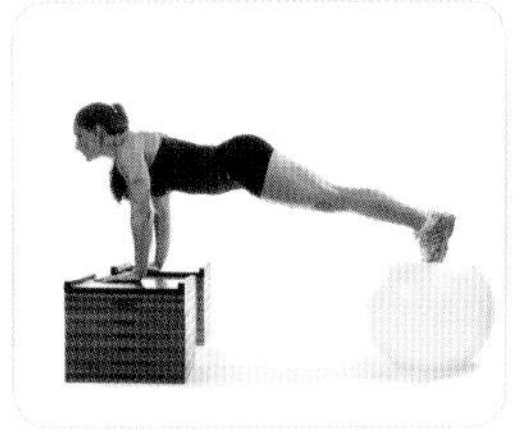
On Physio Ball & Blocks
page 64

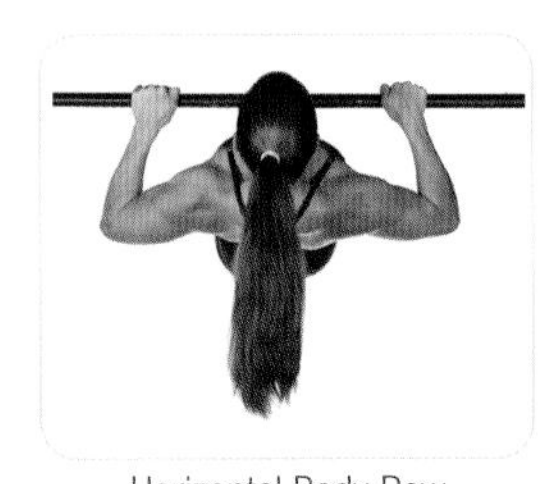
Horizontal Body Row
page 92

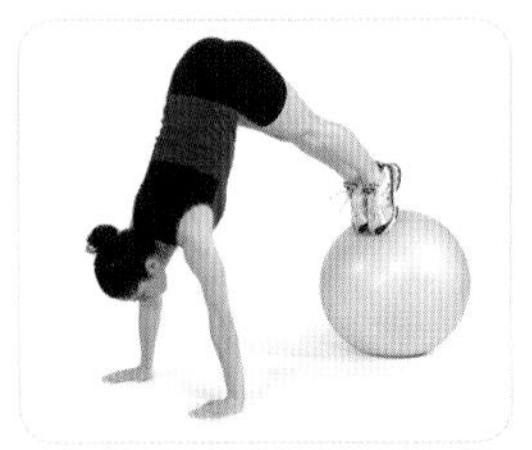
Plank to Pike
page 128

PROGRAM V • INTERMEDIATE

E
weeks 2, 4, 6

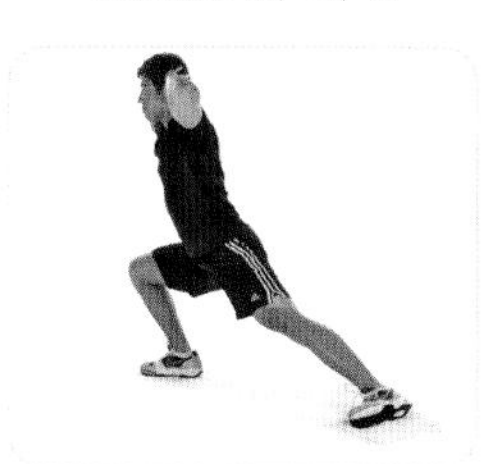

45º Towel Slide
page 44

Push-up & Roll-out
page 62

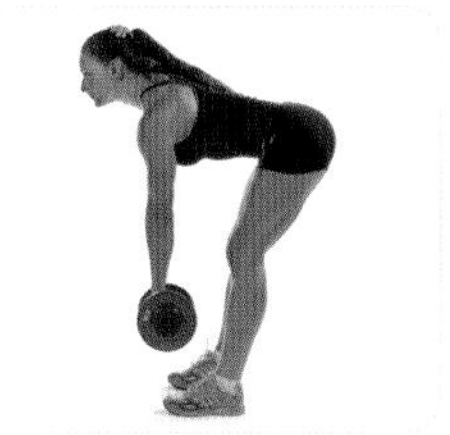

Straight-leg with Dumbbell
page 22

Plough with Rotation
page 114

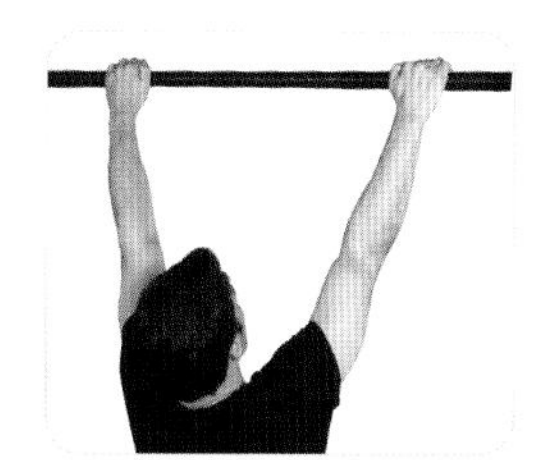

Pull-up Grip
page 88

F
weeks 2, 4, 6

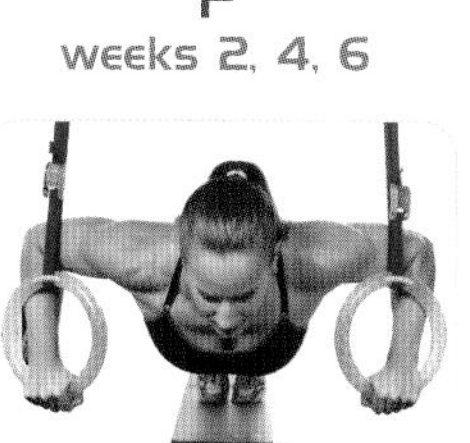

Hands on Rings
page 80

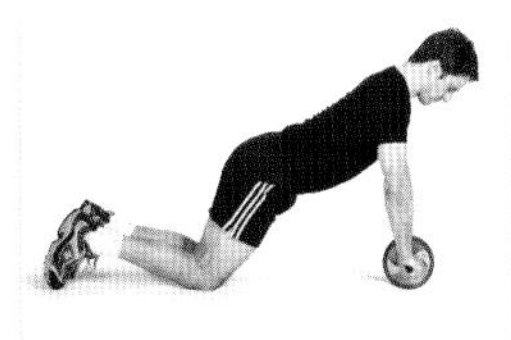

Ab Wheel
page 110

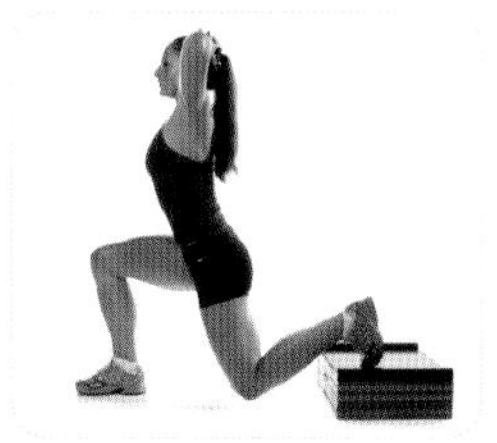

Off Box
page 56

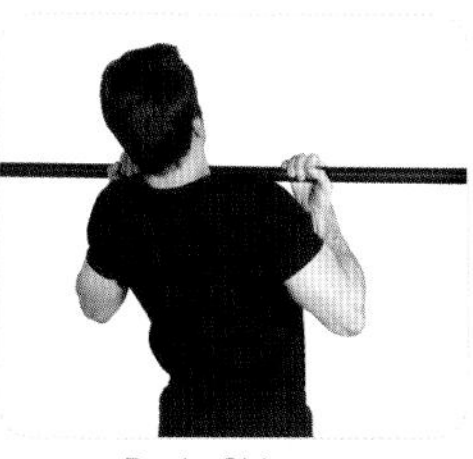

Basic Chin-up
page 86

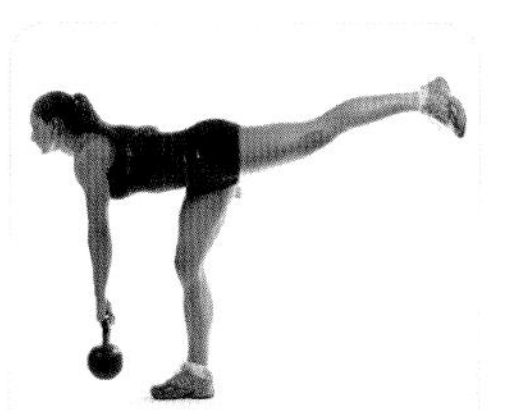

Single-leg / Straight-leg with Kettlebell page 24

PROGRAM: V DURATION: 6 WEEKS

Days per week: 3
Total weeks: 6
Type: Intermediate Endurance

Weeks	Day 1	Day 2	Day 3
1	A	B	C
2	D	E	F
3	A	B	C
4	D	E	F
5	A	B	C
6	D	E	F

PRESCRIPTION

Week	Sets	Repetitions	Weight/Progression	Rest Set/Exercise
1	3	10	T.B.D.	:75 / :90
2	3	10	T.B.D.	:60 / :75
3	4	8	Same as week 1	:60 / :75
4	4	8	Same as week 2	:60 / :75
5	4	10	Same as week 3	:60 / :60
6	4	10	Same as week 4	:60 / :60

EXERCISE SEQUENCE

Order	A	B	C	D	E	F
1	Dead Lift	Lunge	Push-up	Dead Lift	Lunge	Push-up
2	Lunge	Push-up	Ab Wheel	Lunge	Push-up	Ab Wheel
3	Push-up	Dead Lift	Lunge	Push-up	Dead Lift	Lunge
4	Chin-up	Ab Wheel	Chin-up	Chin-up	Ab Wheel	Chin-up
5	Ab Wheel	Chin-up	Dead Lift	Ab Wheel	Chin-up	Dead Lift

Notes: Due to the volume and intensity of work, a 2-day rest between workouts is acceptable, with variability week to week depending upon the body's ability to recover.

ADVANCED

PROGRAM VI

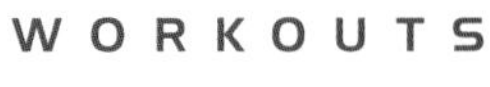

D
weeks 1–4

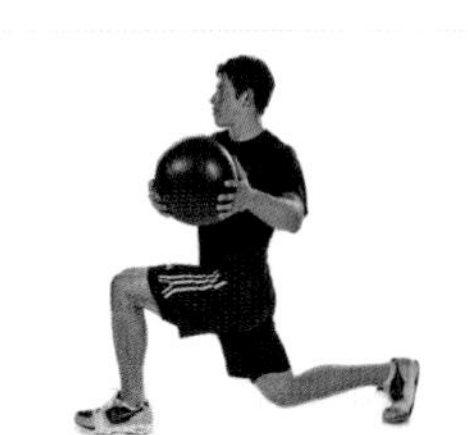
Walking with Rotation
page 40

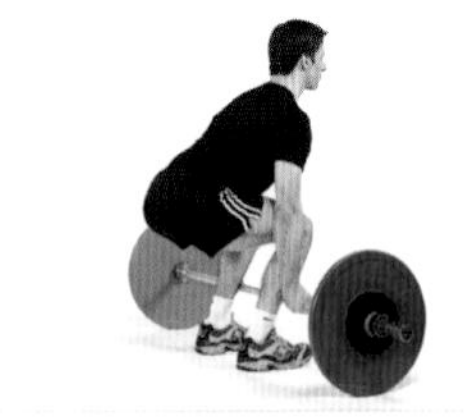
Full with Barbells
page 14

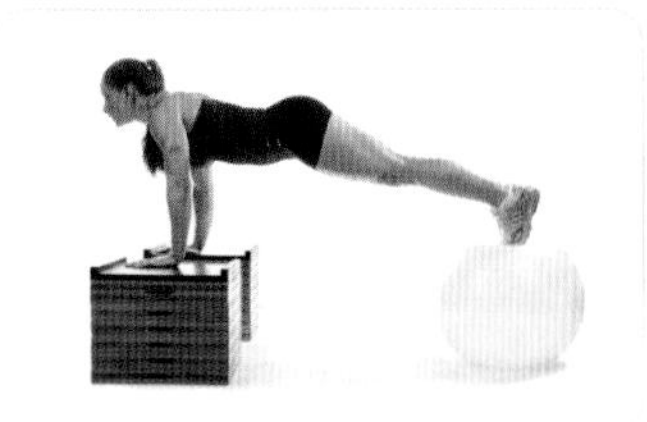
On Physio Ball & Blocks
page 64

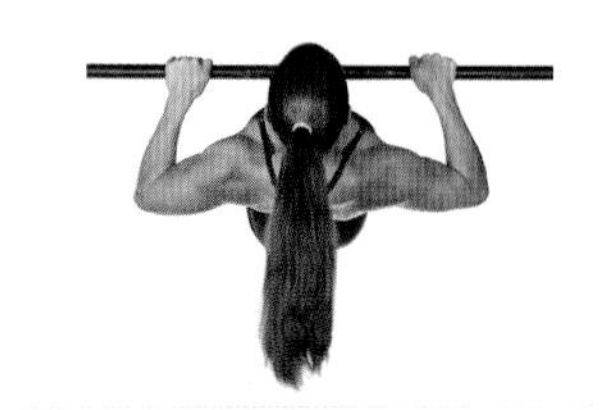
Horizontal Body Row
page 92

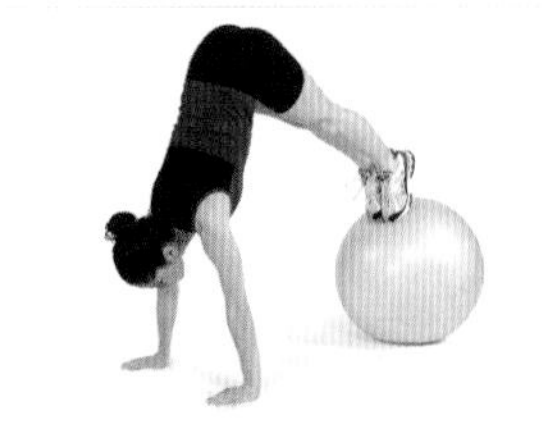
Plank to Pike
page 128

E
weeks 1–4

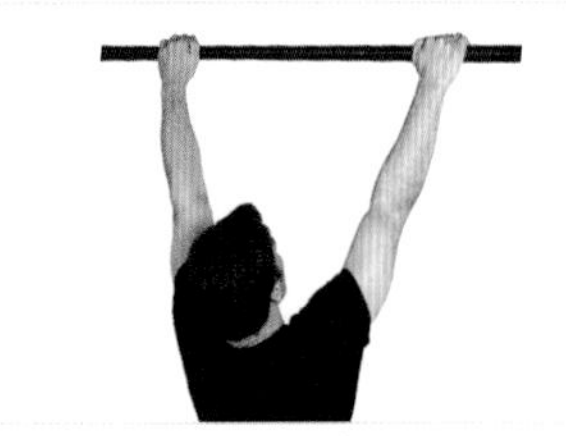
Pull-up Grip
page 88

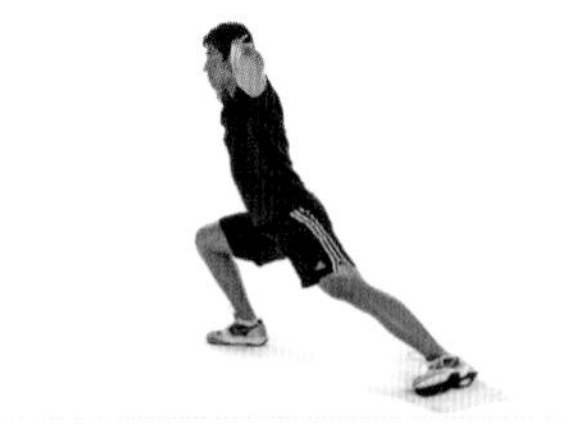
45º Towel Slide
page 44

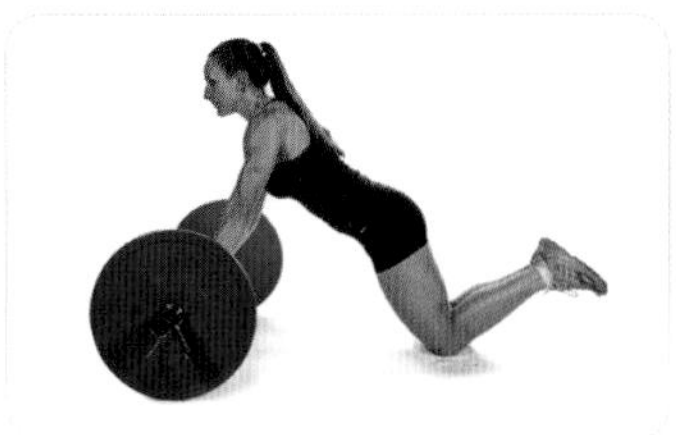
Push-up & Roll-out
page 62

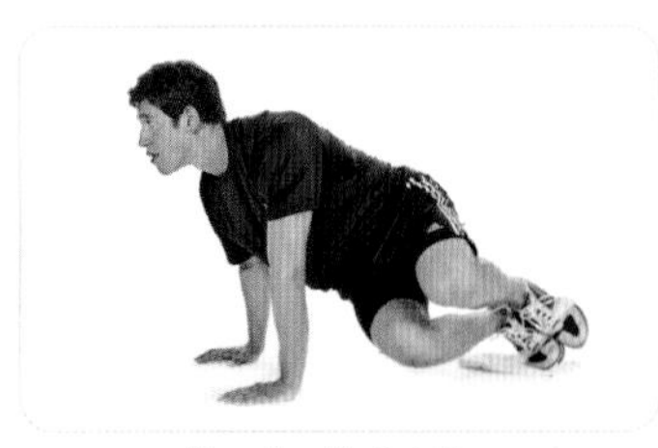
Plough with Rotation
page 114

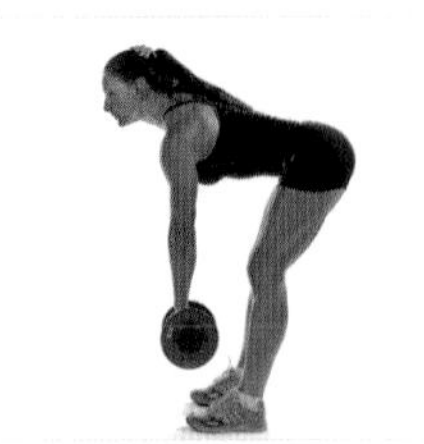
Straight-leg with Dumbbell
page 22

F
weeks 1–4

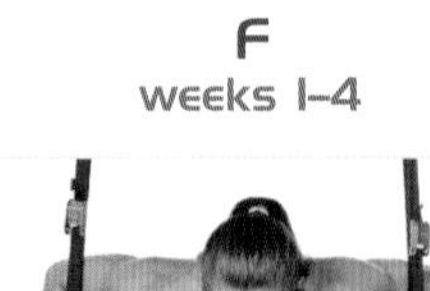
Hands on Rings
page 80

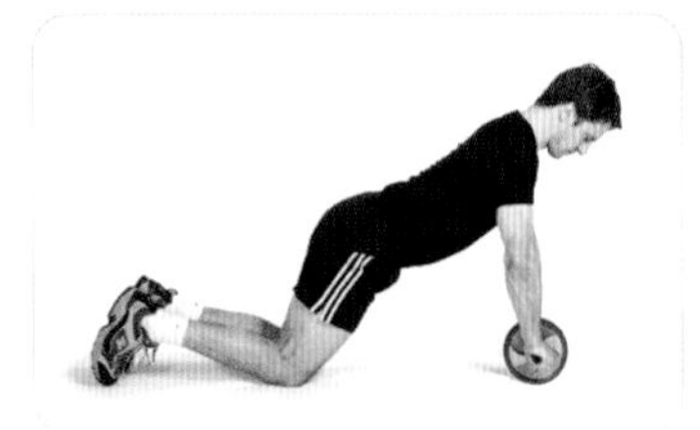
Ab Wheel
page 110

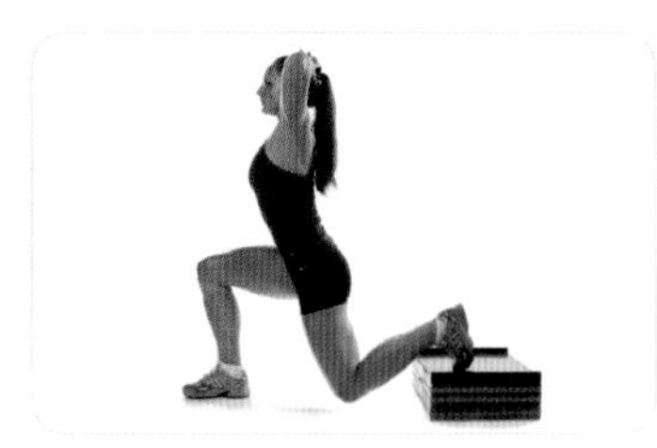
Off Box
page 56

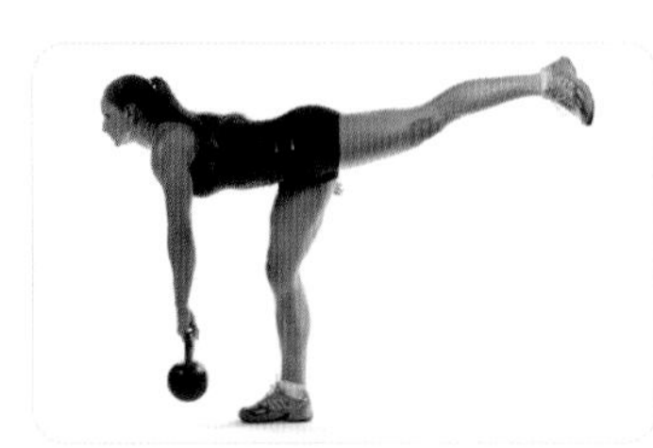
Single-leg / Straight Leg with Kettlebell
page 24

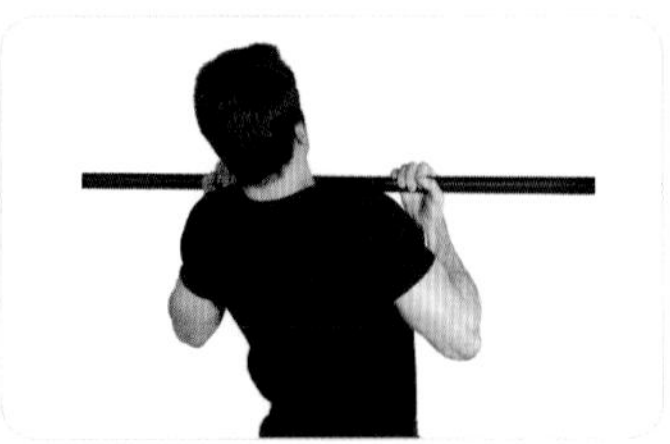
Basic Chin-up
page 86

USER NOTES

PROGRAM VI • ADVANCED

PROGRAM: VI DURATION: 4 WEEKS

Days per week: 3
Total weeks: 4
Type: Advanced Strength

Weeks \ Days	1	2	3
1	D	E	F
2	D	E	F
3	D	E	F
4	D	E	F

PRESCRIPTION

Week	Sets	Repetitions	Weight/Progression	Rest Set/Exercise
1	5	10	T.B.D.	:90 / :120
2	5	8	Up weight by 15% BW 5 reps	:90 / :120
3	5	6	Up weight 10–15% BW 5–10 reps	:120 / :120
4	5	10	Same as week 1	:90 / :90

EXERCISE SEQUENCE

Order	Workout D	Workout E	Workout F
1	Lunge	Chin-up	Push-up
2	Dead Lift	Lunge	Ab Wheel
3	Push-up	Push-up	Lunge
4	Chin-up	Ab Wheel	Dead Lift
5	Ab Wheel	Dead Lift	Chin-up

Notes: Due to the volume and intensity of these workouts, a 2-day rest between workouts is acceptable, with variability week to week depending upon the body's ability to recover (e.g., Week 1: Mon-Wed-Sat; Week 2: Mon-Thurs-Sun; Week 3 Tues-Thurs-Sat, etc.).

PROGRAM VII

BEGINNER

WORKOUTS

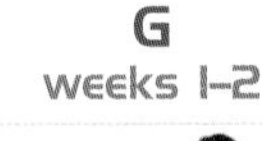
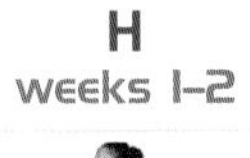

G weeks 1–2	H weeks 1–2	H weeks 3–4	G weeks 3–4
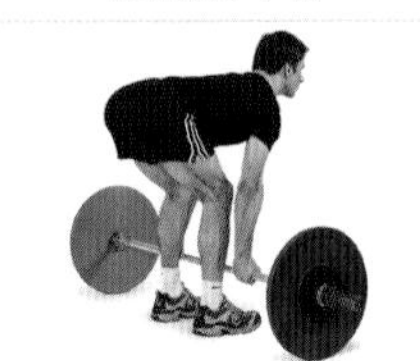 Straight-leg with Barbells page 16	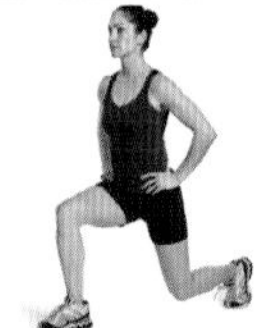 Stationary Lunge page 38	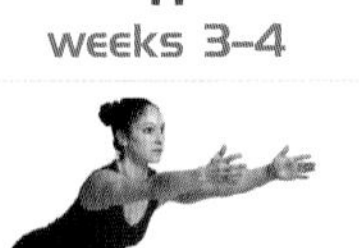 Lateral Lunge page 42	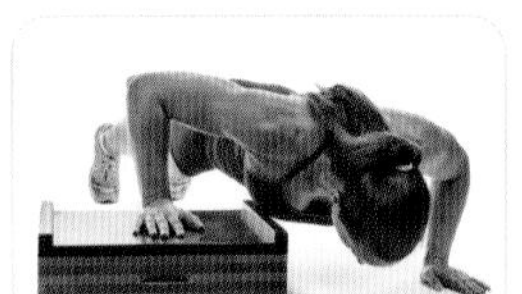 Hand Walkover page 78
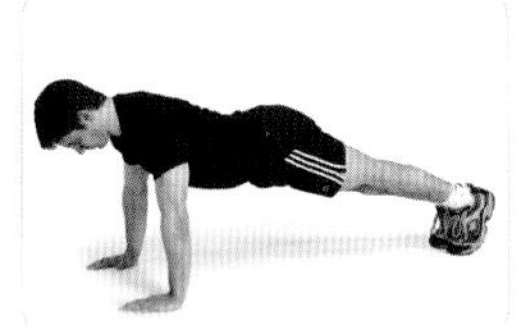 Basic Push-up page 60	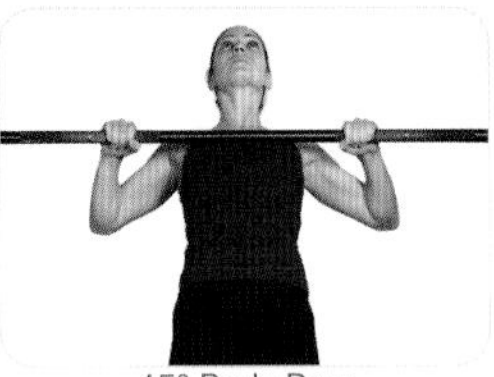 45º Body Row page 90	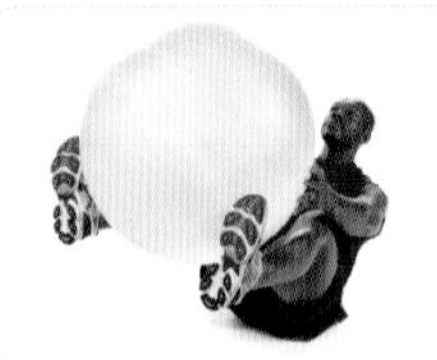 V-ups with Physio Ball page 122	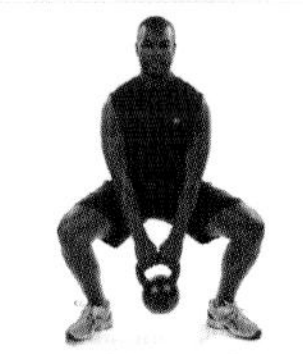 Sumo with Kettlebell page 18
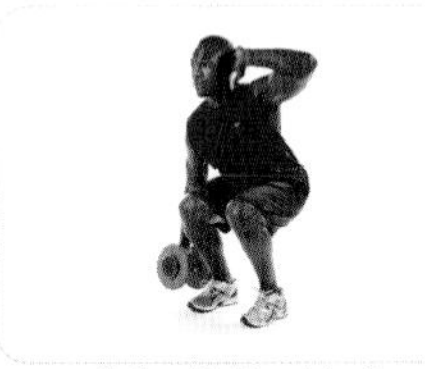 Full with Dumbbell page 34	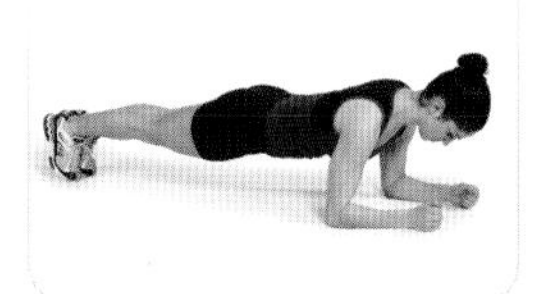 Front Plank page 126	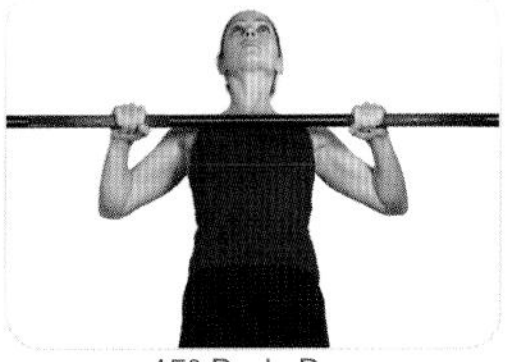 45º Body Row page 90	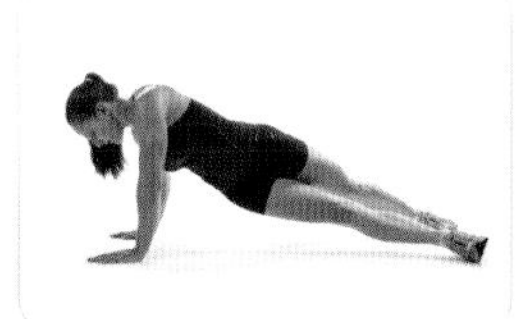 Lower Body Rotation page 72
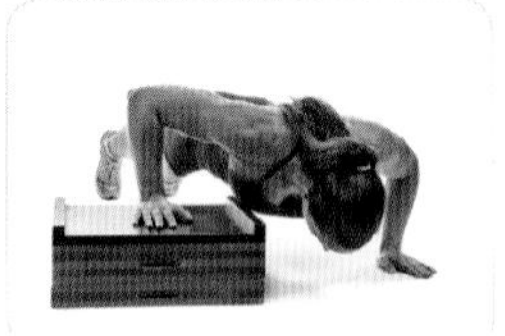 Hand Walkover page 78	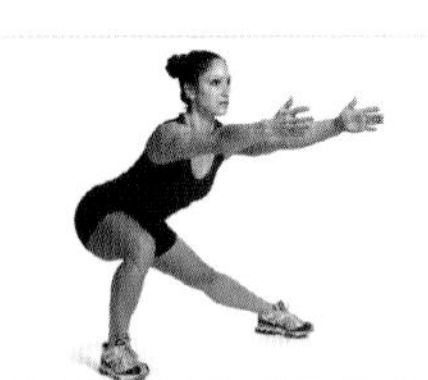 Lateral Lunge page 42	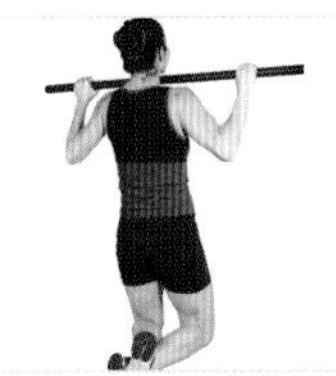 Pull-down Neutral Grip page 96	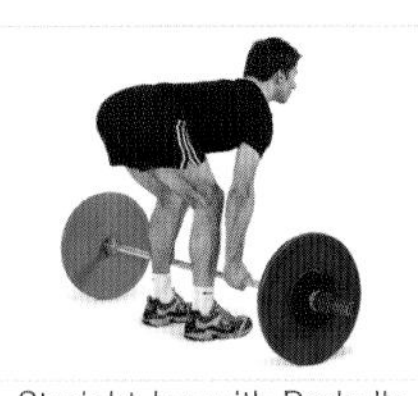 Straight-leg with Barbells page 16
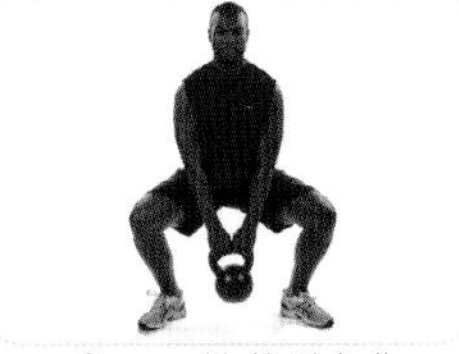 Sumo with Kettlebell page 18	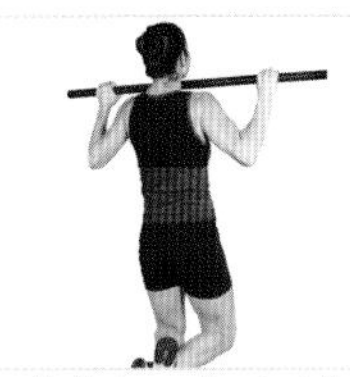 Pull-down Neutral Grip page 96	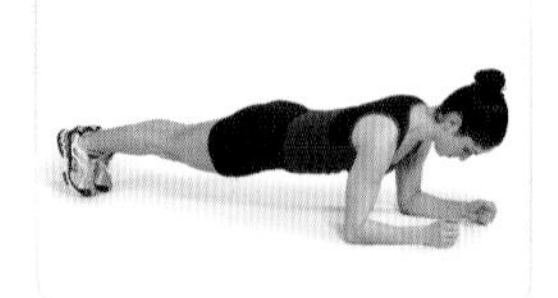 Front Plank page 126	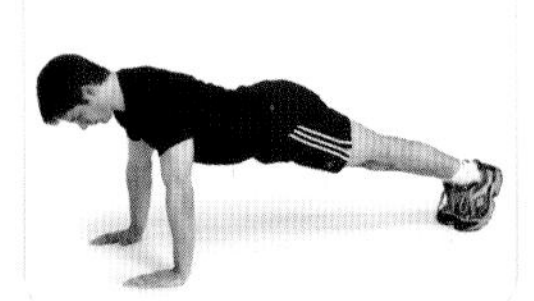 Basic Push-up page 60
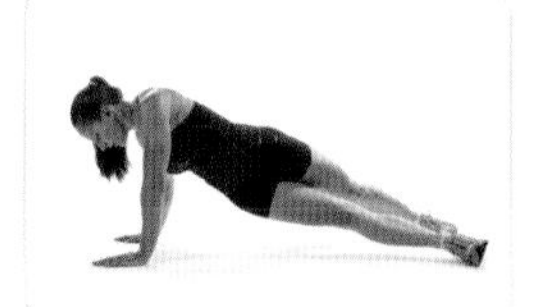 Lower Body Rotation page 72	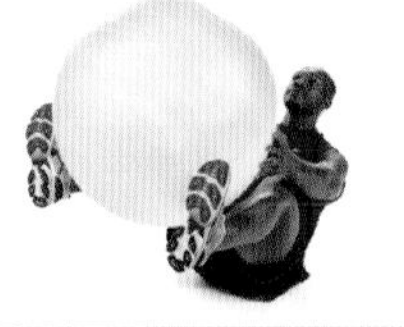 V-ups with Physio Ball page 122	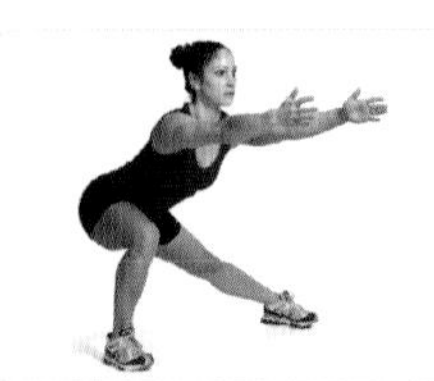 Lateral Lunge page 42	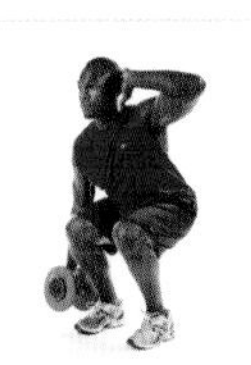 Full with Dumbbell page 34

PROGRAM VII • BEGINNER

USER NOTES

PROGRAM: VII DURATION: 4 WEEKS

Days per week: 4
Total weeks: 4
Type: Beginner

Weeks \ Days	1	2	3	4
1	G	H	G	H
2	G	H	G	H
3	H	G	H	G
4	H	G	H	G

PRESCRIPTION

Week	Sets	Repetitions	Weight/Progression	Rest Set/Exercise
1	2	10	T.B.D.	None / :60
2	2	12	Weights remain the same throughout program.	None / :60
3	2	15		None / :60
4	2	20		None / :75

EXERCISE SEQUENCE

Order \ Workout	G	H	H	G
1	Dead Lift	Lunge	Lunge	Push-up
2	Push-up	Chin-up	Ab Wheel	Dead Lift
3	Dead Lift	Ab Wheel	Chin-up	Push-up
4	Push-up	Lunge	Chin-up	Dead Lift
5	Dead Lift	Chin-up	Ab Wheel	Push-up
6	Push-up	Ab Wheel	Lunge	Dead Lift

Notes: Exercises are to be performed in pairs, or "supersets."
Complete 3 sets of the first two exercises, then 3 sets of the third and fourth exercises, and then finally move on to the fifth and sixth exercises.

PROGRAM VIII

WORKOUTS

I
weeks 1–4

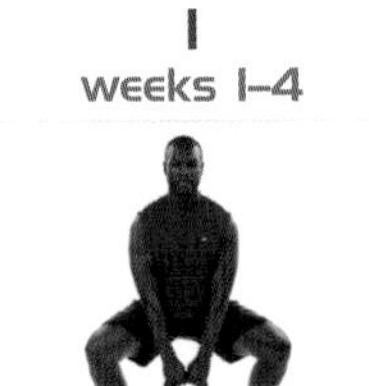
Sumo with Kettlebell
page 18

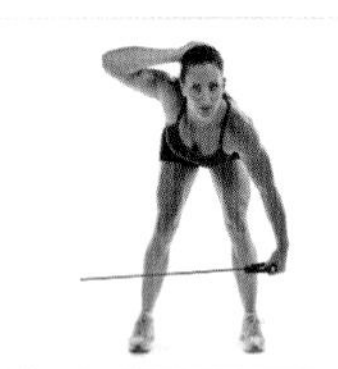
Straight-leg Cable
page 30

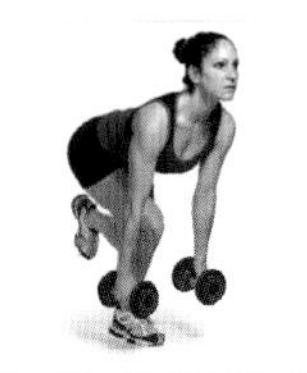
Full Single-leg with Dumbbells
page 20

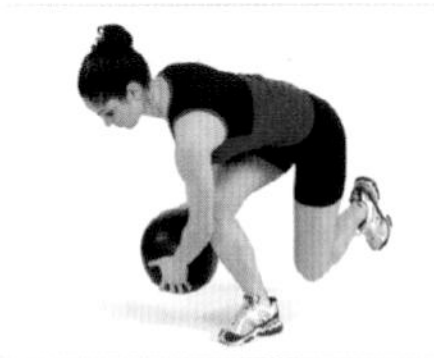
PNF Raise with Medicine Ball
page 26

J
weeks 1–4

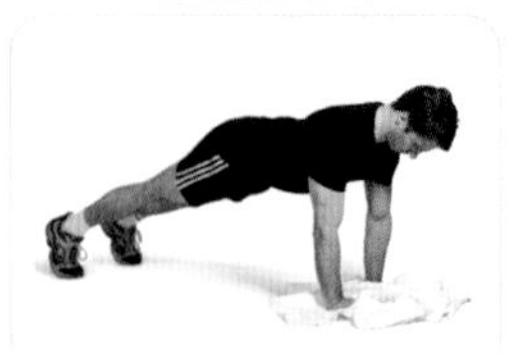
Towel Fly
page 68

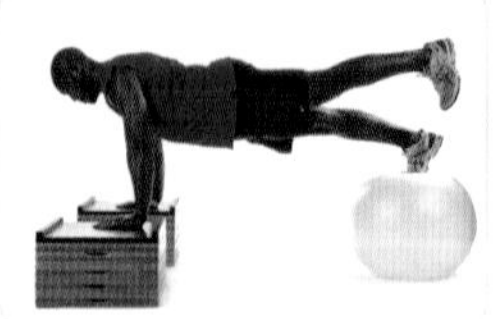
On Physio Ball & Blocks
page 65

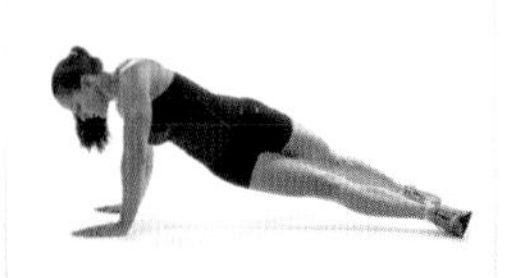
Lower Body Rotation
page 72

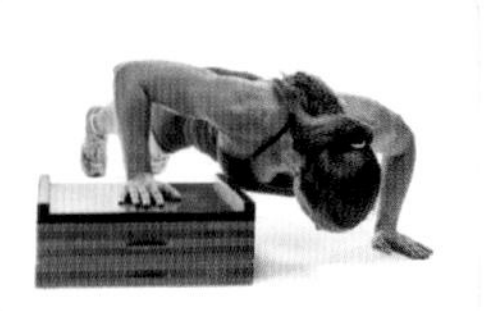
Hand Walkover
page 78

K
weeks 1–4

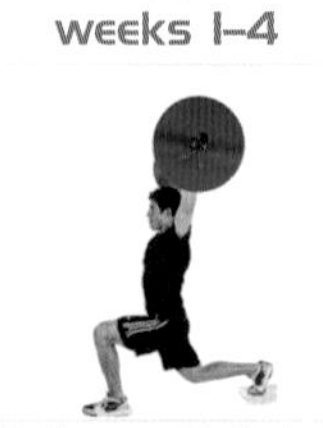
Stationary with Barbell
page 39

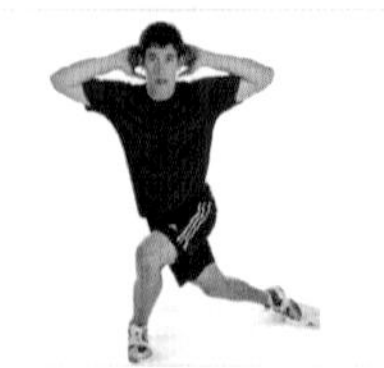
Cross-body Towel Slide
page 48

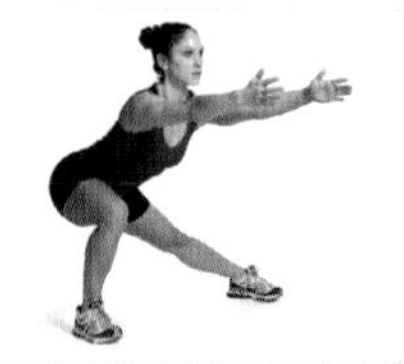
Lateral Lunge
page 42

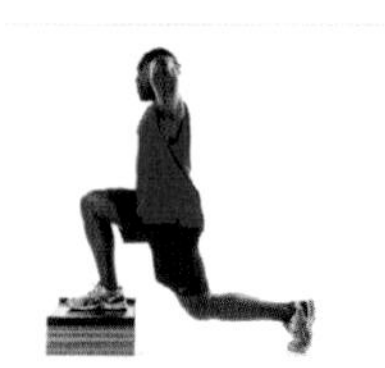
Up to Box
page 54

L
weeks 1–4

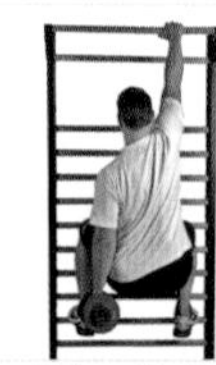
Step Chin with Dumbbell
page 101

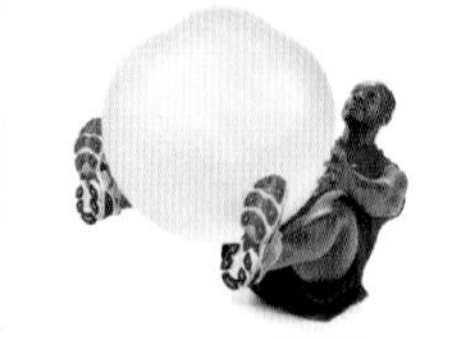
V-ups with Physio Ball
page 122

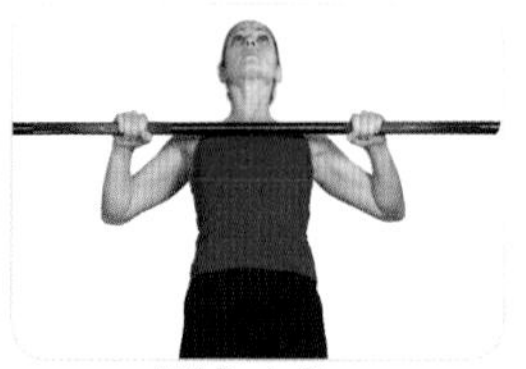
45° Body Row
page 90

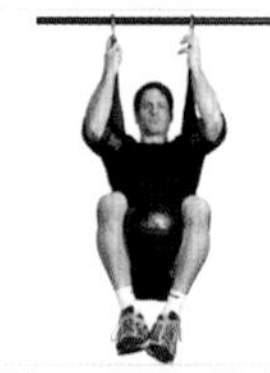
Bent-knee HKR with Medicine Ball page 126

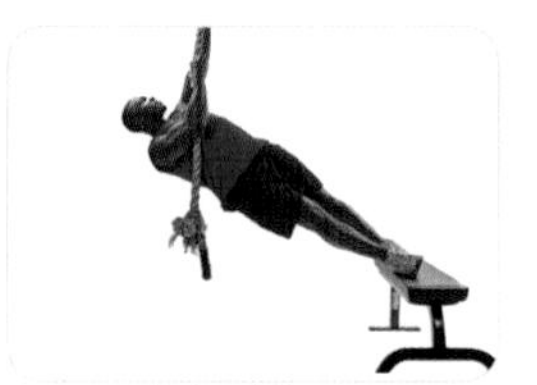
Lateral Rope
page 94

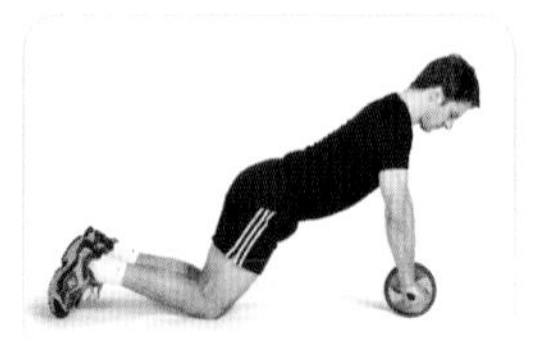
Ab Wheel
page 110

PROGRAM VIII • INTERMEDIATE

USER NOTES

PROGRAM: VIII DURATION: 4 WEEKS

Days per week: 4
Total weeks: 4
Type: Intermediate
Stability and Strength

Weeks	Day 1	Day 2	Day 3	Day 4
1	I	J	K	L
2	I	J	K	L
3	I	J	K	L
4	I	J	K	L

PRESCRIPTION

Week	Sets	Repetitions	Weight/Progression	Rest Set/Exercise
1	3	10	80–85 % max	:90 / :90
2	3	8	Up weight 5% / BW 3 reps	:90 / :90
3	3	6	Up weight 5%/ BW 3 reps	:90 / :90
4	3	10	Original weight	:90 / :90

EXERCISE SEQUENCE

Order	Workout I	Workout J	Workout K	Workout L
1	Dead Lift	Push-up	Lunge	Chin-ups / Ab Wheel
2	Dead Lift	Push-up	Lunge	Chin-ups / Ab Wheel
3	Dead Lift	Push-up	Lunge	Chin-ups / Ab Wheel
4	Dead Lift	Push-up	Lunge	Chin-ups / Ab Wheel
5				Chin-ups / Ab Wheel
6				Chin-ups / Ab Wheel

Notes: This program is 2 days on, 1 off, 2 on, followed by a 2-day rest. Optimally Mon, Tues, or Wed off; Thurs, Fri on; and weekend off. For body-weight exercises, reps should increase in weeks 2 and 3 until close to failure.

PROGRAM IX

ADVANCED

WORKOUTS

M weeks 1–4	N weeks 1–4	O weeks 1–4	D weeks 1–4
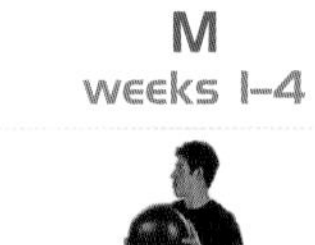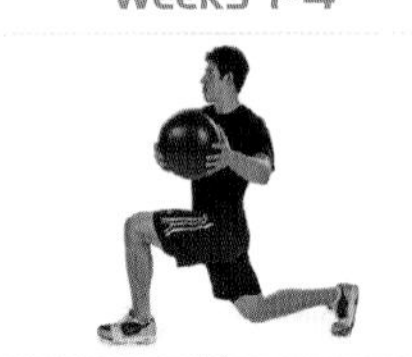 Walking with Rotation page 40	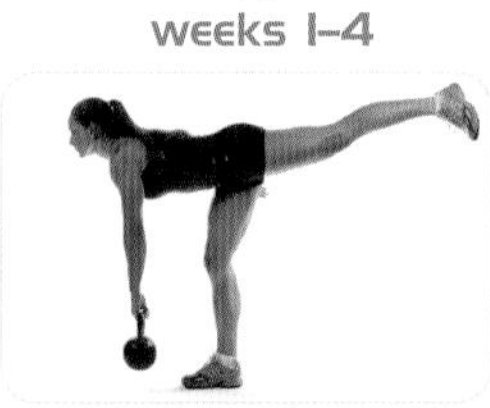 Single-leg/Straight-leg with Kettlebell page 24	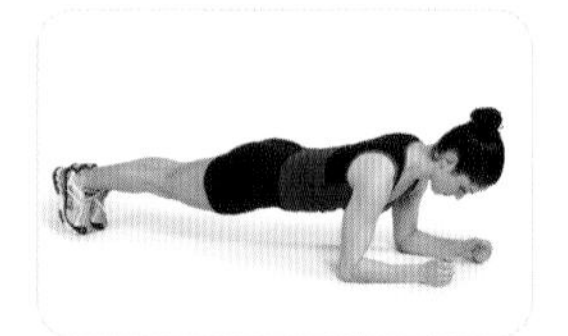 Front Plank page 126	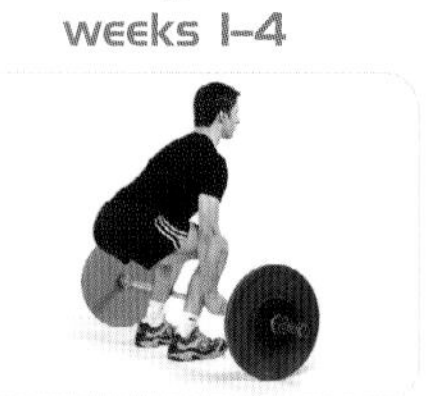 Full with Barbells page 14
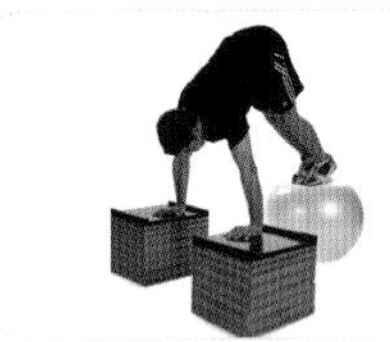 Pike & Press page 70	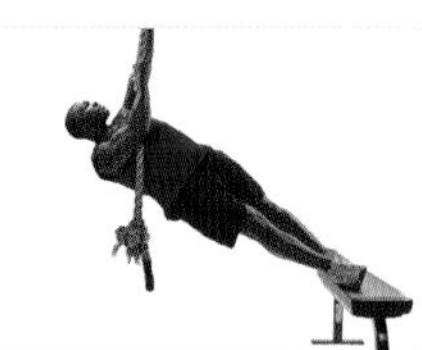 Lateral Rope page 94	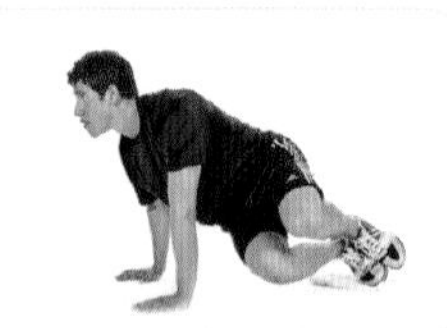 Plough with Rotation page 114	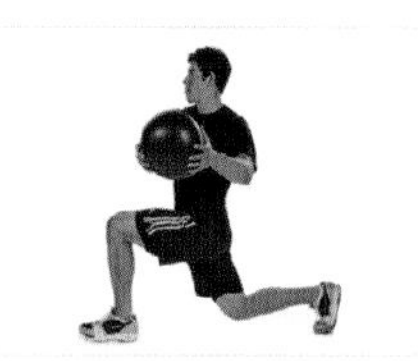 Walking with Rotation page 40
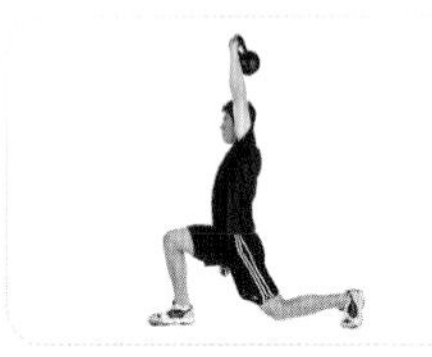 Reverse with Overhead Kettlebell page 52	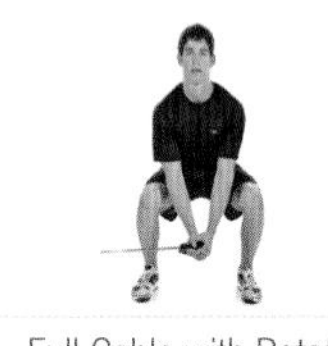 Full Cable with Rotation page 28	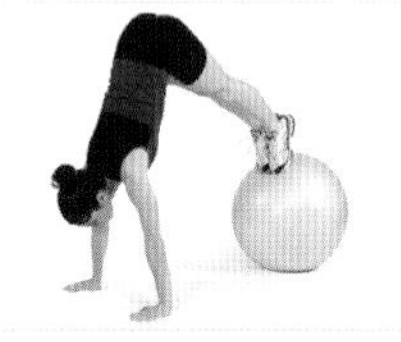 Pike to Plank page 128	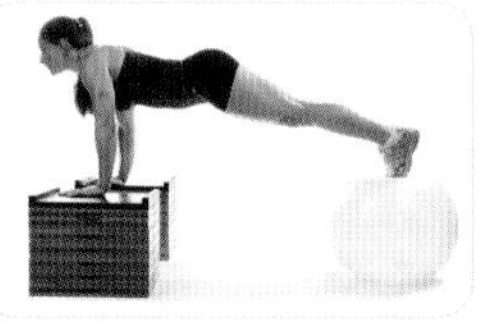 On Physio Ball & Blocks page 64
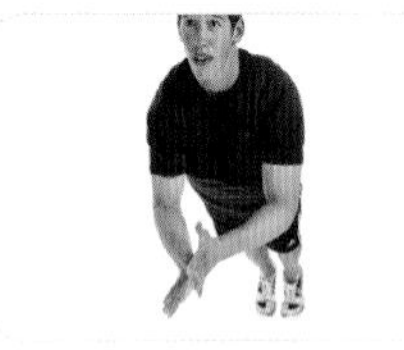 Clap page 74	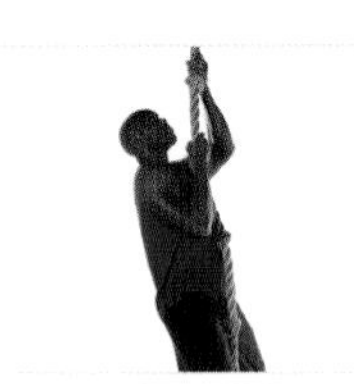 Rope Chin page 107	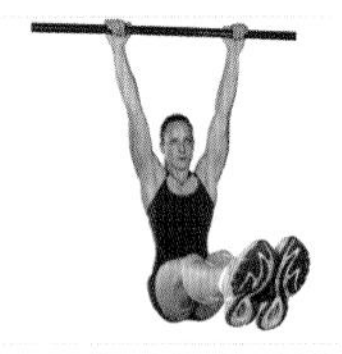 Straight-leg HKR page 116	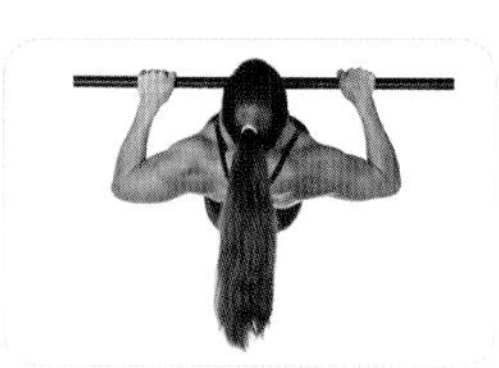 Horizontal Body Row page 92
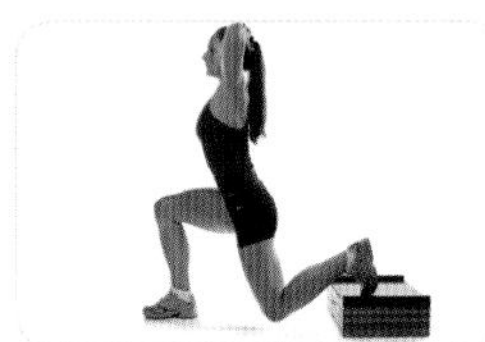 Off Box page 56	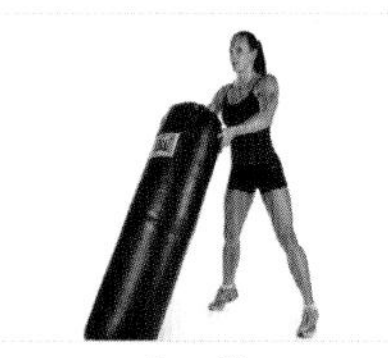 Bag Flip page 32	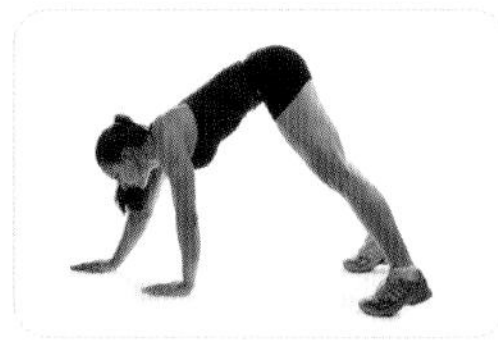 Hand Walk-out page 124	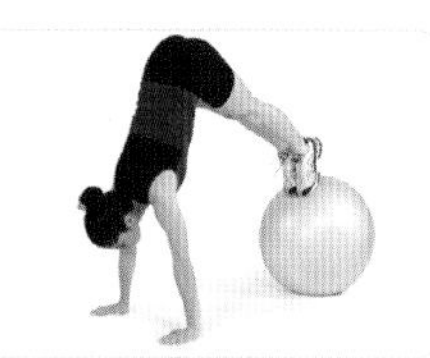 Plank to Pike page 128
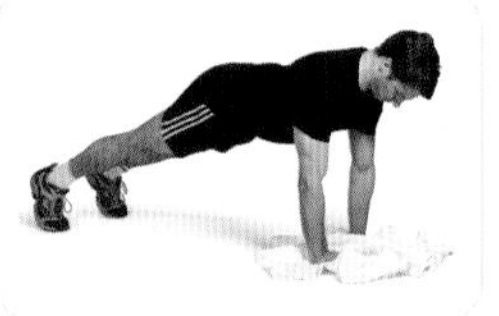 Towel Fly page 68	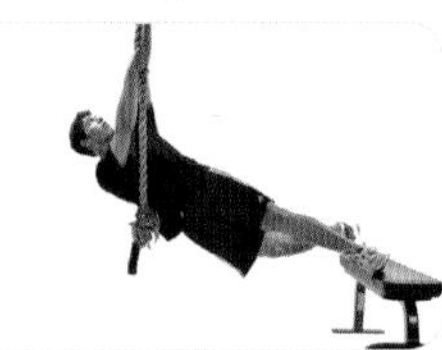 Drop and Pull page 104		

PROGRAM IX • ADVANCED

USER NOTES

PROGRAM: IX DURATION: 4 WEEKS

Days per week: 4
Total weeks: 4
Type: Advanced

Weeks	Day 1	Day 2	Day 3	Day 4
1	M	N	O	D
2	M	N	O	D
3	M	N	O	D
4	M	N	O	D

PRESCRIPTION

Week	Sets	Repetitions	Weight/Progression	Rest Set/Exercise
1	3	8	T.B.D	:75 / :75
2	3	10	Same	:75 / :75
3	4	8	Same	:75 / :75
4	4	10	Same	:75 / :75

EXERCISE SEQUENCE

Order	Workout M	Workout N	Workout O	Workout D
1	Lunge	Dead Lift	Ab Wheel	Dead Lift
2	Push-up	Chin-up	Ab Wheel	Lunge
3	Lunge	Dead Lift	Ab Wheel	Push-up
4	Push-up	Chin-up	Ab Wheel	Chin-up
5	Lunge	Dead Lift	Ab Wheel	Ab Wheel
6	Push-up	Chin-up		

Notes: This sequence is 3 days on, one or 2 days off. There are 2 days that are split, one Ab Wheel–only day and one full-body day. The days before and after full body must be rest days.

PROGRAM X

BEGINNER

WORKOUTS

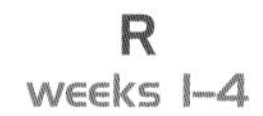

Q weeks 1–4	R weeks 1–4	S weeks 1–4	T weeks 1–4
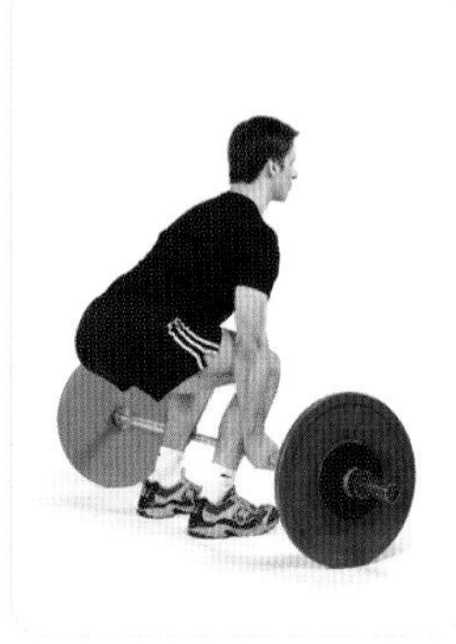 Full with Barbells page 14	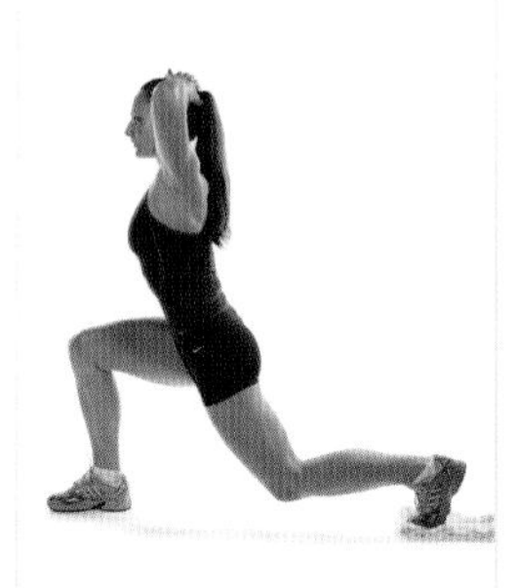 Backward Towel Slide page 46	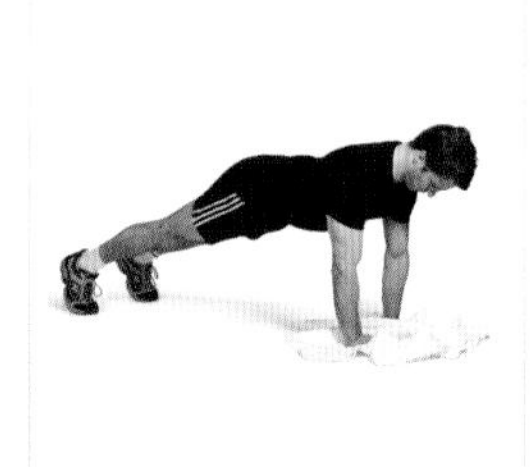 Towel Fly page 68	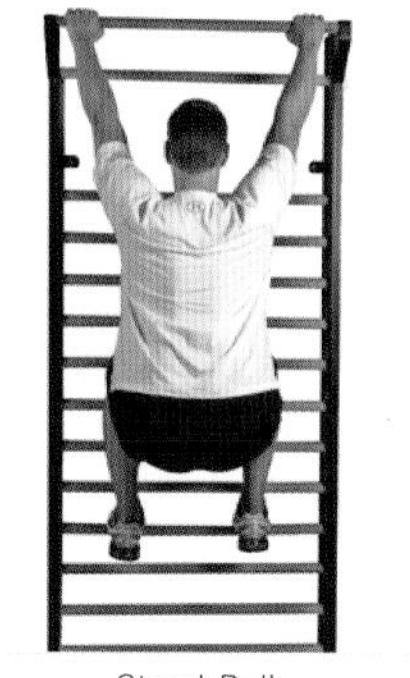 Stand-Pull page 98
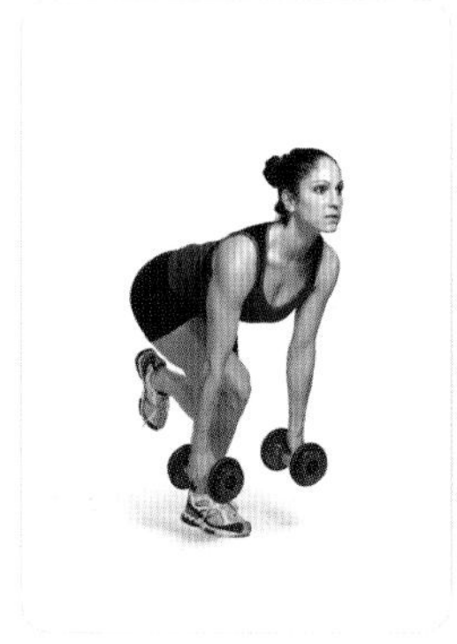 Full Single-leg with Dumbbells page 20	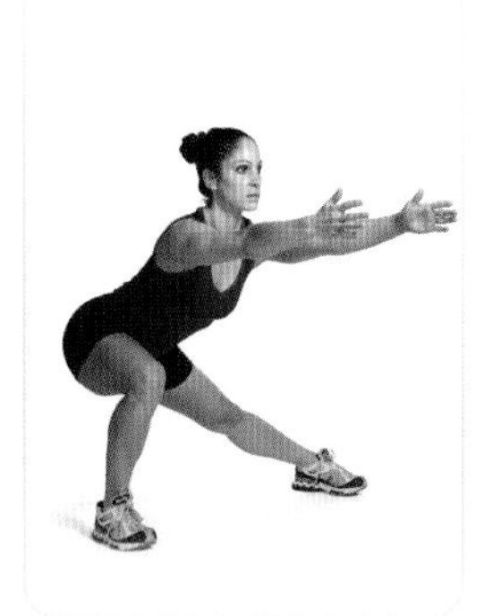 Lateral Lunge page 42	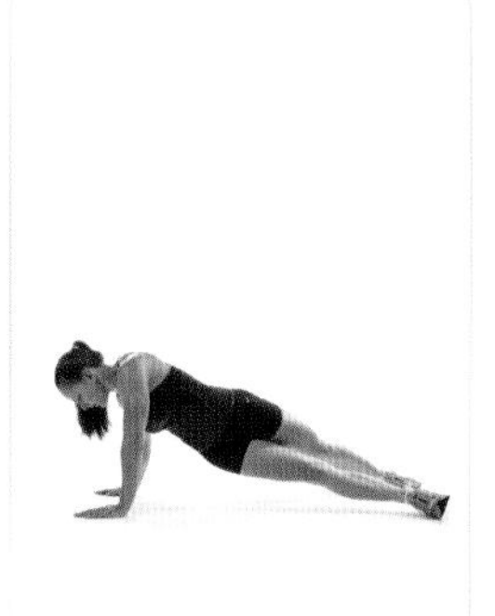 Lower Body Rotation page 72	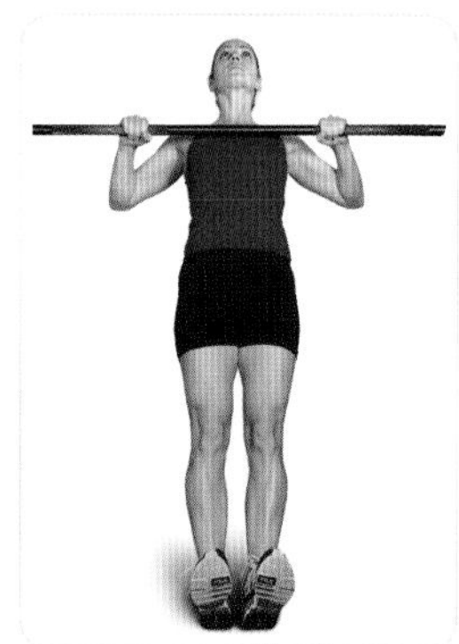 45º Body Row page 90
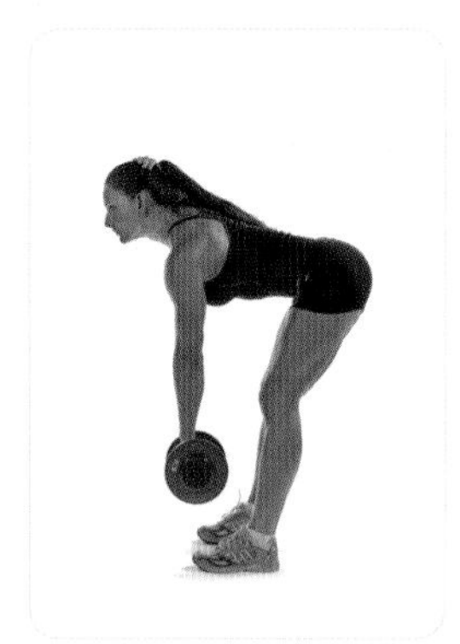 Straight-leg with Dumbbells page 22	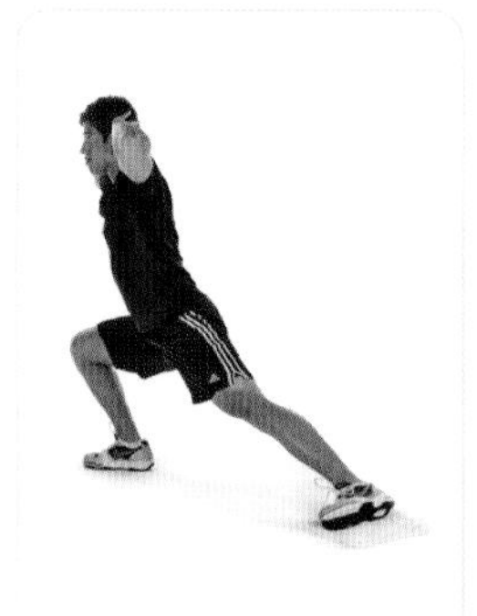 45º Towel Slide page 44	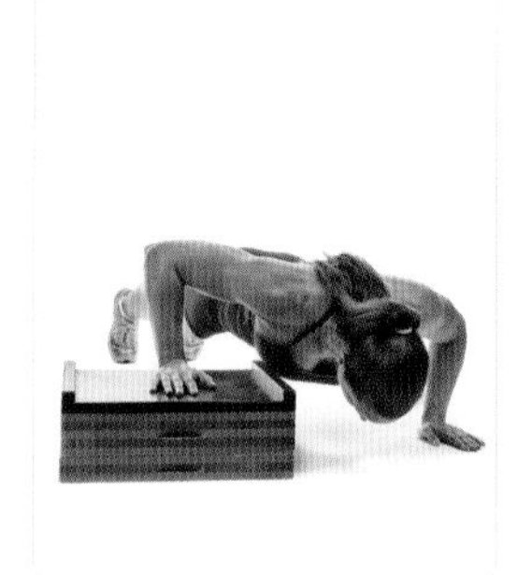 Hand Walkover page 78	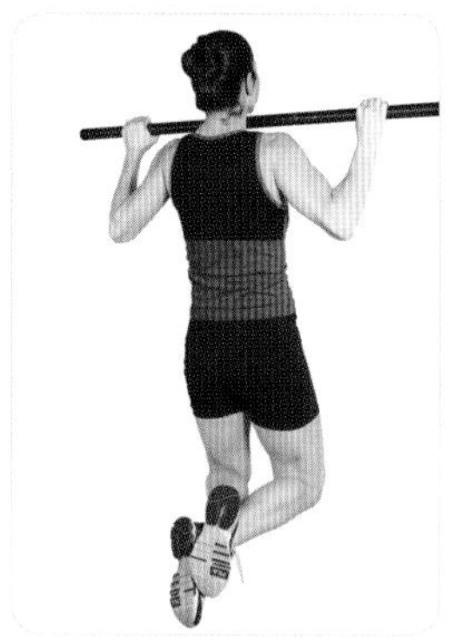 Pull-down Neutral Grip page 96

U
weeks 1–4

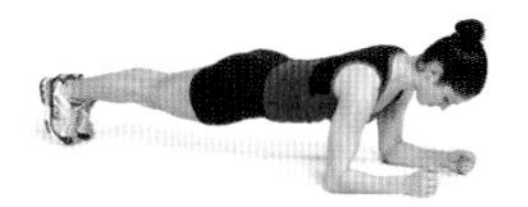

Front Plank
page 126

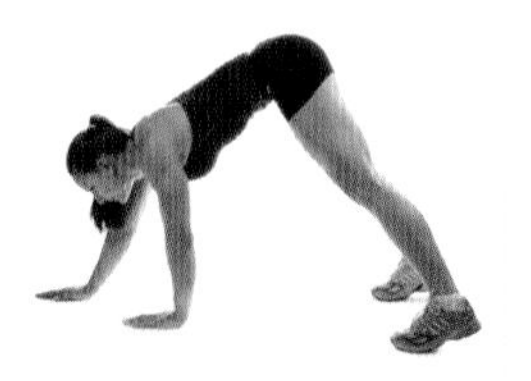

Hand Walk-out
page 124

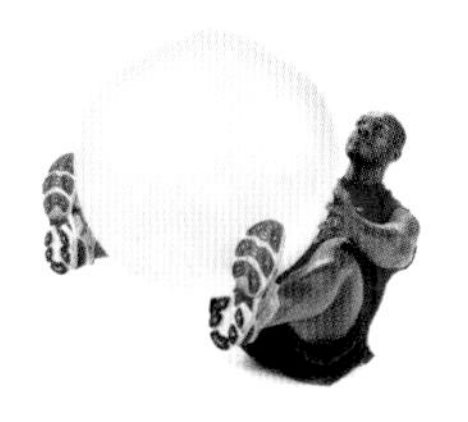

V-ups with Physio Ball
page 122

PROGRAM X • BEGINNER

PROGRAM: X DURATION: 4 WEEKS

Days per week: 3
Total weeks: 4
Type: Beginner
General Conditioning

Weeks \ Days	1	2	3	4	5
1	Q	S	R	U	T
2	Q	S	R	U	T
3	Q	S	R	U	T
4	Q	S	R	U	T

PRESCRIPTION

Week	Sets	Repetitions	Weight/Progression	Rest Set/Exercise
1	3	6	T.B.D	:75 / :90
2	3	8	Same	:75 / :75
3	3	10	Same	:75 / :75
4	3	12	Same	:75 / :90

EXERCISE SEQUENCE

Order \ Workout	Q	R	S	T	U
1	Dead Lift	Lunge	Push-up	Chin-up	Ab Wheel
2	Dead Lift	Lunge	Push-up	Chin-up	Ab Wheel
3	Dead Lift	Lunge	Push-up	Chin-up	Ab Wheel

Notes: Exercise sequence should be completely rearranged for every workout in weeks 3 and 4.

PROGRAM XI

INTERMEDIATE

WORKOUTS

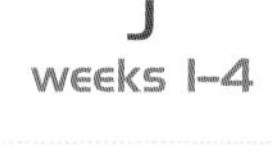

I weeks 1–4	J weeks 1–4	K weeks 1–4	P weeks 1–4
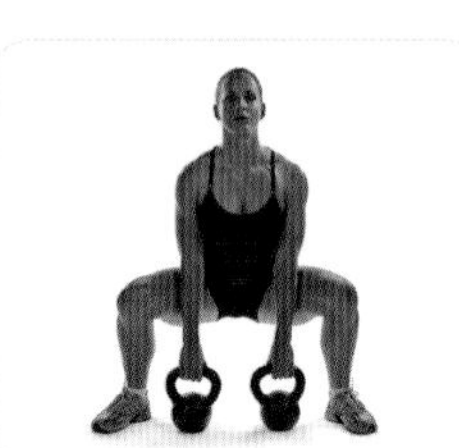 Sumo with Two Kettlebells page 19	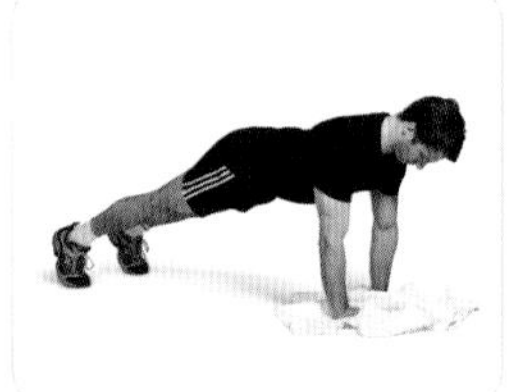 Towel Fly page 68	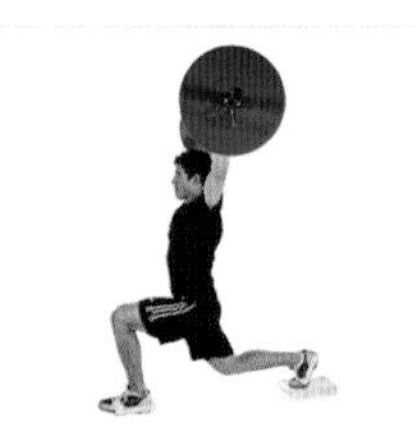 Stationary with Barbell page 39	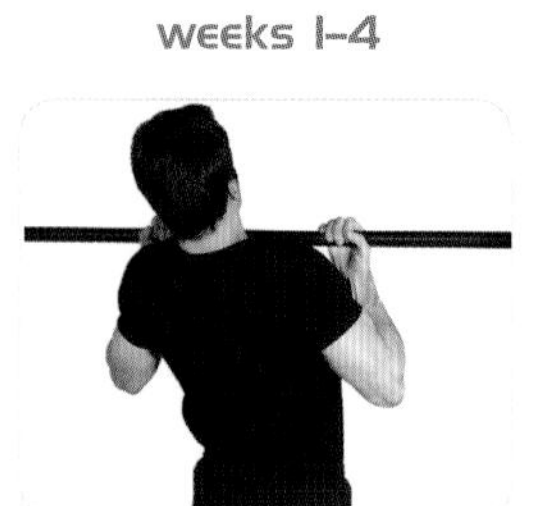 Basic Chin-up page 82
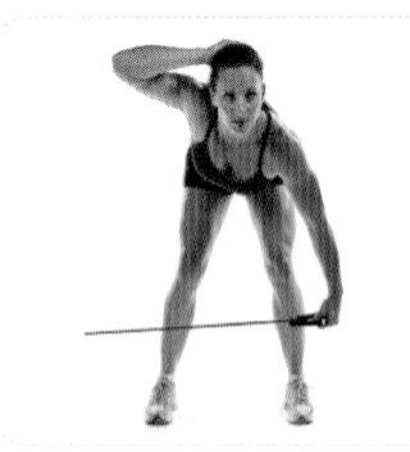 Straight-leg Cable page 30	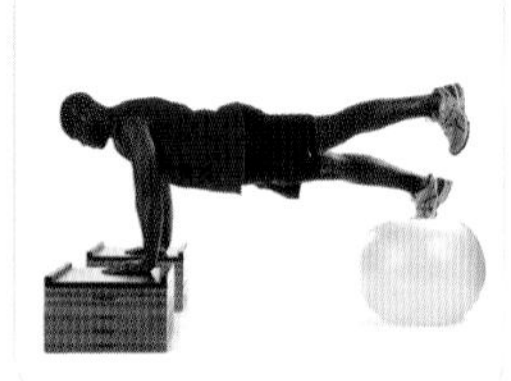 On Physio Ball & Blocks page 65	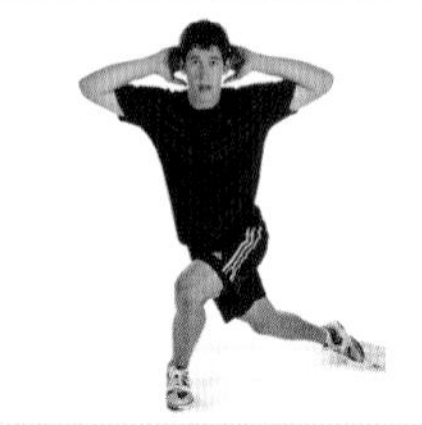 Cross-body Towel Slide page 48	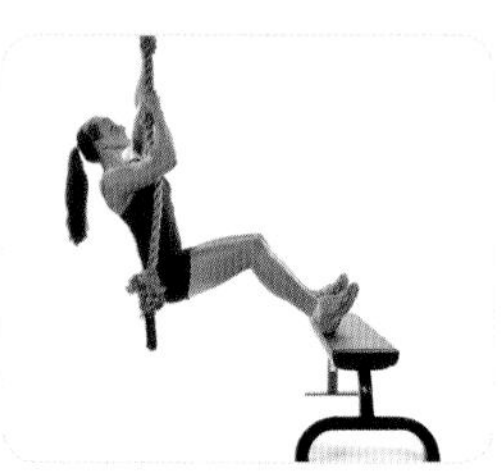 Vertical Rope page 102
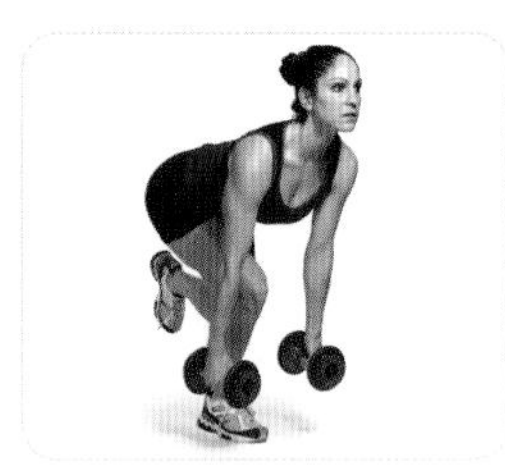 Full Single-leg with Dumbbells page 20	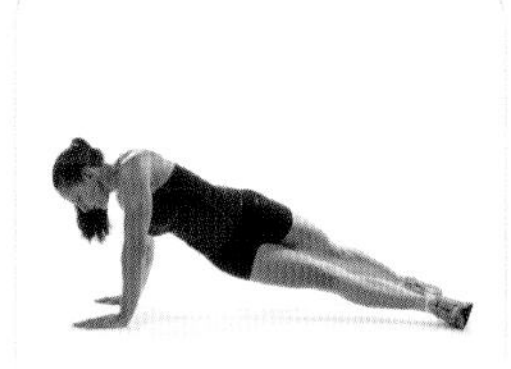 Lower Body Rotation page 72	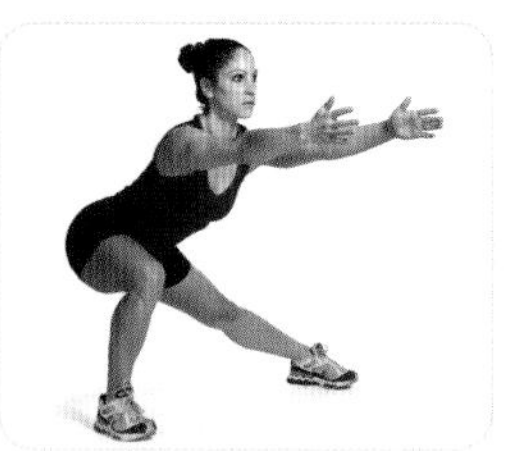 Lateral Lunge page 42	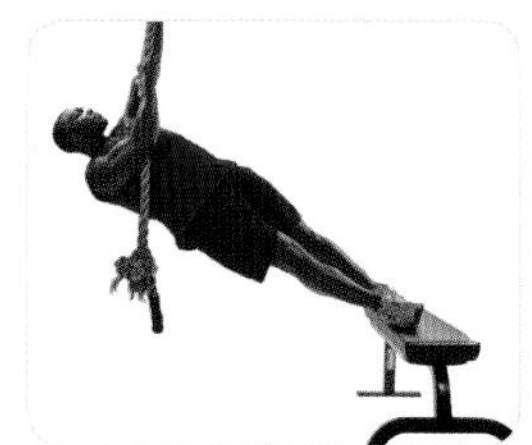 Lateral Rope page 94
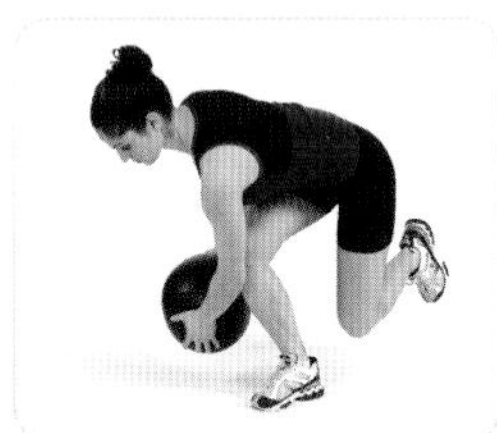 PNF Raise with Medicine Ball page 26	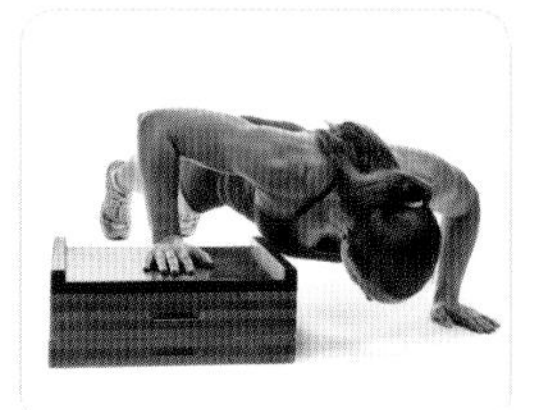 Hand Walkover page 78	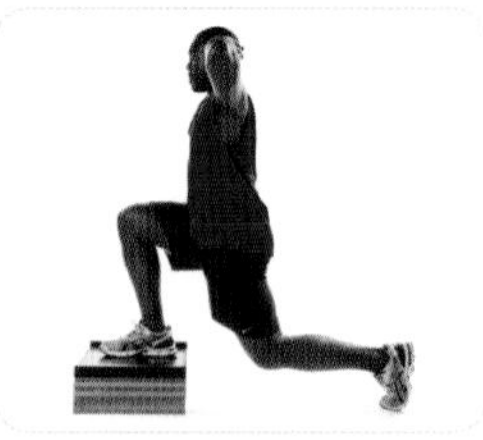 Lunge Up to Box page 54	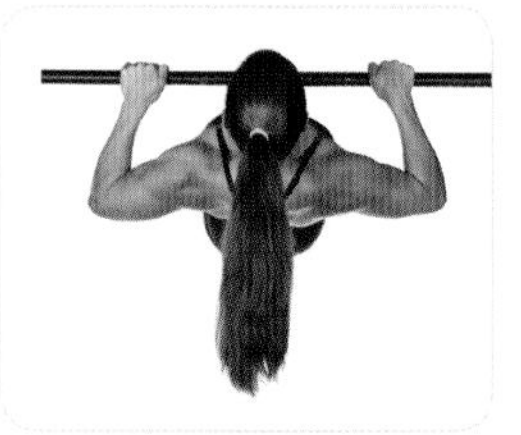 Horizontal Body Row page 92

PROGRAM XI • INTERMEDIATE

Z
weeks 1–4

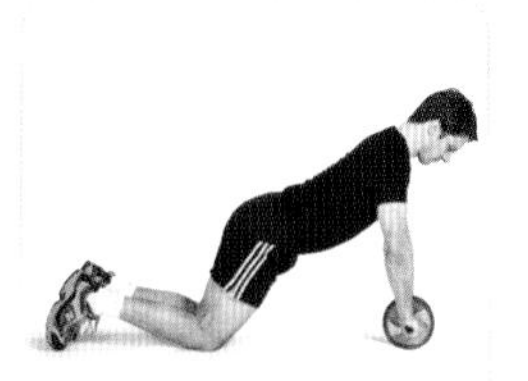
Ab Wheel
page 110

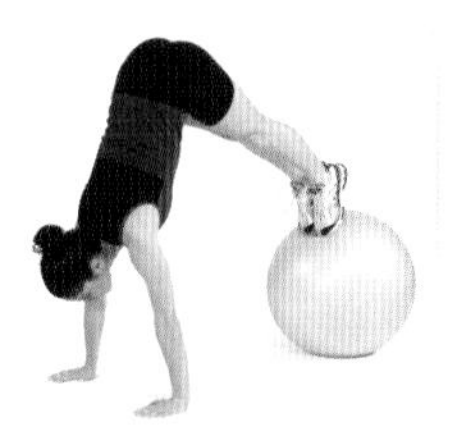
Plank to Pike
page 128

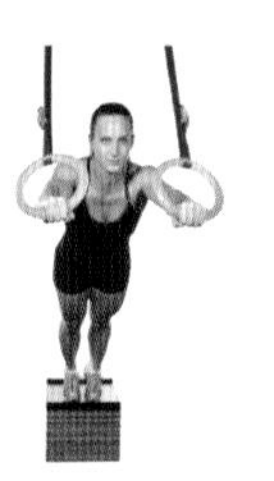
Layout on Rings
page 130

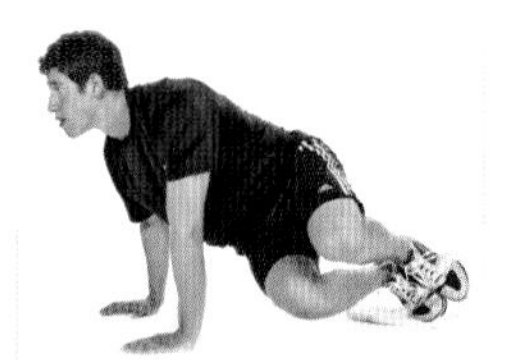
Plough with Rotation
page 114

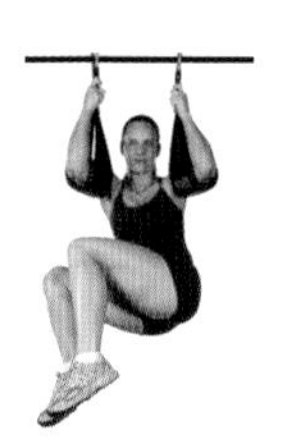
HKR with Rotation
page 120

PROGRAM: XI DURATION: 4 WEEKS

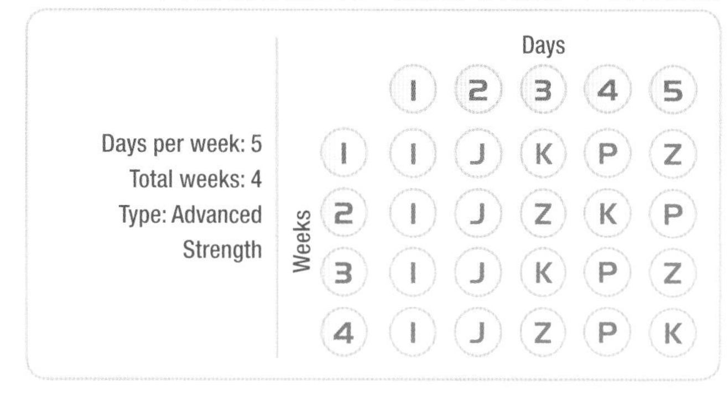

Days per week: 5
Total weeks: 4
Type: Advanced Strength

Weeks	Day 1	Day 2	Day 3	Day 4	Day 5
1	I	J	K	P	Z
2	I	J	Z	K	P
3	I	J	K	P	Z
4	I	J	Z	P	K

PRESCRIPTION

Week	Sets	Repetitions	Weight/Progression	Rest Set/Exercise
1	4	8	T.B.D	:120 / :120
2	4	8	Increase weight 10% BW (2–5) reps	:120 / :120
3	4	8	Increase weight 15% BW (2–5) reps	:120 / :120
4	4	8	Increase weight 10% BW (2–5) reps	:120 / :180

EXERCISE SEQUENCE

Order	Workout Q	Workout R	Workout S	Workout T	Workout U
1	Dead Lift	Push-up	Lunge	Chin-up	Ab Wheel
2	Dead Lift	Push-up	Lunge	Chin-up	Ab Wheel
3	Dead Lift	Push-up	Lunge	Chin-up	Ab Wheel
4	Dead Lift	Push-up	Lunge	Chin-up	AbWheel

Notes: For all workouts in this program, the sequence of a given day should never be the same.

PROGRAM XII

ADVANCED

WORKOUTS

V weeks 1–4	W weeks 1–4	X weeks 1–4	Y weeks 1–4
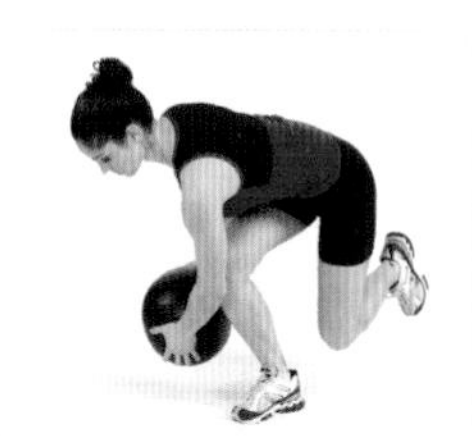 PNF Raise with Medicine Ball page 26	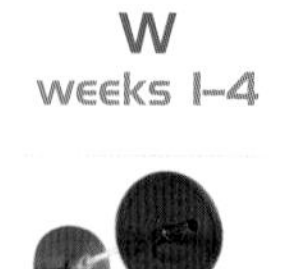 Reverse Barbell Slide page 50	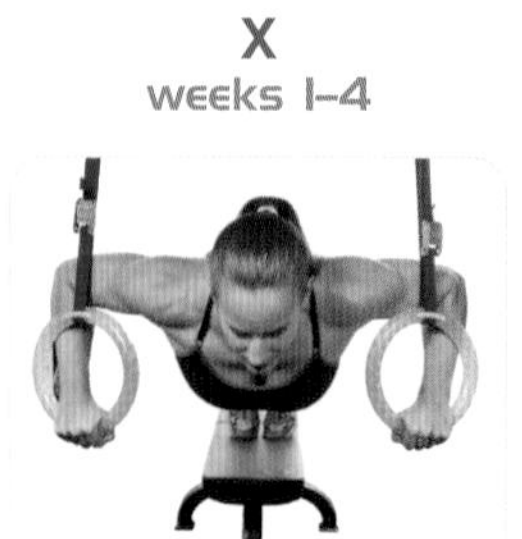 Hands on Rings page 80	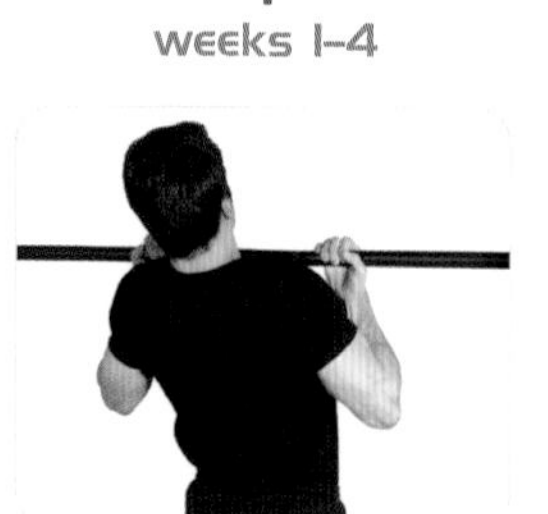 Basic Chin-up page 86
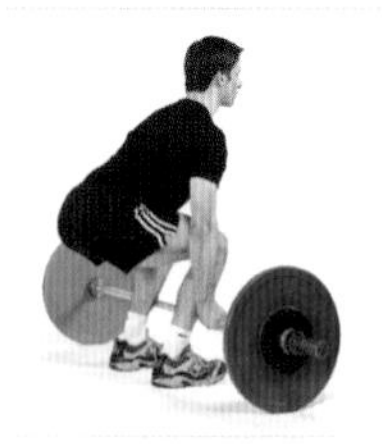 Full with Barbell page 14	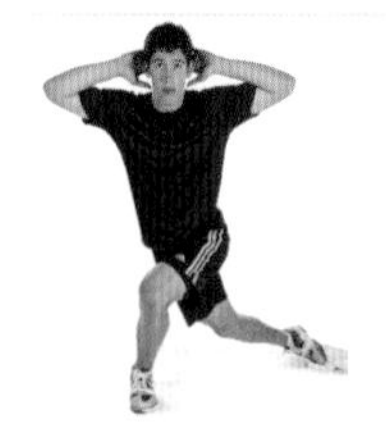 Cross-body Towel Slide page 48	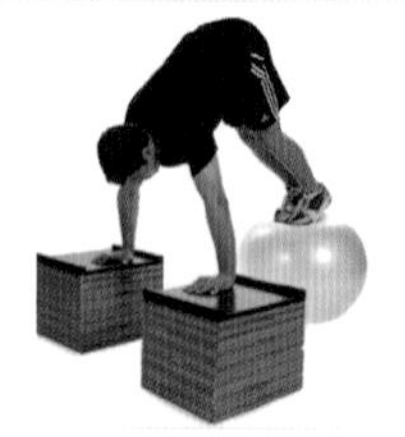 Pike & Press page 70	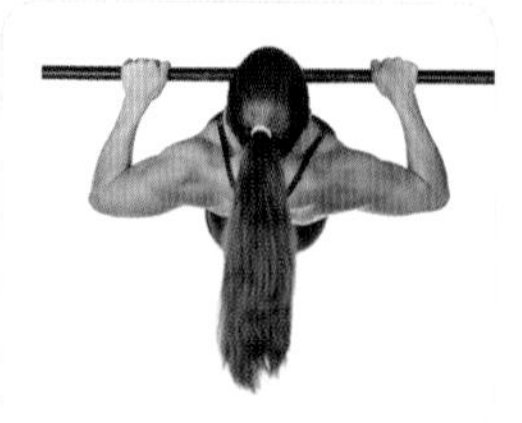 Horizontal Body Row page 92
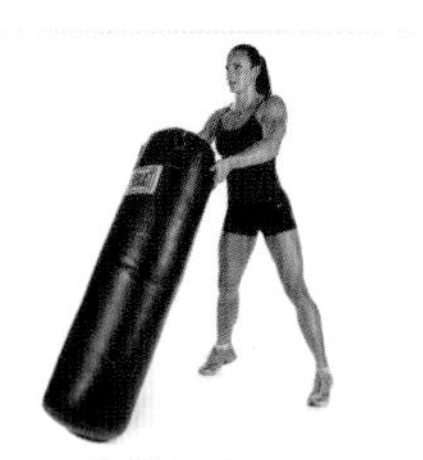 Bag Flip page 32	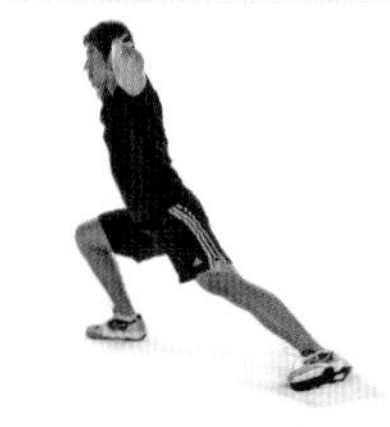 45° Towel Slide page 44	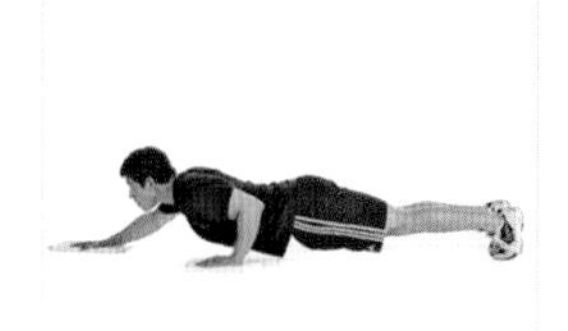 Single-arm Forward Slide page 82	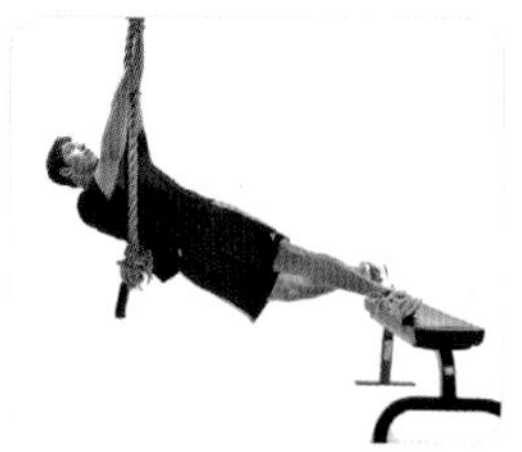 Drop and Pull page 104
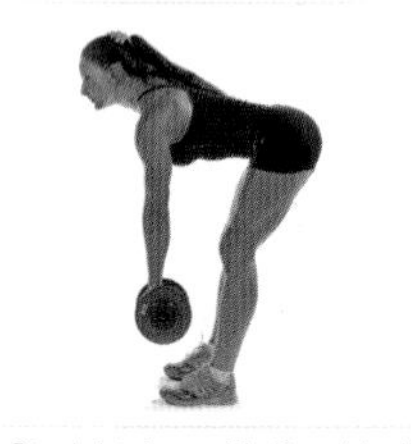 Straight-leg with Dumbbell page 22	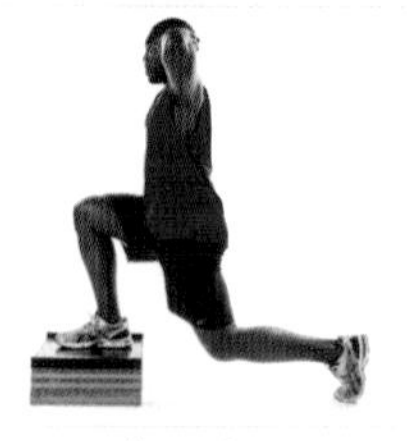 Up to Box page 54	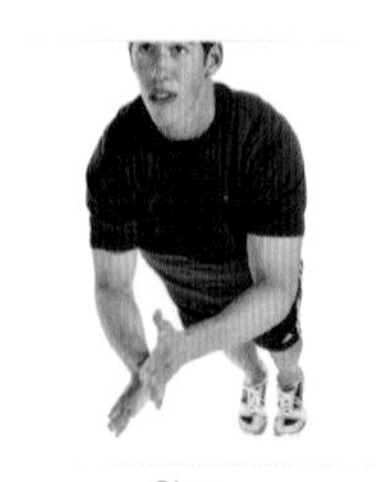 Clap page 74	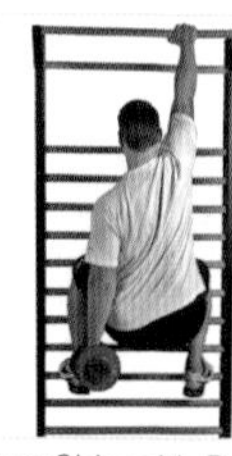 Step Chin with Dumbbell Page 101
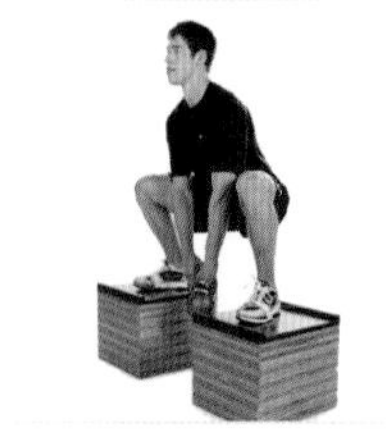 Sumo off Block page 19	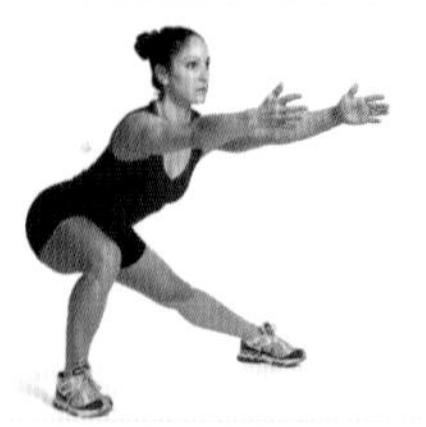 Lateral Lunge page 42	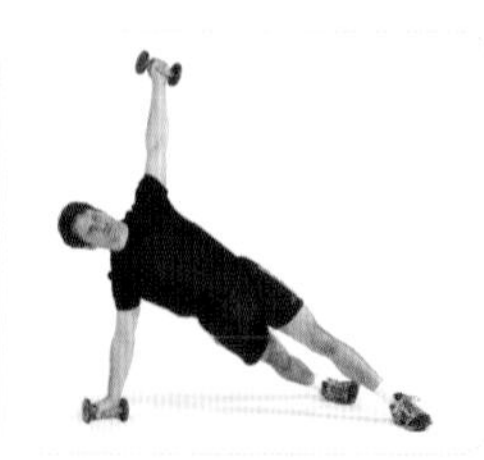 On Dumbbells with Rotation page 64	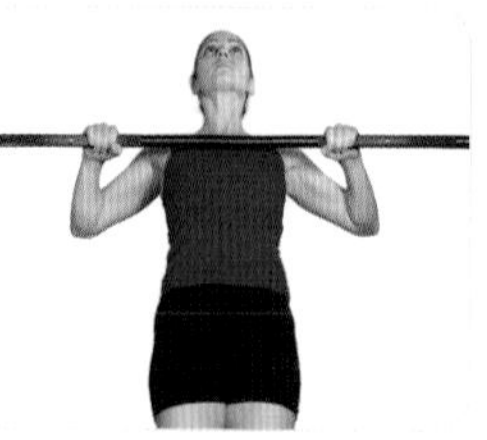 45° Body Row page 90

PROGRAM XII • ADVANCED

Z
weeks 1–4

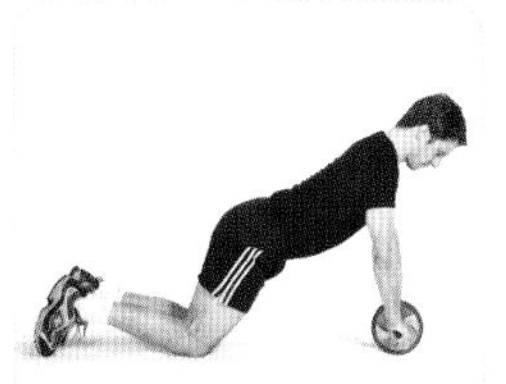

Ab Wheel
page 110

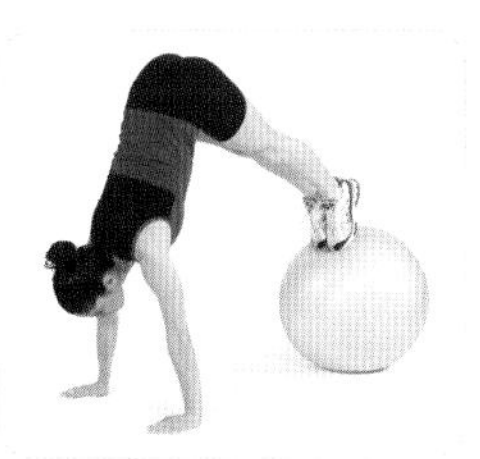

Plank to Pike
page 128

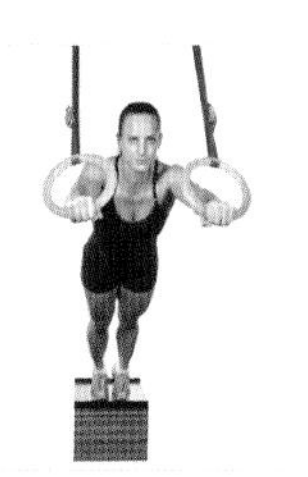

Layout on Rings
page 130

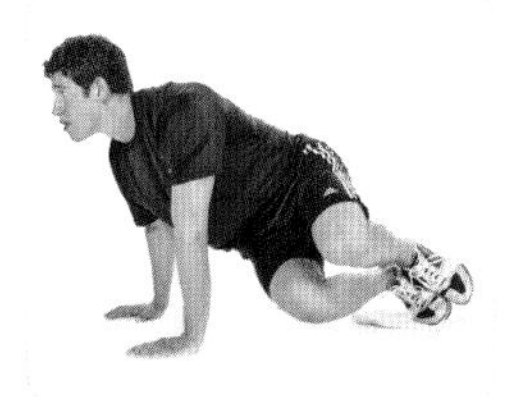

Plough with Rotation
page 114

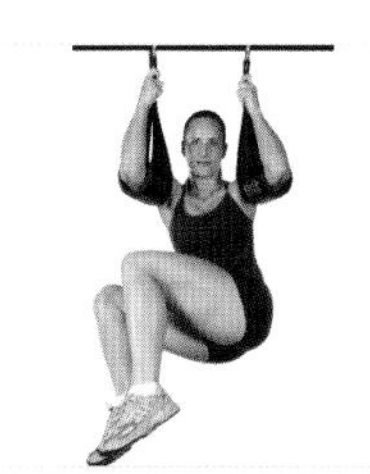

HKR with Rotation
page 120

PROGRAM: XI DURATION: 4 WEEKS

Days per week: 5
Total weeks: 4
Type: Advanced Endurance and Stabilization

Weeks \ Days	1	2	3	4	5
1	V	W	X	Y	Z
2	V	W	X	Y	Z
3	V	W	X	Y	Z
4	V	W	X	Y	Z

PRESCRIPTION

Week	Sets	Repetitions	Weight/Progression	Rest Set/Exercise
1	5	6	T.B.D	:75 / :75
2	5	8	Weight remains the same throughout program.	:75 / :90
3	5	10		:90 / :90
4	5	12		:90 / :90

EXERCISE SEQUENCE

Order \ Workout	Q	R	S	T	U
1	Dead Lift	Lunge	Push-up	Chin-up	Ab Wheel
2	Dead Lift	Lunge	Push-up	Chin-up	Ab Wheel
3	Dead Lift	Lunge	Push-up	Chin-up	Ab Wheel
4	Dead Lift	Lunge	Push-up	Chin-up	Ab Wheel
5	Dead Lift	Lunge	Push-up	Chin-up	Ab Wheel

Notes: In this section, training occurs 5 times per week, so exercises are grouped to 1 ingredient per day, 5 exercises per ingredient. It is not recommended to change the entire order of each group, week to week; however, it is suggested to change the order of 2 exercises per day, on a weekly basis.

GLOSSARY

abduction. Movement away from the body

adduction. Movement toward the body

alternating grip. One hand grasping with the palm facing toward the body and the other facing away

anterior. Located in the front

concentric (contraction). Occurs when a muscle shortens in length and develops tension, e.g., the upward movement of a dumbbell in a biceps curl

curvilinear (movement path). Moving in a curved path

dynamic. Continuously moving

eccentric (contraction). The development of tension while a muscle is being lengthened, e.g., the downward movement of a dumbbell in a biceps curl

extension. The act of straightening

flexion. The bending of a joint

iliotibial band (ITB). A thick band of fibrous tissue that runs down the outside of the leg, beginning at the hip and extending to the outer side of the tibia just below the knee joint. The band functions in coordination with several of the thigh muscles to provide stability to the outside of the knee joint

isometric. Muscles contracting against an equal resistance, resulting in no movement

lateral. Located on, or extending toward, the outside

lordosis. Forward curvature of the spine and lumbar region

medial. Located on, or extending toward, the middle

neutral position (spine). A spinal position resembling an "S" shape, consisting of a lordosis in the lower back, when viewed in profile

PNF (proprioceptive neuromuscular facilitation). Refers to a neuromuscular pattern of contraction that utilizes the greatest efficiency regarding positional awareness.

posterior. Located behind

scapula. The protrusion of bone on the mid to upper back, also known as the shoulder blade

static. No movement; holding a given position

LATIN TERMINOLOGY

The following glossary explains the Latin terminology used to describe the body's musculature. Certain words are derived from Greek, which has been indicated in each instance.

NECK

scalenes. Greek *skalénós*, "unequal"

splenius. Greek *splénion*, "plaster, patch"

sternocleidomastoid. Greek *stérnon*, "chest," Greek *kleís*, "key," and Greek *mastoeidés*, "breast-like"

CHEST

coracobrachialis. Greek *korakoeidés*, "ravenlike," and *brachium*, "arm"

pectoralis (major and minor). *pectus*, "breast"

SHOULDERS

deltoid (anterior, medial, and **posterior).** Greek *deltoeidés*, "delta-shaped"

infraspinatus. *infra*, "under," and *spina*, "thorn"

levator scapulae. from *levare*, "to raise," and *scapulae*, "shoulder [blades]"

subscapularis. *sub*, "below," and *scapulae*, "shoulder [blades]"

supraspinatus. *supra,* "above," and *spina*, "thorn"

teres (major and **minor).** *teres*, "rounded"

UPPER ARM

biceps brachii. *biceps*, "two-headed," and *brachium*, "arm"

brachialis. *brachium*, "arm"

triceps brachii. *triceps*, "three-headed," and *brachium*, "arm"

LOWER ARM

brachioradialis. *brachium*, "arm," and *radius*, "spoke"

extensor carpi radialis. from *extendere*, "to bend," Greek *karpós*, "wrist," and *radius*, "spoke"

extensor digitorum. from *extendere*, "to bend," and *digitus*, "finger, toe"

flexor carpi radialis. from *flectere*, "to bend," Greek *karpós*, "wrist," and *radius*, "spoke"

flexor digitorum. from *flectere*, "to bend," and *digitus*, "finger, toe"

CORE

obliquus externus. *obliquus*, "slanting," and *externus*, "outward"

obliquus internus. *obliquus*, "slanting," and *internus*, "within"

rectus abdominis. adj. of rego, "straight, upright," and abdomen, "belly"

serratus anterior. adj. of *serra*, "saw"; therefore "saw-shaped," and *ante*, "before"

transversus abdominis. *transversus*, "athwart" and *abdomen*, "belly"

BACK

erector spinae. *erectus*, "straight," and *spina*, "thorn"

latissimus dorsi. *latus*, "wide," and *dorsum*, "back"

quadratus lumborum. *quadratus*, "square, rectangular" and *lumbus*, "loin"

rhomboid. Greek *rhembesthai*, "to spin"

trapezius. Greek *trapezion*, lit. "small table"

HIPS

gemellus (inferior and **superior).** adj. comp. of *super*, "above," and *inferus*, "under," with *geminus*, "twin"

gluteus medius. Greek *gloutós*, "rump," with Latin suffix, and *medialis*, "middle"

gluteus maximus. Greek *gloutós*, "rump," with Latin suffix, and *maximus*, "largest"

gluteus minimus. Greek *gloutós*, "rump," with Latin suffix, and *minimus*, "smallest"

iliopsoas. ilia, variant of *ilium*, "groin," and Greek *psoa*, "groin muscle"

iliacus. ilia, variant of *ilium*, "groin"

obturator externus. from obturare, "to block" and *externus*, "outward"

obturator internus. from *obturare*, "to block," and *internus*, "within"

pectineus. *pectin*, "comb"

piriformis. adj. of *pirum*, "pear"; therefore "pear-shaped"

quadratus femoris. *quadratus*, "square, rectangular," and *femur*, "thigh"

UPPER LEG

adductor longus. from *adducere*, "to contract," and *longus*, "long"

adductor magnus. from *adducere*, "to contract," and *magnus*, "major"

biceps femoris. *biceps*, "two-headed," and *femur*, "thigh"

gracilis. *gracilis*, "slim, slender"

rectus femoris. adj. of *rego*, "straight, upright," and *femur*, "thigh"

sartorius. from *sarcio*, "to patch" or "to repair"

semimembranosus. *semi*, "half" and *membrum*, "limb"

semitendinosus. *semi*, "half" and *tendo*, "tendon"

tensor fasciae latae. from *tenere*, "to stretch," *fasciae*, "band," and *latae*, "laid down"

vastus intermedius. *vastus*, "immense, huge," and *intermedius*, "that which is between"

vastus lateralis. *vastus*, "immense, huge," and lateralis, "of the side"

vastus medialis. *vastus*, "immense, huge," and *medialis*, "middle"

LOWER LEG

extensor hallucis. *extendere*, "to bend," and *hallex*, "big toe"

flexor hallucis. from *flectere*, "to bend," and *hallex*, "big toe"

gastrocnemeus. Greek *gastroknémía*, "calf [of the leg]," and Latin suffix

peroneus. *peronei*, "of the fibula"

soleus. *solea*, "sandal"

tibialis anterior. *tibia*, "reed pipe," and ante, "before"

tibialis posterior. *tibia*, "reed pipe," and *posterus*, "coming after"

ACKNOWLEDGMENTS

There are several people who have made very direct and substantial contributions to this book who I want to personally thank. Since I handwrite all of the text in this book (and my handwriting has deteriorated to "barely legible"), I want to recognize Shannon Plumstead, who has again masterfully and expeditiously put my cursive into the typed page. Greg Cimino for getting the "deal done," as he always seems to be able to do in a way that is agreeable to everyone.

I want to also thank these people for their contribution to the content: Rico Wesley for his help with the text and Gillian Gauthier for her contribution to the development of the sample programs. A huge thanks to Noah Emmerich, a client and friend, and my wife, Deborah, for their immensely helpful contributions of time and advice on how to literally lay the programs out so that they would be both understandable and user-friendly.

I also would like to mention Lisa Purcell at Hylas Publishing for her patience in helping put this book together and Sean Moore, who took the idea and ran with it.

Finally, I want to let my family know that without them, Ma, Mary, Jen, Tony, Milena, and Deb, none of this would have meaning. As always, this is for you.